*Fatherless
Children*

WILEY SERIES IN CHILD MENTAL HEALTH

Joseph D. Noshpitz, Editor

FATHERLESS CHILDREN

by Paul L. Adams, Judith R. Milner and Nancy A. Schrepf

FATHERLESS CHILDREN

PAUL L. ADAMS
University of Texas Medical Branch

JUDITH R. MILNER
University of Louisville School of Medicine

NANCY A. SCHREPF
Spalding College

A Wiley-Interscience Publication

JOHN WILEY & SONS

New York / Chichester / Brisbane / Toronto / Singapore

Library of Congress Cataloging in Publication Data:

Adams, Paul L., 1924–
   Fatherless children.

   "A Wiley-Interscience publication."
   Bibliography: p.
   Includes indexes.
   1. Children of single parents—United States.
2. Child mental health—United States.   3. Fathers—United States.
4. Father and child—United States.
I. Milner, Judith R.   II. Schrepf, Nancy A.   III. Title.

HQ777.4.A33   1984   306.8′742   83-21894
ISBN 0-471-88765-X

Printed in the United States of America

10 9 8 7 6 5 4 3 2

Foreword

Until recently, the father has been like the weather—much talked of, but nobody did anything about him. With this work by Paul Adams, Judith Milner, and Nancy Schrepf, someone has done something at last, and something very considerable at that. The authors are a scholarly group; they have assembled data from a variety of sources, and have asked: What, in fact, do we know about fathers and the meaning of fathers to children in contrast to what we opine, or prefer, or have been told? What are the data, and how do we distinguish fact from opinion? Their answers to these questions comprise the content of this work, and a curious and fascinating work it is.

As in all matters that touch on family roles and relationships, there is no end to myth and confusion. Many theorists have pronounced their views, and there are schools of thought with powerful opinions and unequivocal assertions. In all these instances the authors take a dry and somewhat ironic position; they try to represent the several stances as objectively as possible, but they also raise the many questions that such positions evoke, and they refuse to accept any doctrinaire assertions that are not supported by some degree of objective research.

Since the authors' scope is wide and their spirit courageous, this is a book of rare breadth, power, and impact. It faces the ambiguities of human relationship squarely, and recognizes the enormous variability of patterns that the forms of interpersonal connectedness can assume. Its essential conclusion is that children can develop well with fathers or without; withal, however, the importance of the role a positive form of fathering can play in the lives of children does not escape its full and thorough recounting. All in all, in my opinion, in this work the nature of fathering, whether the father is present or absent, gets its clearest exposition as well as its most convincing and thorough presentation to date.

One significant aspect of the writing for which the reader should be prepared is that it is the work of an angry man. This is not meant to have shock value; it is a serious and considered statement. Adams, the senior author, is one of the few child psychiatrists in the United States to have had a cross burned on his front lawn. He is, to be sure, a first-class professional and teacher, but before that he is a human being with a sense of principle so deep that he is in a state of permanent protest against the cruelties and the stupidities of his times. In particular, he finds it unforgivable when those who are trained, those who are professionals, those who should know, and, knowing, care, make themselves unknowing and uncaring so that the children who should be their first concern then fall by the wayside. That makes Paul Adams permanently and uncompromisingly angry. He has remained angry for years, a rare gift, and he is as ready to castigate the medical or the governmental as he is the religious or the university establishment when it betrays the smug unknowingness that is his personal antagonist. Adams is an exorcist who has for a professional lifetime fought the powers of darkness wherever and whenever he has encountered them, be it on the streets, in church, in the halls of academe or in city hall. And he has fought with scholarship, with truth, and with the irony born of ethical passion. In many ways this is a passionate book, so reader, beware. It will not leave you untouched.

JOSEPH D. NOSHPITZ

Washington, D.C.
March 1984

Series Preface

This series is intended to serve a number of functions. It includes works on child development; it presents material on child advocacy; it publishes contributions to child psychiatry; and it gives expression to cogent views on child rearing and child management. The mental health of parents and their interaction with their children is a major theme of the series, and emphasis is placed on the child as individual, as family member, and as a part of the larger social surround.

Child development is regarded as the basic science of child mental health, and within that framework research works are included in this series. The many ethical and legal dimensions of the way society relates to its children is the central theme of the child advocacy publications, as well as a primarily demographic approach that highlights the role and status of children within society. The child psychiatry publications span studies that concern the diagnosis, description, therapeutics, rehabilitation, and prevention of the emotional disorders of childhood. And the views of thoughtful and creative contributors to the handling of children under many different circumstances (retardation, acute and chronic illness, hospitalization, handicap, disturbed social conditions, etc.) find expression within the framework of child rearing and child management.

Family studies with a central child mental health perspective are included in the series, and explorations into the nature of parenthood and the parenting process are emphasized. This includes books about divorce, the single parent, the absent parent, parents with physical and emotional illnesses, and other conditions that significantly affect the parent–child relationship.

Finally, the series examines the impact of larger social forces, such as war, famine, migration, and economic failure, on the adaptation of children and families. In the largest sense, the series is devoted to books that illuminate the special needs, status, and history of children and their families within all perspectives that bear on their collective mental health.

JOSEPH D. NOSHPITZ

Children's Hospital Medical Center, and
The George Washington University
Washington, D.C.

Preface

Fatherless Children was drafted originally when we were working together at the University of Louisville. Drawing on our shared interests in child mental health and our individual origins in education (Milner), sociology (Adams and Schrepf), and psychology (Schrepf), we meant to write a useful guide about fatherless children for members of the helping professions. As it evolved, our practical guide had to include a review of research; some consideration of what a father could mean and be, if present and vibrantly participatory in the lives of his children; specification of the major varieties of father-absence; and some conclusions about research methods, public policy, and psychotherapy concerning fatherless children. In that enlarged process we have attempted to provide not only clinicians but also researchers and policy makers with some guides and suggestions for working with fatherless children.

As we end our work for the book, we are impressed that a father may or may not be a vital part of the child's world and that, whether he is in or out of the household, he may be helpful, harmful, or a matter of indifference to the child. The book itself lays out the evidence for such a general conclusion.

Many persons have helped us in the project. Early help from Joan Kogelschatz and Daniel Tucker must be cited, with later contributions from Evelia Valdés-Rodriguez Adams, Charles E. Holzer, Stephen Nadeau, Christine Adams-Tucker, Jeffrey Horovitz, Roosevelt Walker, Joy Cofer, the computer centers at the Universities of Louisville, Miami, and Florida, Vivian Peterson Martin, Patricia Laffey Smith, John O'Brien, Ann Seiden, Susan Barrows, Linda Crouch, Sue Anderson, Marjorie Potter Grubbs, Mohammad Mian, Daryll Anderson, the University of Louisville library staff, and the numerous fatherless children who have shared with us their ideas and feelings. Administrative and moral support were given by Robert L. Williams, James N. Sussex, John J. Schwab, and Robert M. Rose, who chaired the departments of psychiatry and behavioral sciences in which one, two or all three of us have been employed, and from Arthur Keeney, former dean at Louisville. Grants to Paul Adams from research funds of the University of Miami and the University of Louisville, and to Judith Milner through a medical student summer fellowship from the National Institute of Mental Health, also require our grateful acknowledgment.

PAUL L. ADAMS
JUDITH R. MILNER
NANCY A. SCHREPF

Galveston, Texas
Louisville, Kentucky
Louisville, Kentucky
February 1984

Contents

CHAPTER ONE

The Father's Meaning to the Child

The families of about 11 million fatherless children contrast sharply with traditional families, but we must examine what fathers do when they are present in order to discover what their absence means to children. The traditional family, including a wage-earning man, a housekeeping and child-rearing woman, and their offspring, persists as an ideal for some and inspires criticism from others, but it is actually pretty rare, an institution of the past. It is not easy to describe a typical family today. Bane and Masnick (1980) report that although three-fourths of all U.S. families were "traditional, nuclear types" in 1960, by 1990 two-thirds of all households will be childless, and one-third of all families, say others, will be fatherless by 1990. Later we'll discuss the new typical families, but for now, let's look at the traditional family with a father present but consider especially the father's role from the child's point of view. An added reason to look at nuclear, intact, traditional families is that most child development theories are based on those families, and most clinical approaches postulate the growth of children in such families. As clinicians we know that all children do not have fathers available, but it is "easier" to think as if they do.

For twentieth century children and probably for many before them, the father in a traditional family plays a fairly unimportant role. That sounds off-key, particularly to a reader who habitually thinks father is central to the child's growing up. Erma Bombeck, the newspaper columnist, describes a father's lack of duties in a traditional family: "Daddy just didn't know how to show love. It was Mom who held the family together. He just went to work every day and came home and she'd have a list of sins we'd committed and he'd give us what-for about them" (*Courier-Journal and Times*, Louisville, Kentucky, June 15, 1980, p. G-5). The father keeps busy out in the world; the mother manages the household. Because of this division of labor, infants, even those with fathers, often are fatherless during most of their waking hours.

Newborn babies need to form close and binding attachments to a caring person who helps them survive the risky first year of their lives. Many infants do not live through the first year. The United States itself ranks seventeenth from the top in infant deaths among nations reporting infant mortality to the World Health Organization, a

2

record showing our adult-centered refusal to care for the lives, not to mention the liberties and pursuits of happiness, of infants (Adams, 1981b).

A lucky baby makes a stable attachment, a genuine bonding, to a nurturing person soon after being born. In a traditional family, the mother is the nurturing person, and father cannot help out even when the baby needs more tender care than the the mother alone can offer. However, a strong and passionate, bodily and earthy, libidinal attachment forms between mother and infant. This symbiotic attachment differs from the one-way, parasitic relationship that existed before the baby's birth (Rank, 1924; Benedek, 1949; Mahler & Goslinger, 1955), and both mother and baby enjoy it. The father may enjoy vicariously the symbiotic bonding between his wife and her baby, but he doesn't actually participate much.

Why does the infant nearly always form this relationship with the mother rather than the father? Most theorists, including Otto Rank, Therese Benedek, Anna Freud, John Bowlby, David W. Winnicott, Sidney Bijou, and Donald Baer and O. Hobart Mowrer, disregard the father completely and simply assume that the infant–mother bond is the most important relationship in infancy, with continuations into adolescence and adulthood. Most authors believe that this close liaison develops because the mother encourages it, and the infant, wanting the mother to gratify its needs, cooperates. John Bowlby (1958, 1969) proposes an additional reason for bonding—that an infant who stays close to a protecting adult gains an evolutionary advantage. Schaffer (1971) suggests that the bond results from the infant's attempt to prolong and repeat sensory stimulating experiences. Despite their differences, these several theories—of psychoanalysts, learning theorists, and ethologists—ultimately agreed that, because she spends the most time with the infant, the mother is uniquely important in the infant's life. With a few exceptions—Andry (1962) and Layman (1961), for example—researchers have largely ignored the father's possible roles, but none of these theories of bonding actually requires the caretaker adult to be the mother rather than the father.

Michael Lamb's (1976a) closer critical look at infant attachment reveals that the infant–mother bond need not be the extreme affinity that many authors describe. Lamb suggests that the quality of interaction, not the extent, is what matters to fathers, mothers, and infants. After extensively reviewing the literature, Lamb concludes that infants do prefer mothers to fathers, though many of the studies he surveyed take place in artificial laboratory settings. His own research indicates that infants prefer mothers when distressed; when not distressed, and when both parents are available, infants show no preference.

Infants also behave differently toward fathers and mothers. In another work, Lamb (1976c) reported that 18-month-old infants show more affiliative behavior toward fathers and more attachment behavior toward mothers. He found that fathers of infants merit attention:

> *The results of my study reinforce the belief that fathers are indeed salient persons in the lives of their infants and that there is a great deal of interaction between fathers and infants. Furthermore there is evidence that the characteristics of mother–infant interaction differ substantially. [p. 324]*

Lamb studied 20 white children, 6 from Jewish and 10 from Catholic families, groups that traditionally stress paternal authority and family closeness. His sample was too small and culturally restricted to predict American patterns generally, but further work partially substantiates his findings.

The psychiatrist Felton Earls (1976) reviewed the evidence from clinical psychiatry attesting to the father's importance. Pedersen et al. (1979) report "that the father is a significant influence on development as early as the first half year of life for male infants" (p. 59), though not for females. Like Lamb, the psychoanalyst Meerloo (1968) differentiates the fathers' and mothers' roles, claiming that mothers teach infants to feel secure and safe and that fathers at first influence infants by loving and protecting their mothers because infants aren't ready for a relationship with fathers until between 8 and 18 months.

Herzog (1980) falls into an old psychoanalytic tradition when he opines that children "need" an adult male from whom they learn rough-and-tumble play as a prelude to their greater ease in dealing with aggression in selves and others. He postulated that children without a father would experience "father hunger." By late 1982 Herzog extended his ideas as follows, according to the *Houston Post* (E. Bennett, 1982): "Without this play, a child might be less able to manage anger, love, sadness . . . and also with unexpected developments and having to shift gears (later in life)." Amplifying his viewpoint, he was quoted as stating that children without fathers have more trouble with aggression. "They attack, they get into more fracases." In contrast, when there is a father present who spends time playing with his 2-year-old child the father complements the mother's traditional mothering role of "following the child's lead in play" by taking up a "kamikaze role"—"interrupting regular play, imposing his rules on the game, stirring things up with the child." The child must incorporate both the calm and composed mother-derived view of self and the father-derived aggressive but in-control self. "The father helps to build a piece of the child's mind differently from the piece built by the mother, and it's built by different ways of playing."

In the revised edition of his book, Michael Lamb (1981) showed a mellower attitude about the role of the father in child development, acknowledging that the father, whether present or absent, may or may not have high salience for the child's development and if salient may have an advantageous, disadvantageous, or neutral influence. The trend in most research is to confirm that father, when present, may affect advantageously the child's cognitive and academic achievement, moral or conscience development, sex-role development, and overall psychosocial competence or lack of psychopathology; when absent he may contribute to the obverse in all the spheres mentioned. Lamb and his contributors all took cognizance of the multiplex nature of child development and fathering, showing that a father may have influence directly on the child, indirectly through the mother or through the family system as a whole.

Some post-Freudian writers also assert, as did Meerloo, that the father relates to a young infant either with the mother or through the mother. Patricia Drogos O'Donoghue (1978) concludes her survey of literature on the father's role in a child's pre-Oedipal development thus:

> The father has a specific role in the preoedipal period of the child's development. Initially, the responsibility is that of provider and support for the mother–child dyad; most of the literature points to a definite relationship between father and child forming in the latter half of the first year. The father's specific function is to provide for

the child a reality base and relief from the stresses which are inher-
ent in the separation from mother. The father's own pathology and/
or absence has great impact on the overall personality of the child.
[pp. 160–61]

She agrees with the Freudians that the father assumes increasing importance as the child nears the Oedipal period. Leo Bartemeier's
(1953–54) views presaged O'Donoghue's:

To give consistently to her child the love he needs, a woman needs
the consistent love of her husband and the certainty of his love for
their child. From a psychological point of view she and the child are
one, the disinterest on the part of her husband toward their child is
experienced as a lessening of his love of her. The fathers' influence
on the mother–child relationship has been too frequently overlooked,
in our evaluation of the factors contributing to the dissatisfaction
that so many infants and little children experience at the hands of
their mothers. [p. 278]

If the father can form a mutual attachment with the infant and
can play an important role in loving and caring for the infant, why
doesn't he? *Research indicates that babies can bond to fathers,* but
that mothers rarely give them the chance. David Lynn's (1974) review
of studies shows that fathers spend very little time with newborn infants (Rebelsky & Hanks, 1971; Field, 1978; Moss, 1967; Rebelsky,
1967; Goldfarb, 1945; Pedersen & Robson, 1969). According to Rebelsky and Hanks (1971), the fathers of seven male and three female,
full-term, white, winter-born, middle-class babies spent a mean of
37.7 seconds daily interacting with the infants during their first 3
months, and the father who spent the most time spent only 10 minutes, 26 seconds daily. Mothers, in contrast, increase their verbal interactions with infants over the first 3 months (Moss, 1967; Rebelsky,
1967).

In the little time fathers spend with infants, they often play games
rather than caring for infants or holding them. Field (1978) reports
that fathers "engage in more game playing and less holding of their
infants" (p. 183) than mothers, and Richards, Dunn, and Antonis
(1977) similarly report that fathers prefer playing with children to
taking care of them or being tender and close to them. Pedersen and

Robson (1969), studying 45 fathers of 8- to 9-month-old infants through mothers' reports, discovered that only 6 performed two or more caretaking tasks daily. Only 9 of 45 fathers patiently tolerated fussy, irritable babies, and 10 became irritable themselves around them.

Fathers traditionally don't feel as comfortable as mothers around babies. Dorothy Burlingham (Freud & Burlingham, 1944), a child analyst, studying children in residential nurseries during World War II, observed that visiting mothers fit quite naturally in the nursery setting, but visiting fathers, awkward and shy, remained passive. "They feel uncomfortable in this world of women and children, are at a loss in the face of overtures made to them by their children's playmates, and many of them are obviously glad when visiting time is over" (p. 101).

So fathers generally feel awkward with infants and spend little time interacting with or caring for them, even though surveys show that they like their babies and wish to care for them. Leonard (1976) and Reiber (1976) found that the fathers were willing to nurture their infants. In Leonard's study of 52 primarily Caucasian, middle-class fathers of normal, full-term infants, most fathers scored positively in these six areas:

1. Identifying with the child as a separate human being
2. Touching and holding the infant
3. Assuming a parental role
4. Beginning an affectional system with the infant
5. Looking forward to being a father during the pregnancy
6. Changing feelings about self, life style, and marriage

Reiber, observing nine American families and their firstborn children, theorized that fathers with basically positive attitudes toward their infants naturally want to help nurture, but that mohers who relish and cling to their status as primary or only nurturers won't let them help. Reynolds (1978) agrees that mothers jealously guard their special positions. According to Philip Wylie (1942), the American mother, confined to the home and angry about her captivity, uses her position to dominate the world through embittering her sons and training her daughters in the cult of "momism." In the 1980s, however, growing numbers of liberated men want very much to participate in child care instead of leaving all the fun to women (Lott, 1973). According to a study conducted by Nettelbladt et al. (1980), fathers who experience their children in a positive way are more acitve in the care of the children, less "authoritarian," and more physically intimate.

Division of labor according to gender of parent is greater in working-class families than in upper-middle-class ones. Hence, a working-class infant sees its father, even if present, in a more aloof traditional role. The liberated man, called a "sensitive man" by the writer Anaïs Nin, is less frequently a product of a working-class than of a middle-class family. Psychiatrists and other mental health workers occasionally overlook that basic fact of life.

Another overlooked fact is that children are not always the crux of parent–child gatherings. Pediatricians who are sophisticated about parents and infants often counsel a young mother whose spouse (or common-law husband) cohabits with her and the child: Allow the father to have his own time with the baby, in a room comfortable for the infant, but a room exited by the mother so that the baby will not perpetually be looking at the mother while held by the father. Mothers do that, finding that children do form bonds of loving attachment to their fathers. However, when both mother and father are present with the baby, empirical studies (e.g., Clarke-Stewart, 1978; Parke & O'Leary, 1976; Pedersen, Anderson, & Cain, 1980) inform us that the parents may become fixated on the mother–father interaction (or the conjugal relationship) to the exclusion of attending to the infant. When the two parents are together with baby, they smile more at baby but decrease all other interactions. In such circumstances, the child with a single parent, or two parents experienced one at a time, is in a more advantaged position. But even the much idealized and romanticized bond between mother and infant is not always completely idyllic and enchanted; for when mothers spend long hours with their babies, cuddling is done and dispensed with fairly promptly. Thereupon, the mother goes on with vacuuming, reading, phoning friends, and so on, leaving the infant in considerable isolation.

Richards, Dunn, and Antonis (1977) found that because caring for children is seen as women's work, little participation is expected of fathers. Wisdom (1976), a Kleinian analyst, explains that fathers themselves avoid spending time with their infants. One of the earliest introjections for infants is the breast, followed much later by the penis, which poses no problems for girls, even strengthening their feminine identification. But for boys, this early focus on the breast begins a sex-role conflict never fully resolved. The father avoids the nursery where breasts and nurture really matter, fearing his feminine yearnings stirred by the milieu, fearing that his femininity can't compete with his wife's:

> *In his dealings in the nursery, the man's deepest envy is aroused, . . .*
> *he loses the battle—if there is one—over the nursery, takes second*
> *place, and is a sort of second-rate mother, because he wants to avoid*
> *any indication of femininity . . . feeling uncertain of masculinity*
> *and having a deep-seated identification with motherhood provide*
> *him with a problem, whereas women can feel more secure having the*
> *breast introjection from the beginning. [pp. 233–234]*

So though the experts agree that a baby can attach to the father, given the opportunity, it rarely does because both men and women view infant care as women's work. In Reiber's opinion (1976), men exclude themselves, simultaneously afraid of their own femininity, or ability to nurture, and envious of their wives' ability to nurture. In contrast to these fearful men, Bartemeier (1953–54) describes men raised without fathers who identified with their mothers and treated their children quite maternally.

Learning and maturing in the relationship with the caring person, an infant develops a sense of confidence and trust in the world. Weaning from breast or bottle is a milestone of crisis in the relationship. If weaned while teething, the baby feels ambivalent toward the mother, and indeed toward anyone else. Some writers view this postambivalent phase as a fall from an Edenic state (Coriat, 1946; Adams, 1963). Biting added to sucking may disenchant the mother, and a loving baby may turn to a loving father for comfort if a father is available. The baby sits unsupported by 6 or 7 months and walks at about a year: In the traditional family, the homebound parent, the *Hausfrau*, succors and caresses throughout this first year. The father remains aloof and disconnected from mother's and child's activity or perhaps serves as an *éminence grise*.

Lourie (1971) among many others points out that the 8-month-old baby who shows stranger anxiety can crawl away from its mother and identify strangers and strange places since by that age some separation has occurred already. This separation anxiety organizes the infant's personality according to Spitz (1945, 1972) and Bowlby (1969). In the first stage, the infant both desires and fears autonomy; an inappropriate resolution may cause persistent fears of novelties and strangers as well as later depression. During this critical time, if fathers look like strangers, an infant can turn only to the mother for reassurance.

Writers disagree about whether the mother or the father influences the infant's future relationships more. Bowlby (1958) portrays the infant–mother relationships as the prototype for all later love relationships. Schaffer (1971) urges caution: "Whether a child's first relationship is in any way the prototype of all future relationships we do not as yet know; the clinical material bearing on this point is hardly convincing" (p. 151). Other writers believe that the relationship with the father is the telling one. Some raise it to the power of the tie to mother; others go beyond that. According to Abelin (1971), between 8 and 18 months, the infant begins to notice the father who becomes the second specified object who is "different from the first but equivalent to it." Meerloo (1968), for one, finds this second relationship extremely important:

> *The father is the bridge to the vast world outside. The first transfer of the baby's feelings from the mother to the father becomes the model for many subsequent social relations and involvements. The mnemic imprint of this first shifting of emotional expectations determines the direction of later trial relationships and transference possibilities. This is true for girls as well as boys. [pp. 102–103]*

By 18 to 36 months, the baby begins to talk, to manipulate words, names, and symbols in true interaction with others. By 2½ years (between 18 and 30 months), marvelous self-identification transpires in both gender and self-esteem. Each child knows and values his or her gender, information basic to one's sense of body and self even in a nonsexist society. At the same time, each child also knows his or her worth and acceptability as a person among the significant others in the world. In short, the child knows, describes, and defines the self, evaluating it as profoundly good or, pity be, bad.

These grand intrapsychic and interpersonal processes spin out, generated by the mother and child's symbiotic relationship. The father in a traditional family usually misses his opportunities, fewer than the mother's, to influence the child, because, as an intermediary between home-hearth and marketplace, he doesn't involve himself emotionally with his child and works almost solely through a surrogate, his wife. Through his wife, a traditional father may have elaborate patriarchal fantasies, and his wife may even share them, but the mother expresses both her own and the father's love; she is the conduit for transmitting messages and values directly to the infant. Another kind of father, detached from the "borning and suckling" of infants, feels embarrassedly exposed as he identifies with the new baby. While he greedily fantasizes nurturing the baby, the mother actually does nurture the baby; the father's imagination is more narcissistic than empathic. His projective identification supplants the empathic, interactive identification that a father in a not-so-traditional family might enjoy, a family whose mother and father share the jobs and responsibilities of child rearing. This nontraditional family should not be confused with its parody described by Adams (1983) and Gordon (1975): a family whose "liberated" wife and mother works full time but also retains complete responsibility for home and children.

All told, the traditional family fails to provide infants with contributing fathers. Boys learn, in close relation to mother, to be boys: to enjoy penile erections, to think of themselves as males with obvious, outer genitals, and to begin learning socially prescribed and socially induced gender-appropriate roles. Girls, borrowing many sentiments and values from the mother, learn to be girls: to feel pleasure in the clitoris, to experience orgasm sometimes, to think of themselves as female with cathected genitalia and body images. The mother's ministrations, precepts, and examples forge self-concept and gender identity in the first 30 months, without much help from the father.

Father's role in a traditional family becomes more direct and weighty in the years following infancy, leading to the Freudian exaggerations of Oedipal conflicts, and paternal narcissism diminishes slightly, if ever, in the child's fourth and fifth years. Harry Stack Sullivan (1972) noted that fathers who do not empathize with their sons may drive them back to intensified mutual dependence with their mothers, which can be seen as the interpersonal explanation of the Oedipus complex. If this logic also accounts for Oedipal conflicts in girls at age 4 or 5, a fault in the mother's empathy for her daughter sends the girl to her more understanding father for affection and interest, bringing about the Electra complex.

Traditional families notoriously spawn Oedipal conflicts more than other families. A trio, not a twosome, is the *dramatis personae* for Oedipal conflicts, a basic fact for discussion of fatherless children. Sigmund Freud, aware of the Oedipus kernel of neurosis in family dramas, or romances, found Oedipal trios fitting and proper, eminently human, universal, and phylogenetically programmed. Concentrating on Oedipal triangles, Freud gave fathers a central place in the family drama, and he objected in 1924 to Otto Rank's birth-trauma theory that the mother is paramount:

> *The exclusion of the father in your theory seems to reveal too much the result of personal influences in your life which I think I recognize and my suspicion grows that you would not have written this book had you gone through an analysis yourself. Therefore I beg of you not to become fixed but to leave open a way back. [Taft, 1958, p. 99]*

Chapter 2 considers further how patriarchal all classic Freudian theorizing is.

Normal children come to grips with their fathers by the time they start elementary school. And a study done 25 years later shows they have so inducted themselves into maternal and paternal roles that most kindergarteners can foretell, quite accurately, whether they will marry and have children by 30 (Broderick, 1968). Elementary-school children in traditional two-parent families see their fathers as full-fledged human beings, as encyclopedic funds of information and practical skills, or perhaps as standoffish people rarely at home. Schvaneveldt, Freyer, and Ostler (1970) report a child's description of a good father:

> *A good father does not spank, does not lock doors, and feeds you when your mother is not home. He washes the dishes, helps Mother,*

and picks up the garbage; he is to be sat upon and fought with. He reads stories, sings, and does things for you; he kisses and hugs and helps you get dressed. He works with Mother, sleeps with Mother, and likes her. He does not steal, he is nice to people and helps them get in and out of cars.

A child who can say these things has incorporated many values of a conventional, good-enough father and of an intact nuclear family, integrating the paternal image with his or her own self-picture and blending both perceptions with mother's role in the family. If two parents are better than one, such a child probably has inestimable advantages over one with no father.

Similar flattering accounts of fathers appear in newspapers mainly on Father's Day (Louisville *Courier-Journal and Times*, June 17, 1979):

> *We love our daddy because he loves us. He is very nice. He takes us fishing, sailing and riding. When we are sick he helps us get well.*
>
> Daniel and Matthew Cohen
> Murray, Kentucky

> *My father is an unusually nice father. For example: he bandages cuts. Mom just kisses them a lot. He lets me punch him all the time. Mom won't.*
>
> Beau Janzen, 9
> Danville, Kentucky

> *My daddy is nice to me and loves me. He takes me places. He fixes my bike and does lots of other things.*
>
> Jennifer Jon Stettler, 7
> Louisville, Kentucky

> *It is fun to love my dad, because he gives me pencils and pads. Sometimes he is fun. Sometimes he takes me for walks in the sun. That's why I love my dad.*
>
> Melissa Ann Stettler, 9
> Louisville, Kentucky

Many children, even fatherless ones, accept similar pictures of fathers.

Fathers can easily offer their empathy to elementary-school children. Early in elementary school, according to our clinical experience, a normal girl often believes that her mother is not on her side, so if she feels that her father has her best interests at heart, she is lucky. Somebody loves her. Similarly, a boy with problems in school, unable to trust grownups who aren't relatives, is lucky if his father supports, reassures, and encourages him. Some children, without the father's help and comfort, crash on the rocks of inferiority, incompetence, or inadequacy, those ever-near perils of schoolchildren.

Late in elementary school, some children reach puberty and some start dating and petting, shifting their sights permanently to people outside the family. Some children, instead of venturing into heterosexuality, form close bonds of loving affiliation with friends of their age and gender. Both kinds of relationships are exquisitely validating because children love and are loved by others who aren't relatives, nothing even remotely incestuous; but the other child makes simply possible a radical step upward in children's love lives. The luckiest preadolescents may have both "homosexual" and heterosexual loves. In a middle-class child, heterosexual love, with interstimulation to orgasm, often doesn't occur until adolescence or later, and some parents of preadolescents do not permit chumships, perhaps believing that only kin are good enough for such close associations. Frequently, middle-class fathers, more than mothers, liberate children to loving intimacies with agemates outside the tribe and family. Mothers represent rectitude and control by late elementary school; fathers can represent broader experimentation and outreach, more flexibility.

By preadolescence, children have moved toward social positions considerably independent of the family. They increasingly feel that they belong with others, with those who have no kinfolks' claims. Fathers can serve well as role models for self-realization outside the family. That is where they are so often expert. Mothers, of course, can also encourage friendships, and sometimes fathers do it quite badly: Many fathers we know monitor their children's love relations too closely, particularly their daughters'. Whether parents encourage them or not, children mature sexually, and in adolescence they may turn to or away from their fathers. Fathers only rarely and with difficulty do anything with positive meaning in adolescents' lives, so when they do, it is a special treat for both. When youths emancipate themselves in adolescence, fathers get their last chance to be primary and benign figures in their children's lives; some, of course, erroneously see this opportunity as an invitation to intrude.

Father's meaning to the child, when the former is present, covers wide spectrum of real interactions and unreal fantasies. The actual place of the father within families, and in the mental representations held by children, is one of largely unrealized possibilities. Our definite impression is that the traditional family may have been more restricting and coarcting of the father's potentialities than will be newer family types in which fathers are more nurturant, more equal, and more fully participant members. Our review of the father from the child's standpoint has been given to counteract some of the views that only add, in our opinion, to mystification. Our hope is that the clinician will have a demystified and sensible view of both being fathered and being fatherless.

This limited and partial panorama of what fathers do in traditional families gives background and reference points for studying children without fathers, whose lives assuredly differ from those of other children. In the following pages, we continue to confront encomiums to the father's role in the family, particularly those suggesting that without a father, no family life is worth living (Chapters 2 and 3). We review these theories critically, even if they have been supported by no evidence other than random observations, because they have obviously affected the work of many clinicians in mental health. After reviewing general outlooks on fathers and families, we systematically examine the research data concerning families without fathers, which in their several varieties mean different things to the children involved (Chapter 4). We appraise how fatherlessness affects academic progress and sex-role identity (Chapter 5), delinquency and psychiatric disorder (Chapter 6), reporting our own and others' research, making research suggestions (Chapter 7), spelling out social policy principles (Chapter 8) to diminish the very real plight of fatherless children, and summarizing the numerous clinical applications in our final Chapter 9. But the next chapter shows us that *being a father* is not the same as *fathering* in an active, dynamic interaction with a child. In the title of that chapter we use *father* as both noun and verb.

CHAPTER TWO

Father, Father

Anthropological investigations show that, though fathers' options vary widely from culture to culture, their options within a culture are invariably restricted. Hence, fathering is not one simple, universal culture pattern but a fabric of multiple patterns and colors. Indeed fathering is only one thread in the whole context of family and economy—and the values that comprise a culture. Western psychology, theology, and law, predictably bound to traditional Western values, uphold the patriarchal family, forcing fathers into stereotypical roles, ignoring children's rights generally, and assuming that fatherless children are hopelessly handicapped. These views, culturally (not biologically) based, can no longer adequately describe or illuminate family life.

A few examples from other cultures suffice to indicate how varied, yet limited, fathers' roles can be. La Barre (1954) described polyandry in the Marquesas Islands: One woman traditionally married several unrelated men, including a head husband and a secondary husband. The head husband, the main authority figure, disciplined the children and served as sex-role model for male children, while the secondary husband maternally loved, supported, and nurtured the children. Another possibility is for fathers to be concubines (La Barre, 1954). Among the Nayar of Malabar, all the daughters of a family marry the same man before puberty. Their marriage is not consummated, and after 3 days, the daughters legally divorce their collective husband and remain free thereafter to take lovers at will; the mother's brother acts as (our kind of) father to the children. The Trobriand Islanders of Melanesia, studied by Malinowski (described by Parsons & Bales, 1955), similarly do not recognize biological fatherhood. A Trobriand man holds two roles: that of father to his sister's children and that of mother, always subordinate to his wife's brother, to his own children. The endless variety of family structures shows well that culture, not biology, determines fathers' duties, and, though these studies suggest that fathers might ultimately choose from an unlimited array of possible roles, each father's choice is actually severely limited by his culture. Margaret Mead's (1935) work on *Sex and Temperament* remains a classic to warn us as clinical scientists away from sex-role stereotyping but reminds us simultaneously that as participants in any culture we can do little but stereotype.

In our culture, assumptions about the true nature of the family, particularly those revealed in most psychology, theology, and law, represent a cultural inheritance, a perhaps compelling ideal, but one that now unreasonably restricts family relationships by emphasizing the father's rather than the mother's role in child rearing; it is a patriarchal ideal. In truth, it is an ideal in transition from being patrifocal to being matrifocal with an occasional indicator that wholesome family life may become even "filifocal" or filiocentric. In this chapter we want to examine how that intellectual heritage of patriarchal values has imprinted the thinking of psychologists, theologians, lawyers, and possibly mental health workers.

Many psychoanalysts promote the patriarchal family. An excellent review of the psychoanalytic literature regarding the role of the father has been prepared by John Munder Ross (1979). According to Freud, the father, playing a central role in a child's formative years, stimulates superego development and reinforces sex-role identification. His theory centers primarily on the penis, badge of fatherly and male distinction, though some critics complain that the penis is a frail reed for the family to lean on. A boy sexually desires his mother and simultaneously fears his father's retribution, castration, the punishment he assumes fathers inflict on all girls. Boys see girls as suffering a dreaded amputation, not the castration of farmers and veterinarians—loss of testes—but, from Freud's urban perspective, penile amputation. Fear of castration leads a boy to identify with his father and to repress his longings for his mother. Superego development naturally follows because the boy, having learned the prohibition against incest from his father, learns other prohibitions from him as well. Freud's theory predicts maladjustment in adulthood for young men who do not resolve the Oedipal conflict between 3 and 8 years. Freudians have explained with this theory Leonardo da Vinci's bisexuality (Wallace, 1979) and Charles Darwin's denial of God (Greenacre, 1963) as well as the dynamics of many generations of their live analysands.

The penis is similarly prominent in Freudian explanations of girls' development. A girl initially has a love fixation on her mother, but when she discovers that boys have penises, she feels slighted and blames her mother (not the cruel father of the boy's fantasies) for the injustice. Then she moves her love fixation to her father and soon wishes to bear his child. Realizing that, at 4 years old, she cannot, she

suppresses her desire and, because she fears losing her mother's love
she identifies with her mother. Freud claimed that women never full
resolve their Oedipal conflicts, though men can, because the boy'
fear of castration is a much stronger motivating force than the girl'
fear of losing mother's love.

Peter Neubauer (1960) and Margaret Meiss (1952) describe severa
possible disturbances of Oedipal conflicts in young fatherless childrer
of both sexes. According to Neubauer, existing Oedipal conflicts in
tensify when a parent dies during the child's Oedipal period. If th
parent of the same sex dies, the child perceives fulfillment of th
Oedipal wish and feels guilty. If the parent of the opposite sex die
Oedipal longings increase with no chance of requital. A parent's deat
during this period leads to excessive fantasies about the dead paren
idealized or punitive fantasies or both, depending on the parent'
gender, the child's gender, and the child's developmental needs at th
time of the death.

Other explanations of family relationships—psychological and s
ciological—eliminate Freud's emphasis on the penis but continue t
posit a basically patriarchal family. Although many learning theor
ists or behaviorists agree with Freudian views of the father and pe
ceive him as the source of superego development and sex-role ident
fication, they differ with Freud on the mechanisms of these processe
especially those concerning the male child. Identification with th
father, they claim, takes place through reward and punishment rathe
than solely through fear of castration. The son first of all does wh
he learns from the father's direct teaching and also follows the father
model to avoid punishment and to earn continued affection and nu
ture. According to O. Hobart Mowrer (1950), not stridently ant
Freud at that time, the boy imitates the father in order to "reproduc
bits of the beloved and longed-for parent."

Other learning theorists discard Freud's theory totally. Bandur
and Walters (1963), for example, contend that the imitation theor
accounts more accurately than the identification theory for the sam
behavior: A male child imitates the father only because he sees th
the father is rewarded with a glorified position in the home, a rewar
he desires for himself. Direct reinforcement of imitative behavior
not necessary.

According to role theory, whose main original proponents wer
the sociologists Parsons and Bales (1955), the family is a subsyste

within the larger system of society. Parsons and Bales distinguish two parental roles in the nuclear family: the instrumental and the expressive. The father traditionally plays the instrumental role; his primary responsibility is to serve as liaison between the family and society. He represents society's demands and society's values, making major decisions about the family. His love for his children is conditional: He loves them for what they can do, for what they can contribute to the family and to society. The mother enacts the expressive role, keeping the subsystem running smoothly, making peace among the family members. She loves her children unconditionally, no matter what they can do or actually do. This division of roles allows children to grow up, thanks to the mother, in a secure and loving environment that promotes emotional well-being, and at the same time to learn through the father socially appropriate tasks, behaviors, and values, for a life of competence and productivity.

Parsons and Bales validated their theory with cross-cultural research. Of 56 societies, 46 differentiated roles but did not always assign the mother to the expressive and the father to the instrumental role. Zelditch (1955) provided additional evidence that families in many societies differentiate instrumental and expressive roles and that the father usually, but not always, plays the instrumental role. Eisenberg, Henderson, Kuhlmann, and Hill (1967), studying 6- and 10-year-old children in the United States, found that *both boys and girls* perceived the father (and males generally) as more instrumentally nurturing and the mother as more affectionally nurturing. Other studies, however, raise serious doubts about the correctness of role theory. Leik (1963) and Burke (1972) found that parents in reality either share the tasks of the expressive and instrumental roles or they distribute them by competence rather than gender. Collins and Raven (1968) contended that the longer the marriage lasts, the more the mother tends to become equal to the father.

Notions about instrumental and expressive functions have had an eager endorsement in psychiatry largely because of the preachments of the family group therapists. Westley and Epstein (1969) adopted and popularized the model as a way of differentiating the functions of fathers and mothers, and many have followed them. Today family group therapists acknowledge, at least in conversation, that such distinctions are not valid when applied to nontraditional families.

Burton and Whiting's (1961) status envy theory (in following the

Freudian notion that role learning is strongly motivated and involves identification) suggests that the child identifies with the parent who appears to consume the most valuable resources, to receive the most desirable privileges and goods, to hold the most laudable position in the family. The child anticipates achieving this enviable status and practices for the superior part in fantasy. Whiting, Kluckhohn, and Anthony (1958) studied 56 societies to support the status envy theory of sexual identity. They discovered that a male child who sleeps with his mother until weaned envies her apparent high status and longs to be like her. He gets fixated and centered on being like mother. Initiation ceremonies break his identification with mother by marking his entry into masculine society; through initiation rites the boy learns to envy his father's status and thereafter imitates his father's behavior. Young (1962) disputed Whiting's interpretation of initiation rites, saying that they may establish male solidarity but do not specifically resolve crises in sex-role identification.

Anthropology, by giving a cross-cultural viewpoint, can be of real if limited help to the clinician by showing that fatherly behavior distributes into a wide range of involvement and detachment, that fathers in preliterate societies worldwide (compared to ourselves) do very little caretaking of babies, and that "fathering" is a function of economic institutions, division of labor, level of technology, family structure, and "nucleation propensity" of marital pairs—the latter being a tendency for a monogamous couple to split off from extended family and peers (Katz & Konner, 1980).

Patriarchal psychology and sociology argue that private and public well-being result from a perhaps rarely achieved perfect patriarchal family; patriarchal theology, by assuming that God is male, has justified men's preeminence on earth as morally virtuous, the way things should be. Though many scholars no longer believe that God has gender, religious practice remains faithful to men.

Initially defining God as purely male was troublesome. Female deities preceded male ones in Western civilization, and the many strong warnings given by many religions against women and goddesses may indicate their former power. "Venus figures," representations of a motherlike deity made throughout Europe in Upper Paleolithic times, lend credence to the idea that the Great Mother was the earliest deity. Merlin Stone (1976) suggests that the many goddesses who reigned in tribes surrounding the Jews of the Old Testament were the idols that the Jews—imputing their prejudice to their male God—railed against.

The resulting denigration of women was severe, as two modern interpreters of the Garden of Eden myth show. Stone argues that the myth justifies the patriarchal family as divinely decreed:

> *The myth of Adam and Eve, in which male domination was ex-*
> *plained and justified [by the Levite priests who put Genesis together],*
> *informed women and men alike that male ownership and control of*
> *submissively obedient women was to be regarded as the divine and*
> *natural state of the human species. [p. 218]*

Toyohiko Kagawa, according to the memory of one of us (PLA), reinterpreted the Eden myth with more subtle antifeminism than Stone saw: Women urged men to stop gathering fruits and nuts and to cultivate crops. Since cultivated crops deplete the soil more than fruit trees, Kagawa assumed that women's inferior judgment about feeding the tribe, rather than their intrinsic evil, prompted human-kind (males notably) to leave paradise, cut down food-bearing trees, and begin millennia of scratching in the soil. Perhaps Kagawa approved of women's industry, for he sees men as unabashedly prone to idleness. In all events, an agricultural interpretation of the Eden myth scarcely requires that women instigate the fall.

Early Christian condemnation of sex for pleasure derives from and reinforces the patriarchal family. Paul thought it only better to marry than burn, but preferred celibacy and recommended that married women remain quietly subservient to their husbands. He saw women with orphaned children, however useful to the church, as merely pitiable; the Pauline coloring of Christian thought from the beginning bore prejudice against households with no man in charge. Early Christians, dispossessed and poor, gained moral superiority by speaking out against people apparently more fortunate, by condemn-ing sexual freedom, easy divorce, and women's equality. For them, things of this world, including begetting children, lost their impor-tance compared to the imminent Second Coming; heaven, chastely asexual, would more than make up for any mortal inequity or lack of pleasure. We, too, live in apocalyptic times, and many young peo-

ple today refrain from marriage and procreation, from sexuality itself, explaining, somewhat as the early Christians did, that it is cruel
to bring children into a nightmarish world of uncertain future.

One virtue of Christian emphasis on sex for procreation rather
than recreation is to remind adults that childbearing and devotion to
children are at the heart of family life and that, at times, carnal pleasure and the spirit of Satyricon may interfere with children's well-
being. Generally, however, religious protests against sexuality reflect
more fear of women than concern for children and forcefully urge
men to take control of their families and societies.

An image of God as either androgynous or sexless might help correct psychic and social problems arising from severely restrictive patriarchal ideals. Jung generally preferred balanced ambiguity to one-
sidedness and androgynous to purely masculine religious images. He
saw a sign of greater balance in the Godhead when in 1950 the Roman
Catholic Church affirmed the assumption of Mary as the bride
"united with the Son in the heavenly bridal chamber, and as Sophia
(wisdom) she is united with the Godhead. Thus the feminine principle is brought into immediate proximity with the masculine Trin-
ity" (1965, p. 202). Jung's Catholic women patients responded to
Mary's new status positively, finding in it affirmation of their own
worth. Mary Daly (1973) is a Catholic theologian who argues further
for a completely nonsexist theology:

> Unlike the so-called "First Coming" of Christian theology which was
> an absolutizing of men, the women's revolution is not an absolutiz-
> ing of women, precisely because it is the overcoming of dichotomous,
> sex stereotyping, which is the absolutizing process itself. . . . Neither
> the Father, nor the Son, nor the Mother is God, the Verb who tran-
> scends anthropomorphic symbolizing. [p. 97]

She suggests that our gods should depict our best rather than our
narrowest traits, but not that we should merely reinstate ancient female deities: "Far from being a 'return' to the past, it implies a
qualitative leap toward psychic androgyny" (p. 97). The average parish priest probably disagrees with Daly's theology.

What kinds of groups are inclined to female—and what other kind
to male—deities? Michael P. Carroll (1979), studying some of the data

from the Standard Cross-Cultural Sample of Murdock and White (1969), came up with rather fascinating responses to that question. He studied 56 societies in which children were reared mainly by their parents and discovered that *unilineal families* gave greatest importance to *male deities* even when the lineage was calculated as coming through the mother. Double-descent or cognatic families, by contrast, showed a statistically significant leaning toward *female* deities. In Carroll's formulation, parents rear their children immersed in norms about who their progenitors are, and the gender of the deities can be accounted for by the type of descent system actualized in any given society.

Patriarchal ideals, now more firmly established in religious practice than in theology, have been systematically presented in law. Until recently, laws about families protected fathers exclusively, allowing children no rights at all and actively discriminating against fatherless children. Laws codify much of public morality, and their preference for men and fathers, though beginning to wane, is still evident.

Until the twentieth century, men legally owned their wives and children as well as the family property. The Supreme Court first acknowledged children's rights in 1967, and even today the main law protecting children, the Juvenile Court Act, concerns only neglected, dependent, and delinquent children. Children's rights are still extremely abstract: "Nowhere in the standard juvenile court law or the new Model Juvenile Court Act are there any specifications of the rights of a child or the procedures that he may invoke for his protection or to obtain redress for wrongs done to him" (Foree, 1973, p. 450).

The illegitimate child is even less protected by law than children with legal fathers. Family law has dealt with marriage, property, and husbands' and fathers' rights; such laws simply don't apply to families whose husbands and fathers claim no rights. And the problem is widespread: In 1940, 3.5% of U.S. births were recorded as illegitimate; 5.3% were recorded in 1960, 10.7% in 1970, and higher by 1983. Until 1968, illegitimate children had no firm legal identity other than the demeaning status of *filius nullius* or *filius populi*. Offspring of no one or everyone, they could inherit neither surnames nor property. Legal authorities acknowledged for 200 years that such laws punished children without punishing or deterring parents; finally, in the late 1960s, when the ratio of illegitimate to legitimate births reached toward 1 : 7, the Supreme Court acted, reviewing 14 cases involving the constitutionality of state and federal laws concerning illegitimate children, deciding that the Equal Protection Clause of the 14th Amendment must be extended to illegitimate children.

Robert L. Stenger (1978) notes that constitutional rights benefit some illegitimate children, but that rights will not help many welfare families unless the mothers manage to identify the fathers legally. The Parent Locator Service of HEW, set up in 1970 when over half the children receiving Aid to Families with Dependent Children were illegitimate, helps find fathers, establishes their legal paternity, and requires them to support their children. Such a program, an application of constitutional rights, may continue the good work of the Supreme Court and truly help the half-million illegitimate children born each year. However, Skarsten (1974) suggests a modification of this kind of service. A similar program in Canada spent more money locating fathers than it collected for child support; Skarsten recommends that the money be given directly to fathers to pay child support and educate themselves so that they can eventually support their children on their own.

Not all illegitimate children are poor or black or fatherless. Poverty causes more problems for many illegitimate children than fatherlessness does, but not for all. Though 56.1% of mothers of illegitimate children were nonwhite in 1970, many middle-class white women also refuse to marry or otherwise provide fathers for their children. And while many lower-class illegitimate children live with their mothers and grandmothers, many others live with their mothers and men who act as their fathers, men who are not their biologic fathers. Still others live with foster parents or are adopted.

Adoption laws affect primarily two groups of fatherless children: those awaiting adoption in group homes and those adopted by single women. Adoption laws first appeared in the United States in the mid-nineteenth century, treating children as property. An adoptable child, disowned by one or both parents, could become the property of other parents. Until recently, an adoptable child was a well-formed baby WASP, and suitable parents, heterosexual couples only, matched the child in race, religion, and economic status; courts using these criteria preferred relatives to adopt disowned children. Adoptable children now include older children, non-Caucasian children, and those with intellectual, motor, and emotional difficulties.

Adopted children now have the right to know their natural parents; issues being investigated include the effects of interracial adoption, the possible risks of adopting children of schizophrenics and alcoholics, and the effects of adoption by a single or homosexual parent. Legal requirements for adoption are becoming less strict just as the store of adoptable children gets smaller. Single women, including women who work, women over 40, and homosexual women, are increasingly considered suitable parents. In California, single mothers are encouraged to adopt children, particularly black, Chicano, and disabled children. Some states effectively subsidize adoptions so that children may have parents without economic deprivation.

Children as property become important when parents argue over ownership; children of divorced parents have received more legal attention than adoptable or adopted children. Since 80% to 90% of them are given to their mothers' custody, most children of divorced parents are fatherless at least for a time. While divorce may improve a child's life by ending conflict caused by a loveless marriage, children do not always benefit from custody laws. A couple divorcing fairly amicably may fight bitterly over custody, concentrating their hostility on the children. It is a no-fault divorce but the children suffer.

Over a half-million children are caught in divorces each year (DHEW, 1978), most of them, in their mothers' custody, suffering some estrangement and separation from their fathers, and visitation practices are not always arranged for children. Richard and Elissa Benedek (1977) argue that children need to continue relationships with both parents after a divorce, opposing Goldstein, Solnit, and Anna Freud (1973), who would allow the custodial parent to decide whether visitation is appropriate. Divorce and custody laws increasingly consider the well-being of children, reflecting "a gradual shift in the structure of socializing relations." The state intervenes more in family life, and children increasingly can insist on adequate parents (Block, 1980, p. 45).

Psychology, theology, and law are slowly changing to accommodate the many families who differ from the patriarchal ideal, but they still prefer families with the father conspicuously at the head. Sociology, discussed in Chapter 3, usually measures fathers against a less rigid standard.

In medicine a situation exists that is slightly different from that found in theology and law. Medicine condones an ethic of privacy and acceptance of diversity that, even if it does not make tolerant humanists of many physicians, at least serves to dampen the physician's zeal for his or her particular ethnocentric choices. The medical tradition crimps the doctor's tendencies to be partisan and narrow, including, certainly, those times when a stand is called for. The Hippocratic oath made it crystal clear that the physician would not reveal any confidences shared by his or her patient, regardless of how unconventional the topic. The physician grew used to privileged communication with patients, safeguarded by medical ethics, by statute, and by common practice. Doctors long have understood that "scandalous" things can happen within the homes of their patients but have remained muted and muzzled.

Thus, the role of physicians has been confined mainly to one of keeping mum. And silent they have remained. Even when the Nazis used sick children for their "experiments" to determine the child's body's tolerance for burns, for starvation, and so on, German asepsis was maintained. The German doctors kept mum too. Frederic Wertham (1966) put it ironically: The "hospitals," where ghastly experiments were run on children, had beautiful geraniums in the window boxes. Their tidiness was admired by occupying troops from America.

The physician today finds it slightly out of character for her or him to take up a militant stance on public questions, even on matters such as nuclear armaments, and assuredly becomes very modest and shy when there is any public debate about the family styles that serve the welfare of children. Only when social criticism can be phrased as "good prevention," or in terms of the public's health, does the physician unmuzzle herself or himself. There is a large corpus of evidence that some families do, while others do not, actually benefit children but physicians seldom speak out about these taboo topics. In our time, it is obvious that specialists in family medicine, in psychiatry, in child psychiatry, in pediatrics and obstetrics–gynecology might join forces to begin to make medical declarations about what kinds of families can truly serve children, and under what circumstances. The fact that these medical people do not speak up bears tribute to the sorry political realities of medical practice today.

SIGNIFICANCE FOR THE MENTAL HEALTH WORKER

The mental health professions are relatively newer than the tried and true, if not fossilized, professions of theology, law, and medicine. As mental health professionals define their uses to the public, many of them fall into an ·aping, one way or another, of the older and better-established disciplines of theology, law, and medicine. Psychiatry itself, barely an accepted branch of medicine, is falling all over itself today to copy and adopt the medical model. Health insurance carriers join the pressuring to make mental health professionals medicalize their operations. Hence, it seems valid to assert, as goes medicine so goes the mental health multidiscipline field. The medical model may be useful for evaluating, labeling, formulating, and problem solving, but on the contemporary scene more halo than substance seems to exert an influence to medicalize psychiatry. Our point is that mental health clinicians partake of the same ideological and behavioral repertoire as do doctors; the same thing could be said of our fellow professionals in law and theology. Law in particular is exerting pressures on clinicians, but in the process some commentators have protested that we have become a nation of lawyers and guardhouse lawyers, people who adopt litigious and legalistic mannerisms in their work of serving others.

Mental health professionals share many of the cultural axioms and assumptions that order the thought of the three hallowed professions of theology, law, and medicine. In our roles as citizens (parents, coreligionists, club members) we do, think, and feel as appropriate for middle-class professionals. In our professional practices we aim toward less provincialism but our prejudices shine through quite unexpectedly at times, a reminder that we are both human and anti-intellectual, sometimes snobbish. We believe that to the degree that patriarchal values do suffuse thought about children and families, mental health clinicians share in them and will need to undergo occasional exercises in clearing out conventional cobwebs. The sociologist's record, reviewed in Chapter 3, may help us to be more aware and realistic in both our belief and practice.

CHAPTER THREE

Sociological Views
of Fathering

Sociologists who examine the role of the father within his family usually consider variations in socioeconomic status and race, sharpening the camera's focus. They concentrate on our society in the main but point up subcultural and subsystem differences within our society. Researchers in the psychoanalytic tradition have been faulted and deservedly rebuked for failing to give due regard to socioeconomic status when they study gender differences in parents as if all differences are inborn and assume that parenting is the same and has the same effects at all socioeconomic levels (Petrullo & Bass, 1961). Adolescents' attitudes toward fathers, for example, vary with social class; the higher the class, the more the father is esteemed (Smith, 1969). Sociologists and other social scientists may be instructive about what fathering is.

ECONOMIC CONSIDERATIONS

The sociologist Herbert J. Gans (1962) describes in a way that we condense (perhaps too sketchily) the following family types found in different socioeconomic classes:

1. *Lower Class.* In a female-based family, adult males, present only intermittently, are regarded as neither dominant, stable, reliable sources of affection nor child rearers. The dominant female derogates the male (providing a negative referent for male children), yet she takes him as a sexual partner and asks him for some economic support. This family type, a correlate of economic status, not race, is that of slum dwellers and poor people of all racial–ethnic types in the United States. In the Mum-dominated family of the *working class* in England, Dad is more permanently present and respected and shares child-rearing tasks. But in the U.S. lower-class family, though the mother's perspective is like that of the working-class mother, her male partner's status and role stamp the family as lower class. The lower-class male is not so interested in education, for he is action oriented; he is not wrapped up in work, and his work record is highly unstable; his sexual relationships are typically short-lived.

2. *Working Class.* The family circle itself is dominant: Kinfolk

32

are the significant others. Work is obtained and pursued with stability, but it is regarded as a necessary evil, secondary to family living. A family member seeks education only in order to obtain a better job so as to enhance family living and to minimize the considerable poverty lived out in the working-class family. All evaluations of the outer world—and these are often hostile and negative—are based on the paramount value given to the *extended family.*

3. *Middle Class.* The *nuclear family* with only parents and their offspring dominates the family network of the middle class; most extensions of the nuclear family are secondary in value to this primary group. Families seek togetherness; family life centers on child rearing and in that sense is child centered. Generally family prestige derives from the father's occupation; family morale and spirit interact closely with the father's career fortunes. The middle-class family sees itself as a part of the outside world and the world as itself; it participates in the larger society and sees that "whatever is good for us is good for society."

4. *Professional Upper-Middle Class.* For this group the typical pattern is to use the nuclear family for personal growth or self-enhancement. Nuclear family life that serves personal interests is what matters. Professional-class family members are profoundly oriented to the larger society in both work and education. This class views work not only as a means for securing the integrity of the nuclear family, but also as a route to achieve individual fulfillment and to provide social service to the community at large. These attitudes are held by the man (who is most likely to be the breadwinner) and the woman (who is most likely to be the domestic partner) alike. For the woman,

> if she is not interested in a profession, she develops an alternative but equally intense interest in motherhood, or in community activity. Child-rearing . . . gives the woman an opportunity not only to maximize her own individual achievements as a mother, but to develop in her children the same striving for self-development. As a result, the professional upper-middle-class family is not child-centered, but adult-centered. [p. 248]

Gans attributed to the professional class certain sociable skills that are not shared by "members of less educated strata," among them self-consciousness, empathy, and abstraction or generalization. Gans distinguished the professional from the lower and working classes: "The fatalism of the working and lower classes, as well as their lack of education and interest in personal development and object goals, minimizes introspection, self-consciousness, and empathy for the behavior of others" (pp. 248–249).

The poor particularly engage our attention, because the lower socioeconomic classes include more fatherless families and because poverty has biomedical and sociopsychiatric consequences even for newborn children. According to Adams (1972a), poverty is a potent prenatal influence; among poor people there are:

1. Higher infant mortality: neonatal and postnatal
2. Lower "sex ratio" (male/female births × 100)
3. Higher prematurity
4. Higher incidence of neurologic disorders at birth
5. Higher handicap among male survivors
6. Higher fetal loss
7. Lower birth weight for term infants (38 weeks)
8. Lower IQ at infancy, 4 years, and 12 years old
9. More home deliveries
10. Less prenatal care
11. Higher maternal death rate
12. Higher frequency of infectious disease

Few people break the cycle; poor parents usually raise poor children. Fisher (1978), who studied working-class marriages, when asked if the children of her subjects would have different lives from their parents, answered very easily: "No."

> There's no room at the top and little room in the middle. No matter what changes people or groups make in themselves, this industrial society requires a large work force to produce its goods and services— a work force that generation after generation comes from working-class families. These families reproduce themselves not because they are somehow deficient or their culture aberrant, but because there are not alternatives for most of their children. [p. 43]

Gans' (1971) "functional analysis" of poverty listed several economic and social functions of poverty, which could otherwise be fulfilled, but only at the expense of the affluent. Since the affluent wield
the power in this society—as in most—the drastic reduction and ultimate elimination of poverty are unlikely. Gans wrote:

> *Many of the functions served by the poor could be replaced if poverty*
> *were eliminated, but almost always at higher costs to others, particu-*
> *larly more affluent others. Consequently, a functional analysis must*
> *conclude that poverty persists not only because it fulfills a number*
> *of positive functions but also because many of the functional alterna-*
> *tives to poverty would be quite dysfunctional for the affluent mem-*
> *bers of society. [p. 24]*

MYTHS ABOUT THE POOR

Herzog and Lewis (1970) attempted to dispel some of the myths and
stereotypes surrounding the "culture of poverty," including belief in
the low achievement motivation and rampant breeding practices of
poor people. The fallacy exists that poor mothers have low educational aspirations for their children. Female heads of household, too,
are thought to have lower education aspirations for their sons than
mothers in intact families (Parker & Kleiner, 1966). Poor female
heads of households often are thought to have even lower aspirations
for their children than poor mothers in nuclear families (Heckscher,
1967). Another myth is that poor people are apathetic. But apathy
has been shown to be a situational response rather than an inherent
quality, and it is frequently associated with malnutrition and goes
away when nourishment is provided.

In their breeding practices, the poor are not more fertile than the
rich. Neither do they shun the use of contraception when given the
opportunity to obtain and utilize it. Herzog and Lewis (1970) cited
the example of Margaret Sanger, who was prosecuted in the 1920s for
opening a contraception clinic for impoverished Jewish immigrants
in Brooklyn. She was admonished by physicians of the day that "the
people you're worrying about wouldn't use contraception if they had
it; they breed like rabbits" (p. 379). The district attorney, in his case

against her, accused her of trying to do away with the Jews. Even today, when costs are not prohibitive, the poor liberally utilize contraception and abortion, despite myths to the contrary.

Charles A. Valentine's (1968) survey and critique of the polemics
that now have raged about "the culture of poverty" for more than 2
decades remains sharp, fresh reading today. His hopeful conclusion
ended realistically and darkly:

> *Our nation . . . seems little prepared to meet the foreseeable re-*
> *vitalization of the poor with anything other than the reflexes of the*
> *cop on the beat in the ghetto, the posse in National Guard uniforms,*
> *and world policeman. Perhaps there will be no new anthropology,*
> *no creative resynthesis by the oppressed, but only another long night*
> *of blood and pain.* [*p. 153*]

THE POOR FATHER

Stereotypes hold that the poor father feels superior to the mother,
and the mother feels downtrodden. In reality, though, the father in
the lower-class family is much less involved in child-rearing activities, is less of a material provider, and has a much less prestigious
position than the middle-class father. The lower-class father is downtrodden himself at the marketplace and perhaps doubts his masculinity because the rich white man is his boss. The middle-class father
tends to have more autonomy and self-direction in his job, but the
lower-class father lacks these niceties in his work environment and
may feel inferior to middle-class men. He often takes out these feelings of inferiority on his wife and children. Kemper and Reichler
(1976) reported that father's mobility aspirations determine both
father's and mother's punishment of their sons, but not of daughters.
Punishment of daughters is related to fathers' job satisfaction and
power relations with boss and co-workers. Only at home is the lower-
socioeconomic-level father boss, and there often in name only.
Women in the lower class share the responsibility for breadwinning
and dominate financial decisions. They also assume, usually single-
handedly, the task of child rearing (Besner, 1965). The home is
markedly "mother centered." Thus the lower-class family is para-

doxically "mother centered" and lamely "patriarchal" (Herzog & Lewis, 1970). It is not matriarchal in any true sense.

THE POOR MOTHER

We already know that many poor families are fatherless families as well. In the lower-class fatherless family, male figures—father substitutes—are around from time to time. But according to Bell (1965) lower-class women tend to value being mothers more than being wives, so they don't encourage the father's presence, which may entail an added economic liability to the family. Even common-law marriage is penalized (Associated Press, 1979). Courtship is usually short and nonspectacular, and emotional distance prevails between the spouses (Besner, 1965). Also, when the father *is* present the children tend to view him with less esteem than do middle-class children. Smith (1969) indicated that adolescents' reverence for fathers is positively related to social class although reverence for mothers is not. Mothers have a presence across the economic spectrum in America.

Respect for mothers cannot be related to mothers' priorities in child care because these priorities vary among social classes. Lower-class mothers tend to emphasize discipline and conformity more than psychological development (Besner, 1965); they display more restrictive behavior with sons and more contacting and structuring behavior with daughters—at least when the children are preschoolers (Zunich, 1971). Middle-class mothers more often strive for an individuated relationship between child and environment (Brandis & Henderson, 1971). Although lower-class mothers, too, want their children's self-actualization, they lack the concepts and the techniques to promote it because of their own educational deprivation (Besner, 1965).

THE BLACK FAMILY

Moynihan

Some sociologists themselves fail to consider socioeconomic status and other variables when studying racial differences. For example,

the Moynihan Report (1965) described black society as a matriarchate, contending that adult female rule pathologically leads to
emasculation of black men, demise of the black family as an institution, and perpetuation of poverty—a "tangle of pathology." Moynihan used illegitimacy rates, the number of female-headed households, and employment rates as evidence, but has been criticized for
his motives, for his definition of *matriarchy*, for his methodology,
and for his interpretation of history.

Joanne Hahn (1972) denounced Moynihan's work, saying that he
"is more concerned with restoring proper behavior and properly
Catholic fucking than he is with repairing poverty." She described
Moynihan politically as an "archetype fink liberal," that is, a reactionary. In fact, Moynihan ran with neoconservatives and became a
senator before the 1970s ended, winning a large plurality in his sena-
torial race against Reaganomics in 1982.

Others criticize Moynihan less caustically. Adams and Horovitz
(1980a, 1980b) and Herzog and Lewis (1970) disputed Moynihan's
definition of *matriarchy*. Adams and Horovitz studied a group of 454
impoverished families in Miami to determine the relationship of
fatherlessness to children's aggressive behavior problems and to
mother's psychopathology. Using controls for economic status, ethnicity, place of residence, ordinal position, gender, and age group,
the authors found conspicuous similarity among mothers and sons
of diverse ages, ethnic grouping, linguistic heritages, and family types
among poor people. Thus, problems associated with fatherlessness
and blackness result from neither blackness nor fatherlessness but
from the poverty that both fatherless and black families endure.

Adams (1972b) believed that the racist belief that fatherlessness is
a black phenomenon must be rejected. In 1972 only one-fourth of
black families in the United States were headed by women with men
absent. By 1980, according to U.S. census data, the number had risen
to 36%. "It is from these families and the in-and-out street men who
brush them in brief encounters that Moynihan's 'tangle of pathology'
emerges: poverty–delinquency–illegitimacy–desertion–matriarchy–
economic dependency–unemployment–school leaving–sickness–drug
taking–societal dropping out" (Adams, 1972b, p. 8). Adams further
disallowed calling this minority of black families matriarchal:

As a matter of convention, we call "matriarchal" those impoverished partial families in which no adult male is present. The true matriarchate is a complete family—i.e., a unit of male, female, and child or children—but merely a unit in which the wife–mother is dominant. Is it truly a matriarchy when the father is nonresident or nonexistent and when the mother "rules" by default? [Adams, 1972b, p. 9]

He argued that in the father-absent family the mother hardly rules. She tries to make do, *faute de mieux*, as *the parent* in an underclass.

Herzog and Lewis (1970) asserted that perhaps the least of the problems associated with the matriarchy label is that it happens to be incorrect. The term *matriarchal* can be applied to the low-income black family only when it meets two criteria: (1) The woman is dominant over a man, and (2) her earning power is greater than the man's. According to the Bureau of Labor Statistics in 1966, and again in 1970 and 1976, black women who worked earned less than black men who worked, and unemployment was higher among black females than among black males. A survey sponsored by the Carnegie Corporation, released by the Council on Interracial Books for Children, reported that "while 60 percent of Americans are females or members of a racial minority group, white males still dominate business, government, the news media, education and health institutions" (R. Pienciak, Louisville *Courier-Journal and Times,* January 21, 1980, p. A-16).

Herzog and Lewis concluded that to a certain extent the black mother *does* dominate child-rearing activities and responsibilities, but the same can be said about nonblack American mothers. The label *matriarchy,* nevertheless, is reserved for certain ethnic minorities. Such labeling contributes to ineffective social agencies and programs and compounds mutual antagonism.

TenHouten (1970), Hyman and Reed (1969), Valentine (1968), and Wilkinson and O'Connor (1977) all criticized Moynihan's methodology. TenHouten maintained that Moynihan's conclusions did not follow because his evidence was derived from sociodemographic data rather than from data on family dynamics. TenHouten himself used Los Angeles County 1960 census data to support his own different conclusions that lower-class husbands were *not* powerless or emasculated in either their conjugal or their parental roles. Quite to the contrary, the strength of *both* parents was perceived as a positive resource for black youth and as an asset to black families. TenHouten commented on white people's studies of black people:

> *The Moynihan research is a political weapon used to rationalize intervention in black communities, and used for white control of black people. It can certainly be expected that as an integral component of developing political mobilization by black people and poor people, these groups will assert greater control of research on themselves, and be less inclined to give information and the means of control to academia and to the Government. [p. 171]*

Hyman and Reed's (1969) secondary analysis of surveys by the Gallup Poll in 1951, the National Opinion Research Center in 1960, and the Survey Research Center in 1965 also negated Moynihan's findings. Using data on 4,900 individuals, 7% of whom were black, the authors concluded that the differences in parental power and decision making between white and black intact families were small and inconsistent. White and black family patterns, contrary to expectation, were almost identical. Women's influences predominated over men's in several areas, including political persuasion, where men have long been thought to dominate; children, black and white, more often chose *mother's* political affinity over father's. Thus, they discovered little evidence for a uniquely black pattern of mother's influence. King (1969) found that black adolescents see the family power structure as mainly syncretic. Males reported stronger father participation than females, and females reported stronger mother participation than males. Both males and females indicated stronger father participation in decision making than has been present historically.

The Resiliency of the Black Family

Wilkinson and O'Connor (1977), having collected data from 101 black poverty-level female heads of household and their sons, reported that the black female sole-parent system appears to be an extremely resilient family unit—one that benefits greatly from the availability of adequate employment in an environment that limits the black single mother to a life of impoverishment and hopelessness. These findings should be self-evident.

Adams and Horovitz (1980a) also commented on the notable ability of the single-parent family to rebound from humiliation and financial adversity—although not without scars from gross injustice in its rawest and most blatant form. In the concluding portion of their report on black and Cuban poverty-level families headed by women, they stated that the paranoia often observed in poor mothers is probably adaptive and functional. A fighting attitude may go further than guilt:

> *The more paranoid, outer-directed blame-placing done by poor women may be a healthy tendency (utopical insight). Seen humanistically, the paranoid poor may be less wretched than the depressive poor. The depressed ones seem unhappier, less fulfilled, more maladapted. [p. 155]*

Gutman (1976) refuted the Moynihan Report's interpretation of history. Moynihan stated that 300 years of injustice had caused the disorganization and decay of the black family structure, but Gutman asserted that neither slavery nor reconstruction, both harsh, undid the black family. He found that black family ties and associations remained strong and sustained the development of Afro-American culture despite great adversities. Gutman's documentation consisted of plantation birth and death records, census reports, and manuscript sources largely neglected by historians of black family life, which indicate that the ex-slave family included a poor husband, his wife, and their children. It was not female headed. Gutman noted optimistically that in 1976, 73% of black families had a man as head of household, a percentage that dropped to 64%, still a majority, by 1978 (U.S. Department of Labor, 1978).

Crawford's (1976) overview of literature on the black family found two distinct approaches to the topic as early as the last century; the "strength-resiliency perspective," advocated by writers such as Andrew Billingsley, Joyce Ladner, and Robert Hill, and "pathology–disorganization perspective," advocated by authors such as E. Franklin Frazier, Horace Cayton, St. Clair Drake, Gunnar Myrdal, and

Daniel Patrick Moynihan. W. E. B. DuBois (1961) indicated as early
as 1908 that a realistic view of the black family lies somewhere in
between.

Unfortunately, policy makers do not seek out the golden mean;
they base policy on existing opinion and sometimes on existing facts,
which results in inaction. Adams (1973b) summarized the problem
as follows:

> *Many discussions of the partial family in the United States are highly*
> *charged with political sentiments. Some progressives who fear being*
> *anti-black place themselves in the ludicrous position of defending the*
> *partial family so fully that they end up praising it and contending*
> *that members of partial families do not need any special assistance.*
> *Conservatives, on the other hand, are in the position of arguing that*
> *the partial family is patently debased and inevitably pathologic, but*
> *they contend that it must not be coddled and that it warrants no spe-*
> *cial assistance programs. Equally, then, neither the progressive nor*
> *the conservative described becomes an advocate for needy black fami-*
> *lies. Political neglect is an outgrowth of both ideologies.* [pp. 201–202]

Poor People, Poor Programs

Herbert Gans (1965), aiming neither to whitewash nor to damn the
black family, made some practical suggestions in response to the
Moynihan Report. Gans' suggestions, while not geared specifically
to the poor black fatherless family, were intended to relieve some of
the more general effects of poverty, which would benefit fatherless
children immensely.

Initially, Gans suggested that *decent and stable jobs* be provided
for black men. (No doubt, more than 15 years afterward, this suggestion would be viewed as sexist by some black women.) Following the
publication of the 1965 article by Herbert Gans, the government
made some feeble attempts to provide jobs for blacks. Government
programs were established and funded in inner-city areas with the
agreement that the programs would become self-supporting within a
specified amount of time. Program administrators used many of the
jobs offered by these programs as political jobs, often awarding them
to people not even living in the inner city. Unfortunately, after inadequate planning and supervision, and incompetent and opportun-

istic local administration, most of these programs provided easy money to a fortunate few, a few jobs to a less fortunate few, and a phase-out to everyone after a specified number of years. A more recent attempt to relieve unemployment among the poor is the Comprehensive Employment Training Act (CETA), a program phased out in late 1982—at a time of national economic privation and depression—and replaced by small programs (summers only, for example) for youths, principally those aged 14 to 21 years. The CETA program too provided an abundance of political jobs and a dearth of job-training opportunities for those people for whom the program was designed. Its successors have a similar promise since their funds also derive to the local people from an area council and are administered by local politicians, for example, in Galveston, Texas, through the Commissioners Court.

Secondly, Gans recommended a *massive rehousing* program to provide new housing for low-income families in urban areas and to clear and renovate the slums. A limited program of this nature was enacted. Slum areas have been replaced in many cases by housing projects of even poorer quality that confine to a smaller horizontal area the number of people who previously occupied several city blocks. The compacted housing projects are psychologically confining and demoralizing, seedbeds for crime and discontent, serving merely to consolidate and rigidify the ghetto.

Gans recommended providing equal income for people who could not work and could not earn a living wage—meaning the incremental extension of unemployment compensation and the humanization of policies regulating Aid to Families with Dependent Children. Though some efforts toward this have been made, one can hardly call $4,000 per year a "living wage" for a family of three or even for one disabled person.

The updated picture on poverty is bleak still. S. Miller (1980), a professor of sociology and economics at Boston University, bemoaned the fact that social planners are currently "reinventing the broken wheel" by continuing to implement social programs such as these or presenting "inadequate programs of the past as new, helpful programs of the present" (p. 2). While time and money continue to pour into poverty programs already proven ineffective, the real issues of concern to the poor—"unemployment, income distribution, regional development"—have gone untouched in recent years.

Life Styles of Black Families

Glick (1970), comparing marital stability among blacks and whites, found that the marital stability of both whites and blacks (when pooled) improved between 1940 and 1968, but relative to whites, the stability of the blacks weakened over that entire period. Inclination to marry among black Americans in their late twenties and early thirties has declined since the mid-sixties, but so has the inclination to marry among corresponding white Americans. Glick reported differences mainly in degrees. Generally, he found that black Americans living on farms in 1968 consistently tended, less than whites, toward marriage and marital stability at all ages. Young black adults in nonfarm areas delayed marriage more than their white counterparts. Also, older black adults in nonfarm areas showed far less evidence of marriage intactness than corresponding white adults.

The proportion of black children under 18 living with a single parent or with relatives increased from 1940 to 1968 much more than the comparable proportion of white children. According to the Bureau of Labor Statistics Report (1978), approximately 35% of the 11 million or so U.S. children living in one-parent families were black—a disproportionately high percentage, since only 14.4% of the total U.S. population is black. The median income for black single-parent families was $7,262 compared to $14,524 for white single-parent families. Black single-parent families are more likely to be headed by women than white single-parent families, and black single parents are less likely to work. They have higher unemployment rates, lower educational levels, and higher rates of poverty (Brubacher & Rudy, 1968).

Although we concentrate on the female-headed household, which occurs disproportionately in the oppressed black population, the majority of black families *are* intact. We wish to examine the black *intact* family as a reference standard for all the nontraditional family types.

Black family life styles, like the styles of any ethnic group, vary regionally. Rohrer and Edmonson (1964) described the life styles of New Orleans black society, a racial group "in a state of restless change, expansive development, and increasing community-wide integration" (p. 50). The blacks of New Orleans were depicted as "a society in formation, rapidly gaining precisely those elements of stability and continuity of which it was conspicuously devoid in the past. From the threads of this volatile past and dynamic present come the trends, attitudes, and issues out of which individuals and groups in this society weave their lives" (p. 50).

The New Orleans middle-class black family shows relatively stable monogamous marriage rites, neolocal residence, economic dominance by the husband–father, rigid control over children, and strict interpretation of the Judeo-Christian code of sexual morality. Occupationally, the middle class is heterogeneous. People of the upper and middle class prize those values by which they explain their own privileged positions: their economic and social success, their thrift and caution, their inhibition of aggression and sexuality, their ambition, initiative, and manners. They are not revolutionary, but prefer a conservative gradualism to the forcing of risky changes. The ideology of the middle class is overwhelmingly individualistic. Racism is decried on the grounds that a person should be judged as an individual rather than as a person of color. Children in this kind of family show the stabilities and insecurities found in most urban and suburban child guidance clinics.

There is no complete discontinuity between the middle and the lower class. However, generally speaking, the social structure of the lower class is less organized, less stable, and less coordinated than that of the middle class. Its family life is predicated on unstable marriage and frequent desertion. The mother is often the chief breadwinner; matrilocal customs are practiced. Discipline exercised over the children is apt to be harsh and inconsistent, with both parents frequently absent from the home. The men of the lower class are unskilled laborers, often unemployed. The children of the lower class are more like those seen in center-city child psychiatry facilities throughout the United States.

Cole (1970) described four distinctive life styles within the black community generally: street, down-home, militant, and upward-bound. The street life style represents the cool world of hustlers, musicians, entertainers, and others. Basically urban, distinguished by stylized talking, sounding, signifying, shuckin' and jivin', copping a plea, and whupping game, it is a world of severe poverty and hopelessness for most, as described by Liebow (1967), "cool" for only a few. In this group the care of infants and children frequently falls to someone other than the mother and father. Virginia Wilking (1979) is one of the rare child psychiatrists to discuss these street children capably:

> The street child stands as a model for the damage done to all emotionally deprived children. Living on certain city streets and roaming the adjoining blocks and avenues, he is often heard of, but seldom seen; somehow he is always somewhere else. By definition he is hard to know; he is not to be found at home, not in school, not even in family court or in the precinct station house, and very seldom in the child psychiatry clinic. Those seen most often fit the stereotype least well, and those who fit it best are seen least. [p. 301]

> The need is to go back to the beginning of the child (if not of society); there must be money for prenatal care, visiting nurses, community-based social agencies, high-risk infant centers to make up the seven maids with seven mops needed to serve families with young children. Unfortunately there is no substitute for money. [p. 308]

The down-home life style, basically rural and southern, is seen as the traditional way of black people. It centers in the kitchens and on the front porches of black homes, in the church halls for socials, in the fraternal orders of the Masons, Eastern Star, and Elks. "Down home," a common expression among blacks, indicates that for most blacks the point of origin is the south, which is also called the "old country." It represents a simple, decent way of life. Neighborliness permeates the child's growing up. Children are cared for by the extended family group of mother, father, grandparents, aunts, uncles, cousins, older siblings. The primary caretaker may be the grandmother or an older sibling rather than the mother.

The militant life style belongs to black heroes. It is a life style both social and political, centered currently on college campuses, in high schools, and in urban black ghettos, involving adults and youths more than children. It is the life style of cultural and revolutionary nationalists, infused with an urgency to change the plight of black people and the constant search for relief from oppression. It is characterized by dedication, by thumbing one's nose at "the man," by willingness to die, and by separation from the majority culture. In this group, mothers may care meticulously for infants, and adults generally want dominant fathers and many strong, healthy children, but since black revolutionaries appear to have no unified views on women and children, what results for the children is highly varied.

The upward-bound life style, frequently called "bourgy" (for *bourgeois*), centers in the better neighborhoods and in the so-called integrated churches and clubs. It is the style of the black middle class of teachers, accountants, doctors, lawyers, and other professionals who are trying to move up or in. This group behaves like the traditional white middle class in child rearing, use and style of language, and social values.

Llorens (1971) used these several life styles to illustrate that the labeling of black children as "culturally deprived" or "culturally disadvantaged" is mistaken. Obviously, black children have various life styles and cultures. Not cultural deprivation but *racism and poverty* impede the development of the black child, making it excruciatingly difficult if not impossible for black children "to achieve optimal development even within their own value system and certainly more difficult to achieve within the framework of values held by the majority groups" (p. 148).

The Poor and Black Father

The *Report of the National Advisory Commission on Civil Disorders* (1968) delineated the devastating effects of racism and poverty on the black family. A notable consequence is the disproportionate number of female-headed households among poor black people. The report stated the unemployment and underemployment in racial ghettos give statistical evidence that men living in these areas seek employment but are unable to obtain jobs to support a family. The jobs that they can get are at the low end of the occupational scale, and often lack the necessary status to sustain a worker's self-respect or the respect of his family and friends. Wives of these men often must work, and, unable to afford child care, they leave the children unattended to spend the bulk of their time on the streets—the streets of a crime-ridden, violence-prone, and poverty-stricken world. Under these conditions it is hardly surprising that men frequently desert their families, that youth learn to disclaim both work and marriage, that frustration and anger build up to the point of a kind of genocide and racial suicide achieved through violent crime in the ghetto. The pattern reinforces itself from one generation to the next, creating a culture of violence with an ingrained cynicism about society and its institutions.

Liebow (1967, 1970) studied black street-corner society in Washington, D.C., during the years 1962 and 1963. He contributed a perceptive and sensitive portrait of the day-to-day passions, banalities, brutalities, and struggles for life and survival among poor, urban black people.

As described by Liebow (1970), marriage, given status and respectability, is clearly superior to a more evanescent consensual union. In marriage, an institution that claims legitimacy and public recognition, rights and responsibilities are better defined than in the street-corner society that Liebow studied. On the other hand, the financial burden of marriage among the poor, both black and white, is often overwhelming. Marriage for the poor is a luxury, frequently doomed from the outset. To hear the men tell it, they were too manly to stay married. They could not sacrifice drinking, gambling, and chasing other women for the comfort of home and hearth. A more plausible explanation is that these men, facing an overcrowded job market with few skills and little education, could not live up to the expectations of their spouses that a husband would provide for, and be the head of, his family. Here is how Liebow put it:

> *Thus, marriage is an occasion of failure, to stay married is to live with your failure, to be confronted by it day in and day out. It is to live in a world whose standards of manliness are forever beyond one's reach, where one is continuously tested and challenged and found wanting. In self-defense the husband retreats to the street corner. Here, where the measure of a man is considerably smaller, and weaknesses are somehow turned upside down and almost magically transferred into strengths, he can be, once again, a man among men. [pp. 163–164]*

The men and women described by Liebow are real human beings, economically and psychologically devastated by a social system that denies them even the security of an intact family.

Psychological and economic profiles of people suffering the ravages of poverty and racism simultaneously have been offered by several authors. Pettigrew (1964) claimed that both poverty and migration maintain lower-class fatherless families, that the lower-class black man could hardly find a job that would support himself, much less his family. While the intact black family can foster ego strength to help the children cope effectively with racism, unfortunately, the lower-class family is poor both financially and emotionally.

What are some of the sequels of fatherlessness for the black child? Glautz (1976) wrote that father-absent black males are less likely to hold an internal orientation toward their world than father-present black males. Father-absent males are more likely to be punitive and less likely to be revolutionary. Hunt and Hunt (1975), however, comparing black adolescent boys to white adolescent boys on three aspects of orientation toward conventional success goals of early adulthood and two dimensions of personal identity, found damaging effects of father-absence only among the white boys. Father-absence seemed to have a slightly positive effect on black boys. The Hunts suggested that cultural values might explain this phenomenal discrepancy. Again we come upon a basic schism in the research findings about the strengths of lower-class black culture; we reiterate our guess that this problem is one that only the continued efforts of black and nonblack researchers can resolve.

The Negative Self-Concept

The idea of the black negative self-concept goes something like this. Black Americans feel passive and inferior, angry about powerlessness. The "anger shows in delinquent acts, addiction to drugs and excessive gambling. Since they believe they can't achieve their goals, blacks never do achieve them."

Proshansky and Newton (1968), looking at self-hatred in blacks, criticized conclusions about all black people drawn from data about mainly the lower class. Comparisons of self-identity characteristics of lower-class blacks with those of middle-class whites make it impossible to distinguish between effects of race and effects of socioeconomic status. Since most of these data were gathered before the impact of the black consciousness-raising movement, the bias of white middle-class researchers crops up again and again. They take the white middle-class value system as the norm, treating other value systems as deviant and, by implication, sick or bad.

The middle class holds itself as a model yet refuses entrance to its ranks. Rodman et al. (1969) indicated that the greater the pressure to adhere to conventional values, the less likely it is that the members of the group will normatively accept deviant patterns of behavior. But if people cannot enter the middle class because of race, why should they conform to middle-class values? It is less degrading to maintain one's own life style and folkways while simultaneously being allowed the rights and privileges of the minority group. The rich and the poor have always done what they wanted to do, but for different reasons—the rich because they are powerful and untouchable (in a Western sense), the poor because they have no hope for upward social mobility and are untouchable (in an Eastern sense).

Whether blacks have a negative self-concept may be a question with no flat answer, but the idea that blacks have a negative self-concept serves racist purposes, shifting the blame for black under-achievement onto blacks. That lets the dominant group off the hook so that no structural changes will result.

Some of the research that supports the premise of the "negative self-concept" holds on tenaciously even though Carpenter and Busse (1969) and others have found no differences between the races on the variable of "negative self-concept." Differences between races can support equally well the idea that blacks are inherently flawed and the idea that they must tolerate exceptional injustice. Raskin, Crook, and Herman (1975) analyzed psychiatric history and symptom differences in black and white depressed patients, to find that there was a greater tendency toward negativism and the introjection of anger in blacks than in whites. In addition, depressed black males indicated that they were more likely than their white counterparts to strike back, either verbally or physically, when they felt their rights were being violated. There was also a very high incidence of suicide threats and attempts among the black males. Psychiatric patients may not represent the entire population from which they come.

Some authors feel that fatherlessness is more devastating to black children than to white children because black society lacks high-status adult males who can act as surrogate fathers. This viewpoint, however, directly opposes the research findings of Hunt and Hunt (1975), as well as those of Earl and Lohmann (1978). Many ills have been attributed to the black male child's dearth of male role models—delinquency, cross-sex identity, poor school achievement, and impaired mental health, among others. Earl and Lohmann (1978), however, discovered that 53 black latency-age boys from the lower and middle socioeconomic classes had frequent contact with their fathers, as well as with male relatives and members of the community with whom they sustained close relationships. The authors concluded:

> *Contrary to assumptions of much of the literature the black children in this study saw their fathers with surprising frequency. For the boys who had limited contact with their father, other family and community males were available to provide them with loving guidance and attention. Thus, these black children were not as bereft of male guidance as the popular literature would suggest. [p. 415]*

Some authors dispute assigning all the problems of poor blacks to blackness or fatherlessness and prefer to identify poverty as the villain. Wylie (1963) showed that when evaluating themselves, black and white students (when SES was controlled) showed no differences in self-estimates of their schoolwork capabilities or in levels of aspiration. This discrepancy will be discussed in greater detail in Chapter 5.

For Consolers and Policy Makers

Tuck (1971) recommended some ways to work effectively with black fathers who receive agency assistance, ways to help the men provide positive emotional experiences for their children. He lauded the results of a pilot project in which a black male family worker was assigned to work intensively with four fathers and four children by attempting to make the fathers more sensitive to the developmental needs of their children. The suggested model for working with black fathers was based on seven principles or guidelines, among which were the following: Strive to establish trust within the all-male group; actively engage the fathers in recruiting other fathers into the group; assist the group in planning special activities for their children that take the families, including the mothers, away from day-to-day activities at home. This project resulted in a much larger-scale neighborhood involvement that included the fathers' engaging their wives in a neighborhood social event and sponsoring a local business venture, and it culminated in a concerted drive for community control. Such male black resources are seldom sought or cultivated.

*Carkhuff and Berenson (1972) suggested an approach employing "systematic interpersonal training as a preferred mode to facilitate relations between races and generations" (p. 92). In their study a black male and a black female were trained as functional professionals to offer high levels of responsive and initiative dimensions to two fatherless families, one white and one black. The results were favorable although the sample was tiny.

In the current decade specific recommendations have been made to human service agencies for working with select populations of black unmarried adolescent fathers. Hendricks et al. (1981) indicate that appropriate roles for agencies include the provision of psychosocial counseling, vocational guidance, and parenting education. Outreach intervention needs to be aggressively pursued by such agencies.

Although Riessman wrote in 1964, his views on this subject seem to have a timeless quality. He, also, made recommendations for working effectively with the poor—black and white. He accentuated the strengths of the poor, born out of coping with a negative environment, rather than emphasizing their failures and pathology. He simultaneously dismissed the noble-savage ideal of the poor. He called the noble-savage concept false admiration based not on the struggles of the disadvantaged themselves but instead on their relative lack of the disreputable elements of middle-class society—inhibitions, competitiveness, disloyalty, pretentiousness, boredom, or whatever. He railed against comparing the coping efforts of the poor with standard middle-class behaviors, unlikely alternatives for the economically deprived. The strengths of the poor, he stated, were often the reverse side of weakness.

Riessman's indicators of moral fortitude among poor people included greater sibling interaction, greater freedom from intellectualization, less prestige-centered, competitive, individualistic ethos, proclivity for independence and self-education, greater maturity of the children, and greater receptivity to therapeutic techniques (p. 418). These strengths must be taken into consideration by formulators of social policy. Of his opponents, Riessman said, "Recognizing that the poor are not uninhibited, do experience serious strains, and want no part of poverty, this view can only hold that an emphasis on the strengths of the poor is sentimental drivel and naively anti-middle-class" (p. 417). One need not be poor in order to be happy!

WESTERN WORLD AS MATRIARCHY

Moynihan (1965) drew fire for defining black family life as a matriarchy. Yet other authors have defined all of Western industrial society, American society in particular, as matricentric if not matriarchal. This society is not a true matriarchy, some agree, such as can be observed in some East African societies. It is rather a "pseudomatriarchy," because the woman rules by default, with the man absent at work for prolonged times and the mother confined to homemaking and child rearing. That this overassignment of domestic responsibility to women tends to warp the female personality has been pointed out by advocates of the women's movement. Women oppressed in this manner are angry toward men. Their vengeance is taken out on the children, particularly the male children. Thus there emerges another generation of angry women and of men who strive to keep women in their places, men fearful of women, men who experienced a woman's wrath in childhood.

John Nash (1965) compiled a useful survey of the research on matriarchy and female domination, including the views of Gorer (1948), Elkin (1946), Kluckhohn (1949), Josselyn (1956), Ostrovsky (1959), and Rubenstein and Levitt (1957), whose views naturally seem dated now. Gorer (1948), a Britisher who epitomized American society as "the mother-land," stated that in our society the mother has assumed all responsibility for child rearing and father has become vestigial. He claimed that adolescent males have lived throughout childhood in a world totally dominated by female authority. According to Elkin (1946) these young men are exposed primarily to feminine models; they experience great difficulty in accepting mature and socialized concepts of virility. From that arises their need to be supermasculine in adolescence and adulthood. Clyde Kluckhohn (1949) said that the father was archaic because father had abdicated his role as parent in order to pursue the more immediately rewarding phantom of success in the marketplace while mother stayed at home and pampered her children, her housework being done in large part by labor-saving devices. Kluckhohn's concept did apply to many middle- and upper-middle-class mothers and fathers during the 1940s. Even in that decade, a few working-class families actualized this stereotype of mother at home pampering the children and father out wheeling and dealing and bringing home the bacon. During half of that decade, many working-class fathers were absent because of a war.

Irene Josselyn, a social worker turned psychoanalyst and child psychiatrist (1956), wrote that fatherhood is viewed as a social obligation, but motherhood, by contrast, is perceived as a biological state that can afford some psychological gratification to both mother and child. Josselyn asserted that this cultural stereotype impeded fathers in their attempts to form healthy and mutually gratifying relationships with their children. Fathers, probably a bit less so now than when Josselyn was writing, are viewed as effeminate when they give, like mother, tender nurturing care to their young ones. If not seen as sissy, they often are seen as "passive," "henpecked," or "pussy-whipped." Josselyn also noted that in America mother is often maternalistic not only to her child but also to the father, her husband—a view supported more recently by Goldstein (1977). Father is frequently just a big sibling to his offspring and sometimes a serious rival. Illustrative of this quandary is the case of the patient seen by one of the authors who upon the birth of his first child mandated that the baby only be allowed to nurse from the right breast as the left one was his alone (Adams, 1979).

Other authors have remarked that not only the home life but also the school life of children is dominated by women (Ostrovsky, 1959). Ignored is the fact that males rarely seek the low-paying position of elementary-school teacher when times are good. Father limits himself to providing financial sustenance (Rubenstein & Levitt, 1957)—and not even this, among the poor. Ideological support of this viewpoint is seen in contemporary literary works steeped in references to mother—mother's milk, beloved mother, protecting mother, *"la" patrie,* devoted mother, and so on. Some perceive the mother as ruling the household with an iron hand. She makes her husband impotent, emasculates her sons, and traumatizes her daughters. Occasionally, a mother almost does all that. Platt (1970) presented the case history of a family dominated by a she-viper matriarch—though this tends to be the exception rather than the rule. Phillip Wylie (1942), an early writer who saw mother as ruling the household and dominating church and state by means of her divisive manipulations, described the phenomenon of "momism" or "mom-worship," assiduous devotion to the state of momhood equalled in prevalence only by adoration for the flag and the Bible. He wrote, foreshadowing Phyllis Schlafly:

> *Mom got herself out of the nursery and the kitchen. She then got out of the house. She did not get out of the church, but, instead, got the stern stuff out of it, padded the guild room, and moved in more solidly than ever before . . . she swung the church by the tail as she swung everything else . . . she also got herself the vote, and . . . the damage she forthwith did to society was so enormous and so rapid that even the best men lost track of things. [p. 188]*

So what became of the omnipotent father viewed by Freud as the stern, forbidding—almost terrifying—Victorian patriarch? Some believe that father defaulted to mother. Others report that father did not default but was sent away. Until the Great Depression, father was the primary breadwinner for the American family. With the Depression came the valuing of women in the work force for various reasons, mainly for the economic reason that they would do the same job as men for less pay. Following the Depression came the prosperity of war. Numerous unemployed men got jobs but simultaneously many men were sent out of the country. Household *and* country were left to the women, who apparently functioned quite effectively in the men's absence. The first generation in recent times to be exposed almost solely to the influence of women emerged. Other forces eroding the absolute authority of the father in the United States are industrialization, modernity, fearless sexuality, female liberation, the youth movement, kiddie lib, affluence, equalitarianism, and, especially for working-class and lower-class males, the class system (LeMasters, 1972).

A more psychoanalytic explanation for the hegemony of matriarchy was proposed by Erich Neumann (1956), who analogized patriarchy to the tendency of the ego to triumph, of consciousness to prevail. The moon archetype, in Neumann's opinion, is the epitome of matriarchal consciousness, and he foresaw a coming renaissance of spiritual illumination that will restore the moon to full equality with the sun.

> *The ego of the matriarchal consciousness is used to keeping still until the time is favorable, until the fruit of the moon-tree has ripened into a full moon; that is, until comprehension has been born out of the unconscious. For the moon is not only lord of growth, but also, as moon-tree and life-tree, always itself a growth, "the fruit that begets itself." [Neumann, p. 47]*

Having reached fruition, progression out of the unconscious turns into a clinging in desperation to the unconscious. For Neumann, matriarchy is opposed by patriarchy, the latter being epitomized by the sun. Matriarchy represents rule by heart, patriarchy, rule by head. The ideal, a Jung-like union of these opposites, is somehow missed in the vying. The patiarchy, too, conquers, is embellished, and recedes—in absurdity—defeated (Neumann, 1956).

Western culture lies somewhere within this cycle. Deborah Slawson (1979) interpreted Neumann's work as indicating that matriarchal consciousness is the source of ultimate power, the power to give birth. Male power is perceived as being female given. According to Slawson,

> *men, suffering from the acute fear that their women-given power may be lost, make every attempt to insure that woman remains ignorant of her own power. This has been done through a long process of social subjugation. Because men fear what they have never experienced, especially if that experience is a power-source as most experience is, and because men seldom participate in the matriarchal consciousness of creativity, they fear not only the consciousness but the incarnation of that consciousness—woman. [p. 1–2]*

Hence, societal power is patriarchal in nature and women's attempt to share in this power is an expression of their search for a

outlet for creativity. Women's creativity has been confined to reproduction, but the largely male medical profession—to cite only one
example—has denied their total participation even in that. Consequently, women are restricted and frustrated in expressing spiritu-
ality. Yet, stated Slawson, "woman-power cannot be restricted by patriarchal forces at the basic level because the (female) power roots
have no base in patriarchy" (p. 4). The theory laid down appears to
be one of female superiority, an old gynecocentric viewpoint shared
by Briffault, the sociologist Lester Ward, and many other proponents of the matricentric or matriarchal mode. Opponents might say
that woman has taken over the home, the sphere of matriarchal consciousness, and she now seeks to extend her realm to the marketplace with her demands for equal rights. Perhaps matricentrism has
been accomplished in our society, but matriarchy has yet to be attained. As noted earlier, in a matriarchal society women have the
greater power in settings where men are present but do not rule.

SOCIAL CHANGES AFFECTING FAMILY LIFE
FOR ADULT MALES

In the present century several important changes have come about
to (1) *democratize families* in which fathers live, (2) *popularize families with fathers,* and (3) *conjugalize families generally*—to make the
conjugal relationships of the adults the true backbone of the family
life (Sussman, 1978). The father's role as a mate to his wife is his
consolation prize for not being an effective, zealous *father.*

Being an adult male is not as easy a role to play as it formerly was.
Some authors attribute father's decline in status to such societal influences as television, increased specialization, and accelerated work
demands, but we wish to emphasize as well the impact of social
movements and economic forces aimed at achieving equality among
all peoples. The oppression of women will end only when men accept the equality of women. Child liberation is somewhat different,
because children need *not only* greater access to liberty and freedom
of choice, along with more genuine respect from all adults, *but also*
greater protection and greater help owing to their dependence. In
all events, the family is democratizing.

Considerable security, unstudied, unreflected, or even unconscious, accrued from patriarchal views and practices, and institutional change is not a happy experience. Giving up advantages and privileges is not fun for adult men. Risking some losses when no compensatory gains rise into view is frightening. Future shock is a daily diet. The predicament is a shaky one, but many men sense that there is no going back to a time of female inequality. Dr. Sol Gordon (1975) writes:

> *The myth that's operating now is that the family is breaking down, our children are unresponsive and the only cure is a return to that traditional family picture. But as a matter of fact, if we try to go back, the situation will only get much worse. Children won't tolerate it, wives won't tolerate it. We can't go back to something that is no longer viable if, indeed, it ever was. [p. 52]*

No matter how compulsively writers such as the psychoanalyst Voth (1977) decry changes, changes will keep on snowballing, from all indications. Hear Voth whistle in the dark past, extolling the traditional family virtues of Freud and early analysts:

> *The fine concept of equal opportunity for everyone is being misread as meaning that everyone is equal. They are not. Men and women are not equal in ability. They are equal in worth but their worth can only be fully realized by enhancing not blurring their difference. [p. 220]*

> *You men, are you living up to the responsibilities which have traditionally fallen to men? Are you the head of your family? You women, are you doing the same: Are you really committed to your husbands? And above all, are you mothers taking care of your babies and preschool children? [p. 222]*

Democratization of the intact nuclear family means that father no longer has the exclusive voice in decisions for the family, for mother now has chimed in and even children have some say-so. The middle-class family council—with one vote per person—epitomizes an extreme of democratization. But the family's larger surround, a more democratic society, has formed some kind of equilibrium with a multitude of family changes: mothers working away from home, higher divorce rates and more liberalized grounds for divorce, alterations in family laws affecting the custody of the child after divorce, some advance in female liberation so that women are more realistic toward men and more reluctant to revere the specialty of child care as the exclusive domain of women, some increased consciousness of the rights of children to both greater liberty and greater protection and help, the emergence of the concept of parental guardianship (Block, 1980), and at times an extension of equality and personal autonomy to an extreme that is absurdly narcissistic for fathers, mothers, and children.

A *father* in the "me generation" looks out for himself. If one's vote is cast in one's own individual interest, "wife and children be damned," then a father does not do anything for his immediate family except as it enhances his own pleasure or is a trade-off for his individual growth, his orgasms, his male ego, and so on. Nobody lives for others in a group of narcissists—as is evidenced by the increasing incidence of family violence, most frequently seen in the form of child abuse and wife beating (Sussman, 1978).

Although father participation literature is somewhat limited to date (Croninwett, 1982), noteworthy research in the 1980s suggests that father's emerging role is less egocentric and more child focused. Jacobs (1982) considers the breakup of the nuclear family to be a major mental problem in the United States today. He suggests that as some fathers become more involved in family nurturing, they will be more intensely affected by marital disruption, particularly as it involves changes in the relationship to their children. Collins (1979) takes another new look at life with father. In analyzing the current literature on father participation, he states that the crucial impact of the new research should be that "a father's role ought to be an optional choice . . . and with some education and training, they can become parents—but only if they want to be."

Fatherlessness has become more frequent. In the United States today, women head one out of every five households. Many children will be exposed to all the risk factors attending fatherlessness and its correlates, whatever those risks may be. We must be vague about risks in order to be truthful, for we could accidentally attribute to fatherlessness many features of unhealthy childhood that have no intrinsic correlation to father-absence. For example, just as two out of three poor adults are female, most households headed by women are poverty-stricken, so fatherlessness alone does not account for the numerous quandaries that *poor and fatherless* children find themselves immersed in.

For a woman not to marry was a rarity, relatively speaking, in the nineteenth century. But in the twentieth century many choose not to marry, and divorced, widowed, or deserted women do not feel compelled to remarry and reconstitute a nuclear family. Divorced women typically still do remarry—more often than their never-married agemates marry—but more and more they too choose to remain unwed. Unwed, they select a life style of sexual freedom (both lesbian and heterosexual) or masturbation or celibacy, sometimes devoting more of their attention to the needs of young children in the process. Not all of that is pathologic. It is now conceivable that every mother does not need a male companion, yet some men think it incredible. Household size gets smaller and smaller in the United States, partly because, when a man leaves, no one replaces him. Especially among the poor, more and more children are born out of wedlock each year—another expression of the growing popularity of the fatherless household.

A third social trend is *conjugalization* of the family, ranking conjugal relation of the two adults above their relation to children. When concern for his personal autonomy leads an adult male to opt out of family life, he may choose to remarry but remain childless in the new marriage. With personal autonomy and self-realization as basic motives, he realizes that the conjugal family alone serves the self better. Hence, even if pregnancy ensues, the man keeps thinking of his relation to his partner, not of bearing and rearing children. Fortunately for his children, he may become an active father when the baby is born, but, unfortunately for his children, his heart may not be in it because he thinks first and foremost of the conjugal relationship, not of the father–child relationship. It has not always been that way. In fact, in the nineteenth century families were more child centered. The contemporary family is conjugally centered, modern, democratized, and often fatherless.

Men, dethroned from their superior status with respect to wife and children, often choose not to marry and have children or opt for homosexuality and other orientations that put personal pleasure ahead of procreative and child-caring duties. Lower-class men led the way historically in father-absence. Now, through divorce, desertion, and never marrying, men of the working class and even more affluent men are absenting themselves from family living and child rearing so that there are over 11 million children in the United States today who have a lessened daily contact with adult males as fathers. Women do have an impact on the young generation but men, through absence and some forms of unconcern, have little encounter and few interchanges with young children and adolescents.

Finally, then, if the man does marry and have children and takes an interest in their care and upbringing, and does, in short, *father*— most men still do this very thing—the marriage itself is never so underlined and stressed. Complete satisfaction of oneself through a conjugal relation is everyone's right; total satisfaction of one's conjugal mate is everyone's duty. But that is marriage with a conjugal focus, not a child focus. Although Henderson (1980) reports that the experience of fathering is important to the psychological development and further growth of the father himself, this opportunity is sadly missed by many biological fathers who are physically absent and, indeed, physically present, in the American family.

To conclude about our brethren, the sociologists, we have shown that they examine in a sophisticated way the variables of classism, racism, and sexism when they describe the role of the father in today's U.S. family. Sociologists seem to bring increasingly vital contributions to the child mental health field (Adams, 1982), not by uttering eternal verities, but by conducting rational empirical studies. What we learn from sociologists is that, because of sexism, the female-headed household is most likely to suffer the ravages of economic deprivation. Because of sexism and racism, the black female-headed household is more likely than the white to be sorely deprived economically. While some writers mistakenly call the Western world a matriarchy, we see that at best it is a pseudomatriarchy. Women do not even have earning power equal to men—much less, greater earning power. On a more positive note, we see social changes occurring, but with much resistance from many sectors of society, chief of which is white male-dominated power, a force still alive and well in the United States today.

CHAPTER FOUR

Types of Fatherlessness

INTRODUCTION

I am a fatherless child. I have no father as a regular member of my family. Who am I likely to be? Which characteristics outline a statistically correct picture of me? I am more likely to be female than male. The adults in my neighborhood are mostly female too. I am likely to be black since there is a 50.6% chance that, merely by virtue of being black, I will not live with both parents. Since I do not live with both parents, I am ten times more likely to live with my mother rather than with my father; if I am black, I am twenty times more likely to live with my mother than with my father. I am poor, and merely because I am poor, there is a 60% chance that I live with my mother only. If I live in a female-headed family, there is a 66% chance that my mother receives welfare and we barely subsist economically. There is an over 50% probability that my mother works full time, exposing me to motherlessness as well as fatherlessness. She earns 50% to 60% of what her male counterpart receives (U.S. Department of Labor, February 1980). My mental health and my school adaptation may be impaired. (See Chapters 5 and 6.) However, damage to school attainment and social adjustment, when observed, are consequences of poverty rather than single parenthood itself (Schorr & Moen, 1979). I may, if male, be more aggressive than my agemates and may not get on well with them. Probably, given a choice, no one would choose to be a fatherless child.

In this chapter, we try to account for the growing number of fatherless children and to look at the various causes of fatherlessness—death, desertion, divorce, and other circumstances.

INCREASE IN FEMALE-HEADED HOUSEHOLDS

A report from the U.S. Bureau of the Census (1978) carried the news that although there were 5.4 million fewer people under the age of 18 in 1977 than in 1970, the number of children living with only their mother had increased by 3 million. In 1970, 85% of all children under 18 years of age lived with two parents. By 1977, this percentage declined to 79%. The figures also showed that five out of every six people who maintained families with no spouse present were women (Saluter, 1978). Fatherlessness is spreading like an epidemic.

In 1976, an estimated 4% to 8% of the nation's families were fatherless. It was 8.6% in Louisville, Kentucky, a city of keen concern to the authors. Statistics from the Bureau of the Census for 1978 revealed that 10,905,000 blood-related children were living in one-parent families; of those 10,029,000 (92%) were living in families headed by women. The median income of one-parent families headed by women was $6,260—by men, $13,698 (U.S. Bureau of the Census, 1978). These women, on the average aged 30 to 34 years, had an average of 3.07 dependent children (statistical bulletin of the Metropolitan Life Insurance Company, 1970). Black single mothers were twice as likely as white unwed mothers to have *three or more* children dependent on them (Brubacher & Rudy, 1968).

Of the economic inequity between single-parent families headed by women and those headed by men, Waldman et al. (1979) wrote aptly:

> *The wide economic disparity between these two types of families is illustrated by the fact that 42 of 100 families maintained only by a mother had incomes below the poverty level, compared with 15 of 100 of those maintained by the father only. Thus, children in one-parent families maintained by the mother are far more likely to live in poverty, have inadequate housing, receive inadequate health care, obtain insufficient education and training, and experience fewer job opportunities. Often these experiences in their childhood and youth affect them throughout their adult lives. [p. 45]*

Reasons for Increase

What are the reasons for this increase in female-headed households? Klein (1973), who discussed middle-class single-parent families, proposed that the single-parent life style has its roots most deeply implanted in the soil of unfulfilled promises. Perhaps this is more true for middle-class single parents than for lower-class single parents. Many single parents, according to Klein, grew up in families where the parents' marriage seemed loveless and unfulfilling. They were raised in the traditional nuclear family and found it to contain more enmity than intimacy. Thus, they as parents have become deviant, avant garde—dedicated to expanding the concept of the family beyond its old tightly patrolled borders—and they try on alternative family types. We can tell that the parents studied by Klein are middle-class single parents because economic considerations are not of major importance to their choices. Others contend that the general decay of the middle-class nuclear family, and the consequent increase in female-headed households, arise out of the existential alienation of individuals from one another in late twentieth century capitalistic society. But an economic interpretation holds better: So many are poor. The fatherless family all over the world is a lower-class phenomenon especially.

Cutright (1974) examined family patterns sociologically and insisted that it is not a matter of rejecting the isolated, nonextended family, not at all. There is an increased probability that a mother at risk will form a separate family, Cutright held, rather than living as the offspring or other relative of a family head. The upshot is that when she has children a mother does not want to reside in the extended family. Cutright calls this trend the nucleation propensity component in his sociological explanation for the increase in the number of female-headed households. Population growth and changes in fertility patterns and in marital stability are the remaining components.

Contributions to Increase in Female-Headed Families

1. By disproportionate female-to-male ratio (ages 15 to 44)   36%
2. By nucleation propensity of husbandless mothers   32%
3. By greater fertility of married and unmarried   13%
4. By 1, 2, 3 acting in concert   90%
5. By decline in marriage stability only   3%

The above depicts how fatherlessness comes about because there are so many females relative to males, so great a compulsion for a woman to take her children into a separate place away from the extended family, and for women (whether married or unmarried) to have children and provide a home for them.

Thirty-six percent of the total increase in the number of female family heads was due to the growing population of women aged 15 to 44. Incidentally, that trend continued throughout the 1970s so that the female population has continued to grow and to exceed the male population (U.S. Bureau of the Census, 1978). Population growth, in combination with the nucleation propensity component, accounted for 68% of the total increase during this time period. The decline of childlessness (i.e., a greater fertility) among the married, together with rising illegitimacy among the never-married, seemed to account for about 13% of the total increase. The three components (nucleation, population growth, and fertility changes) all together accounted for 90% of the increase from 1940 to 1970. Declining marital stability, independent of other components, accounted for only 3% of the total increase. White and nonwhite populations differed little in the relative weight of these various components.

The Metropolitan Life Insurance publication (1970) presented globally divergent ideas. The insurance company stated, contrary to the conclusions of Cutright, that the increase in the proportion of families headed by women stems *mainly* from more marriage break-ups, more divorce or separation. No cognizance was taken of fertility changes, of the pressure for separate dwellings, or of overall population growth. No statistical study accompanied the Metropolitan Life statement. It has a rhetorical ring, politically conservative but radically undocumented, an odd kind of demography.

From our 1984 perspective, however, we see a somewhat different outline when we try to give a priority ranking to the elements increasing fatherlessness, particularly among poor people. Inflation skyrocketed during the late 1970s, and the cost of raising a family likewise soared. Families who might have made it without public assistance during the fifties and sixties cannot hope to do so now. For these families, it is economically sounder to dissolve marital ties since welfare practices discriminate against the intact family that needs public assistance.

Regarding the U.S. family as we ended the seventies, *Newsweek* (May 15, 1978) said, "Raising children has never been more costly—in time and money—and the interference from outside forces has never been more acute" (p. 64). In 1977, a family of four, earning between $16,500 and $20,000 a year, could expect to spend $54,297 to support a child to the age of 18, excluding the expense of higher education. The $1,000 tax exemption for children and elderly dependents, which once favored larger families, has shrunk to a pittance alongside this inflation-fed cost of nurturing children. Economically, the situation of the fatherless children looks even worse in the 1980s, but their numbers keep increasing.

BOTH POOR AND FATHERLESS

If the middle-class family is hard pressed to meet basic familial needs, how can the poor family meet its needs? Schorr (1966) reported on this, recounting the results of a Cleveland study of 100 families with 446 children. Attributable to "low income . . . only" were substantial vitamin deficiencies, resulting from a diet that was inadequate in milk, vegetables, and fruit. Concerning housing, Schorr commented, "In 1960 about 10 million children lived in houses that lacked a proper toilet, bath or hot water. About 4 million lived in housing that census enumerators called dangerous" (Schorr, p. 13).

As for health care, the fact that children's poverty and poor health reinforce each other has been substantiated by every national health survey ever made. In 1966 the average child in a family with an annual income over $4,000 was the subject of one or more telephone consultations with a doctor during the year; among families with less than $2,000, fewer than one child in five benefited from even one telephone consultation in a given year. Similarly, poorer children made fewer visits to a doctor's or dentist's office. Three out of four of the children living in families with income under $2,000 had never seen a dentist. Although by 1980 Medicaid had brought about some improvement in the medical treatment for the poor, over 27 million still were not covered under this or other programs, many of them members of female-headed households.

Adams and Horovitz (1980a) commented that in health care a little bit does go a long way, however, for they found that physical complaints and health concerns were atypically reduced among the fatherless poor whom they dealt with in Miami. Because of their poverty, the mothers and their fatherless, firstborn sons were eligible for treatment in the Comprehensive Health Care Project administered then by Fred Seligman, M.D. Having comprehensive health care available quickly made both blacks and Cubans feel inordinately secure and reassured about health matters.

When Schorr compiled his statistics in 1966, the estimated number of poor children was 15.6 million. We must assume that by now the number has grown still larger, making Schorr's message relevant today, and even more poignant. He concluded his report as follows:

In short, poor children in the United States are poorly sheltered, many of them do not eat adequately, and their medical care is insufficient. Their right to an intact family is compromised. Their recreational and personal needs are not met. They do not even benefit from proper education. It would be hardly worth saying these things if we could bear to keep them in mind. The children suffering from each of these deficiencies must be numbered in the millions. On the average, families with poor children have about three-fifths of the income required to escape poverty. [p. 15]

Waldman et al. (1979) noted that, of the total single-parent families counted in 1978, two out of every five were living below the poverty level, as compared with one out of every sixteen two-parent families.

The multiple problems spawned by poverty *and* fatherlessness are further elucidated in *Families in Crisis* (1970), edited by Glasser and Glasser. The Glassers' work is characteristic of the sociopsychiatric approach to poverty-related stresses of the 1960s. The relationship between fatherlessness and poverty appears to be blatantly close. They go together. They are mutually reinforcing. Herzog and Lewis (1970) had a similar message:

Even though the majority of inner-city children are in two-parent homes at any given time, a smaller proportion remain in the two-parent home throughout their first 18 years. The relation of income to family composition is well documented but often forgotten. The frequency of one-parent families is inversely correlated with income . . . the difference between income levels is more striking than the difference between whites and blacks with regard to proportion of broken homes. [p. 380]

Orshansky (1968) enumerated the following three groups who bear the greatest burden of privation existing in the United States: black people, aged people, and women heading households.

PUBLIC ASSISTANCE

What public programs do exist to help fatherless families, what is generally thought of such programs, and who uses them? The best-known program began as Aid to Dependent Children (ADC) and has been known later as Aid to Families with Dependent Children (AFDC). According to Brenz (1959) two million U.S. children received aid from ADC in 1958. Of those children 80% lived in homes from which the father was absent, over 66% of them in large metropolitan areas. In over half the families, estrangement of the parents was the reason for the family's needing ADC. Approximately 20% of the families were in need owing to the father's desertion, and about 20% owing to unmarried parenthood. A high proportion of the latter were found in big cities. About two-thirds of the children who received assistance were white and one-third nonwhite; of the nonwhite 94% were black. The children were chiefly of school age or younger, and lived with the mother only. The average number of children was a little under three per family in 1958. The national average for these ADC monthly assistance grants was $103.26 per family and $27.44 per individual.

By 1978, with inflation, this figure rose to a maximum of $256.63 per month. In November 1980, the average nationwide was $286.23 per family. But amounts ranged from $50 per month for a family in Puerto Rico ($87.90 in Mississippi, $185.24 in Kentucky) to $371.40 in New York, $383 in Atlanta, $384 in Hawaii, and a family maximum of $429.20 in California. For individuals the "caps" in 1980 ranged from $29.78 per month (Mississippi) to $147.09 (California). The average length of time that a family received assistance was merely 2½ years in the 1960s and 1970s. But we know better: Children's poverty does not undergo such hasty remediation, nor is $286.00 per family adequate to meet children's economic needs.

By 1973 the grim situation had become discernible: 7,836,000 children were receiving AFDC, and 84.8% of them lived in female-headed households with the etiology presented below.

Trends in Fatherless Families from 1958 to 1973

1958	1973
30+%	21.4% female headed due to divorce
20%	25.5% female headed due to separation (legal and nonlegal)
20%	33.8% female headed, never married 4.1%, other
80% or 1.6 million of those getting ADC	84.8% or 6.64 million of those getting AFDC

Of these AFDC children 77.1% lived in large metropolitan areas. Of the total 3,523,000 families receiving AFDC, 52.6% were white and 43.0% were black (U.S. Bureau of the Census, 1978).

Public assistance, particularly ADC (AFDC), has become a sort of whipping boy for many taxpayers. The conservatives attack aid for dependent children because they feel that the system encourages slovenly living conditions, illegitimacy, crime, and general social decay—particularly among blacks. They depict the welfare mother as less than human, a procreating sloth. The liberals attack AFDC because they feel that the system militates against the intact lower-socio-economic-class family by denying benefits when an unemployed father lives in the home. Liberals depict public assistance as a system that dehumanizes its recipients and keeps them at a minimum level of sustenance with no hope for betterment of their life positions.

Radical economists view the welfare system as a ploy utilized by capitalistic governments, a conciliatory token institution designed to prevent the outbreak of civil disorder and resulting in "the erosion of the work role" and other demoralizing conditions. Piven and Cloward (1971) wrote from a quasi-radical perspective:

When attachments to the work role deteriorate, so do attachments to the family, especially the attachment of men to their families. For all practical purposes, the relief check becomes a surrogate for the male breadwinner. The resulting family breakdown and loss of control over the young is usually signified by the spread of certain forms of disorder—for example, school failure, crime, and addiction. In other words, the mere giving of relief, while it mutes the more disruptive outbreaks of civil disorder (such as rioting), does little to stem the fragmentation of lower-class life, even while it further undermines the patterns of work by which the lower class is ordinarily regulated. [*p. 402*]

Carol Glassman (1970) described welfare as "one of our society's attempts to preserve the traditional role of woman as childbearer, socializer, and homemaker" (p. 102). She enumerated the ways in which the welfare system maintains a patriarchal, condescending, and judgmental stance toward the female welfare recipient. Glassman saw the welfare system as one that deprives its female recipient of privacy and the freedom to choose her companions, to enjoy a social life, and to live in anything but the most squalid conditions of poverty. The recipient, as Glassman depicted her, must live powerlessly and dependently under the perpetual surveillance and mandates of the welfare agency: "The welfare board, like a jealous husband, doesn't want to see any men around that might threaten its place as provider and authority" (p. 102). Glassman generalized as follows: "Throughout the welfare department one finds the combined view that poverty is due to individual fault and that *something is wrong with women who don't have men*" (p. 104). Victim blaming is ubiquitous.

Brenz (1959), like Glassman, defended welfare mothers against the conservatives' attacks. She noted that welfare was hardly a "way of life" for most recipients, but rather a stopgap measure while the children were young, and that most AFDC—ADC in 1959—mothers strove to end their dependence on welfare as soon as possible. She added that, although there was a high degree of social breakdown among welfare families, particularly those living in cities, the mothers of these families did their best to adapt to the meager grants and the social breakdown; they tried to bring up their children with love and adequate care. Evidence for this point of view was provided from a study performed by the Philadelphia County Board of Assistance (1963), which showed that in Philadelphia, only 3% of the ADC children had been involved in child neglect hearings, and only 2% had been involved in court hearings on juvenile delinquency—

percentages no higher than the averages for the city as a whole. Brenz concluded:

> *ADC therefore seems to be fulfilling its function admirably for the majority of families, and the average ADC mother is being most unfairly accused when she is said to be misusing tax funds for the sake of being able to live riotously rather than using them properly for the care of her children. [p. 67]*

Recommendations for Improvement in Public Assistance

Brenz (1959, p. 77) made some recommendations to improve the ADC program:

1. Increase the size of ADC grants.
2. Take active measures to increase community understanding of ADC families' needs.
3. Hire additional and better-paid staff to run ADC facilities.
4. Establish and implement federal standards of service to be given.
5. Obtain assistance from other social agencies in order to enable the public assistance to meet client needs.

Public assistance, if made good, would be good for fatherless children in the nation.

Did the welfare situation improve during the 1970s? According to *Newsweek* (May 15, 1978),

> *the Administration has promised to get rid of the man-in-the-house restrictions and provide firmer income support for families. But by calculating benefits on the basis of "household units" instead of individual need, the President's proposed welfare reform would still penalize related persons living under one roof. An unwed mother, for instance, would lose $66 of her maximum $250 a month if she and her child moved in with an uncle who was ineligible for aid. She would retain her full benefits if she lived with a boyfriend, but would lose part of them if she married him. [p. 74]*

By the early 1980s, therefore, the situation hardly showed improvement. Today, AFDC will provide no benefits to children whose biologic father is married to or cohabiting with their mother unless he is disabled and/or unable to work. The amount, too, is still inadequate. In Louisville, Kentucky, for example, a mother who does receive payments receives approximately $185 to cover her expenses and the expenses of her children, to pay for rent, utilities, transportation, clothing, and so on—for everything except food, covered by food stamps, and medical care, covered by Medicaid.

The existing program is of little more benefit to fatherless children than some of the plans that have been rejected on humanitarian grounds. For example, the Fatherless Child Insurance (FCI) Program, proposed in 1960 by an advisory committee to the commissioner of Social Security, was discussed by Schorr (1966). The committee's proposal was never earnestly considered beyond the early 1960s by those with political power. This program would have applied only to children of families in which parents had been divorced or separated in court. Without court certification of separation, no benefits could have been received. This stipulation would have eliminated automatically all illegitimate children and a number of children who resided in families where separation of the parents was tentative and where the father tended to drift in and out. For lower-class people: "The family is sometimes fatherless and sometimes not, and the mother's planning for herself and her children is apt to be haphazard, a day-to-day affair" (Brenz, 1959, p. 68).

Under the FCI program the mother's benefits would have ended if she remarried; the children's benefits would have stopped if they married before age 18 or were legally adopted; again, the stipulations militated against the intact lower-class family. Schorr criticized the FCI plan because, among other things, as the family size increased, the benefits would not have increased proportionately. Thus, large families who received FCI benefits would still be dirt poor. In addition, small-to-moderate-sized families would still be poor despite receiving FCI benefits if these payments were their only source of income. Schorr reinforced his point with data already collected on children who receive survivors' insurance, a comparable form of public assistance.

Sandra Murphy (1979) denounced legislation that concerns the family generally as too disjointed and remedial rather than preventive. She said, essentially, that this is par for the course in U.S. social policy. The story is one of negatively oriented crisis intervention offered only after the family has failed. Far better would be supportively oriented help—help that would reinforce existing family strengths and prevent failure. The need for social policies that are "criterioned" on family impact will be considered more fully in Chapter 8.

MATERNAL EMPLOYMENT A PANACEA?

So it is no fluke that income and fatherlessness have come to be inversely related. Public assistance programs are not adequate to alleviate the problems raised by the coincidence of poverty and fatherlessness. What other alternatives are available to the afflicted subpopulation? Well, for one thing, we know that poor, single mothers often can provide better for their families by getting welfare than by working at low-paying and degrading jobs. We know also that those mothers for whom welfare is not an option are forced to seek employment. A whole new set of family problems ensues when mother works, but more and more mothers must get paying jobs. Nye reported a 1957 study in Washington: Over 80% of the female heads of household were employed, in contrast to fewer than 40% of women who were not heads of household. A 1978 Department of Labor report showed that the labor force participation rate of women who headed families had risen to 58.9% by March 1978 after averaging approximately 54% through most of the 1970s.

Historically, participation of black women in the labor force has greatly exceeded participation of white women at all ages. Although more recent statistics indicate that the proportion of working white women has risen, it is still exceeded by the proportion of working black women (Johnson, 1979). This situation, however, is reversed in one-parent families, where a higher proportion of black children than white children live with an unemployed mother. National statistics indicate that unemployment rates are higher, and median incomes lower, for black female heads of household than for white female heads of household (Waldman, et al., 1979). It is an unfailingly recurrent phenomenon. Black women are vulnerable and live at high risk.

EFFECTS OF MATERNAL EMPLOYMENT ON CHILDREN

Poznanski, Maxey, and Marsden (1970), reviewing the literature on the effects of maternal employment on children, indicated that much had been written, but few facts derived. They determined that the effects of mother's working probably depend on the developmental stage of the child and on his or her ego maturity. Among boys particularly, they said, an increase in dependency behavior and in sexual identity problems may be seen in the children of working mothers. However, these effects are most pronounced among lower-SES children, so it is extremely difficult to tell whether these characteristics are precipitated by mother's work, father's absence, poverty, or a combination of these variables, perhaps with different weight attributable to each variable.

Poznanski et al. believed that, under conditions of marital strife, "maternal employment escalated many undesirable behavior problems in children, including delinquency . . ." (p. 759). Again, it seems impossible to prove an absolute, linear causation. They did state, however, that in some instances maternal employment appears beneficial. For one thing, school achievement, especially reading, is enhanced by maternal employment. They wrote, "Whereas maternal employment places stress on the family, it can be tolerated, and in some situations even appears beneficial, if the family itself is stable" (p. 759).

McCord et al. (1963) concluded that "maternal employment has different meanings to the child in stable as compared to unstable homes: in the former, it appaers only to equalize status between the sexes and make sex role adjustment more difficult; in the latter [unstable homes], it may be interpreted by the child as rejection" (p. 177). A frequently espoused view is that such children from female-headed households are doubly deprived, suffering more from maternal deprivation than from paternal deprivation.

Regarding other specific effects of maternal employment, Herzog and Sudia (1968) concluded that

> *analysis of available evidence indicates that the effect on her child of a mother's employment depends on a number of other factors, such as her attitudes toward working or not working; the attitudes of other family members; her relationship to her husband; her temperament; her arrangements for child care; and the age, sex, and special needs of the child. [p. 182]*

Harris (1970) noted that maternal employment affects not only the children but also the mother and the family. Harris traced a vivid silhouette of an exhausted mother, attempting to hold down two full-time jobs simultaneously and succeed at both. One of us (Adams, 1981c) previously commented on the paradox of women's liberation when there is merely freedom for a woman to take on additional work, without provisions to lighten a mother's responsibilities:

> *Even if mothers are emancipated, so called, by being set free to work away from home, they are burdened with two jobs instead of the one homebased job that the mother traditionally held. This hokum emancipation of women holds true in capitalist and socialist countries alike. It seems to be a modern way of retaining the vestiges of an outmoded patriarchal system, for the woman is liberated and allowed to work away from home but no provisions are made to take up the full-time job she formerly did at home. With great industry and some facilitating martyrdom, the contemporary woman undertakes to do two full-time jobs. What a price for emancipation it is, to go under the yoke of a double bondage. [p. 6]*

A recent study, conducted under the Reagan administration by the Department of Education, found that children whose mothers work and children from single-parent homes score lower on school achievement tests. However, these results are in direct contradiction to the conclusions drawn by another recent group of investigators working under the auspices of the National Institute of Health (the Louisville, Kentucky *Courier-Journal*, Sunday, June 26, 1983). Obviously, there are still no clear-cut answers in this area.

PROBLEMS OF DAY CARE

A mother who can afford it hires a maid for part-time child care and domestic chores. Sachs (1971) has written on the importance of the maid in child development, but it is a story that has not been told sufficiently: the affluent for centuries have had surrogate mothers. Those mothers less fortunate, who may themselves have to work as maids to other people's children, have to leave their own children unattended and neglected in order to provide adequate child care for the more affluent.

The mother who works full time may have difficulty maintaining family social contacts. She runs into hurdles in providing adequate health care to her children since clinics usually are open only during working hours. The clinics too are run largely by working mothers. Furthermore, the preschool child of the working mother may show developmental effects of deprivation. Responsible for this is the lack of adequate day-care facilities to provide children in this age group with the love and affection conducive to healthy development (Harris, 1970). This problem likely does not exist in Israeli kibbutzim where day care provided is consistent and designed to meet the developmental needs of the children within its domain (Poznanski, Maxey, & Marsden, 1970). Competent day care could help fatherless children.

CHILD-REARING PRACTICES

What about the additional pressures of raising a family all by herself? Those pressures leave an imprint on a mother's child-rearing practices. Of course, a mother's child-rearing behaviors are primarily determined by her own mother's child-rearing behaviors, sometimes with slight modifications (Cohler et al., 1971), and are only secondarily determined by situational stresses. Nevertheless, definite patterns of child rearing have been observed in female heads of households—at least at some of the socioeconomic levels.

Besner (1965) reported that the single-parent family headed by a woman, the most common type of low-income American family, concentrated more on discipline and conformity training than on psychological development of the child. Phelps (1969) studied 38 parents from middle-class two-parent families in Berkeley, California, along with 22 parents from middle-class one-parent families, and found that one-parent families were considerably stricter than two-parent families, accounting for these group differences in degree of authority overprotection in one-parent families, an attitude not overtly present in the two-parent families. For reading by the history minded, David M. Levy (1943) gave a thorough discourse on the topic of maternal overprotection, with case studies included, showing the interrelationships of hatred, guilt, rejection, and pampering but not stressing their economic base very strongly.

An alternative explanation for the differences in child-rearing practices between one- and two-parent families is this: that more restrictive child-rearing behaviors are attributable to the depressed income suffered by fatherless families rather than to fatherlessness per se. A mother on the run needs her kids to shape up quickly. This outlook has been supported by the work of Nancy Donohue Colletta (1979).

PARENTS WITHOUT PARTNERS

Freudenthal (1959) examined material emanating from a project involving a significant number of parents without partners over a prolonged period; he attempted to delineate basic dynamic features that could be considered characteristic of the one-parent family. He observed the following characteristics in the single parents: a sense of incompleteness and frustration, a sense of failure, a sense of guilt, and marked (overt or underlying) feelings of ambivalence between only-parent and child. Gadpaille (1974), a psychiatrist, recommended counseling procedures for frustrated mothers who feel inadequate or cannot relate effectively to their children, particularly male children, due to feelings of ambivalence. This mentalistic approach is often applied to middle-class parents, who appear to welcome it.

Freudenthal did not note the socioeconomic status of the parents studied. However, they sound very much like middle-class mothers from the traits he has described. Fortunately for the children, lower-class mothers tend to be more child focused than "conjugal focused"

(Kohn & Carroll, 1960), so the lower-class mother would not be made to feel inadequate, guilty, and ambivalent toward her children when her marriage dissolved. But she may feel paranoid and almost assuredly feels economically deprived (Adams & Horovitz, 1980a).

A group that has existed since 1957 to meet the social–emotional needs of single parents, although not exclusively female heads of households, is Parents Without Partners, Inc. (P.W.P.), a predominantly white, middle-class, nonsectarian group that has been able to obtain favorable publicity in the mass media and has spread all over the continent (Schlesinger, 1966). These are its aims and purposes:

> *P.W.P. starts with a membership of followers who are troubled, un-happy, deprived, confused, often depressed and hurt. The purposes of P.W.P. are to overcome these painful states by various means, and to strive toward happier, healthier, and better adjusted adults. And indirectly through better adjusted adults, strive to provide a more un-troubled atmosphere for children with single parents. . . . Every new member must be led from sickness to health, from unhappiness to more happiness, from feelings of being lost to feelings of direction and purpose. [Stillman, 1965, pp. 4–8]*

Parents Without Partners in some parts of the United States is used as a dating bureau, referred to simply as a meat market. Principally adult oriented, P.W.P. may offer some recourse to middle-class single parents beset by problems of financing, child rearing, maintaining a satisfying social life, and adjusting emotionally to single parenthood. But P.W.P. does little for single parents who are very poor. For this sector of humanity, Schlesinger recommended that programs similar to P.W.P. be set up in community centers.

TYPES OF FATHERLESS FAMILIES FOR CHILDREN

Let us now look at life in the female-headed family from the child's point of view. We will deal here with six types of fatherless families, originating from divorce or separation, death, desertion, illegitimacy, work demands, and state intervention (because father is unfit or in military service).

To show things from the child's aspect, we have tabulated these six types of father-absence according to whether it is *loss or non-existence* the child feels. Loss connotes conscious feelings, but non-existence means not in awareness.

Examples of Children with No Father

I. Never Had Father	II. Had but Lost Father (child has sense of loss)
a. Father died in child's pre-natal or preverbal period.	a. Father died after being present for two or more years.
b. Father divorced or separated and departed very early in child's life.	b. Father divorced or separated after being present.
c. Parents unwed and never together.	c. Parents did cohabit, then split.
d. Father deserted early.	d. Father deserted after being part of child's and mother's life.
e. Father very early sent to 1. remote job, 2. prison, 3. military, 4. mental hospital.	e. Father sent away in child's second year or later to 1, 2, 3, 4.
f. Father always detached and "psychologically absent" or nonsalient.	f. Father seldom home after initial presence: worka-holic, etc.

Clinicians certainly realize that the child experiencing paternal death inhabits a world that differs both materially and mentally from the private world of the child whose father had little to do with the mother and left the city as soon as her pregnancy became obvious. The clinician leans toward the individual case and makes an effort to empathize with the special circumstances of each case, while simultaneously understanding that there are some structural, institutional uniformities that put their marks on families and households with the varied forms of fatherlessness operating within them. The types that we survey in this chapter are not the complete spectrum of fatherlessness, but they are the ones that seem to have most relevance to clinical practice as well as social policy.

DIVORCE

Divorce is often considered to be a problem between two adults, and nothing more than that. Our interest in divorce, not confined to what happens in the lives of two adults, concerns the lives of children when their parents divorce. More concretely, we are most attentive to divorces in which the mother has custody of the children and the children are rendered fatherless. The material that follows says some broad and general things about divorces in the United States in order to limn the social context in which families are broken up by divorces. Then we examine what divorce means for the children in a household headed by a divorced mother, that is, a fatherless household.

Adults Obtaining Divorces

The divorce rate in the United States is the highest in the world; it rose sharply in the early Seventies and appears to have leveled off since 1976. Historically, the rise in divorce rate was a matter of concern even in the nineteenth century, although death, not divorce, was the prime cause of one-parent families up until the mid-1960s (Skolnick, 1980). Although the current divorce rate has leveled off, 38% of all first marriages fail. Not all divorces end in fatherlessness for children, but a great many do. According to the U.S. Bureau of the Census, in 1978 there were an estimated 8.1 million men and women who were divorced and who had not remarried compared to 48 million married couples; there were 84 divorced persons for every 1,000 persons in an intact marriage in 1977. In 1978, census data showed 1.1 million divorces compared to 2.2 million marriages, making the divorce rate 5.1 per 1,000 compared to 2 per 1,000 as recently as in 1940 (Reinhold, 1979). These figures may be somewhat deceiving, as the divorce rate is figured per 1,000 people—not only married people, but all people, including the never married, children, elderly widows and widowers, and so on. We must assume that if the divorce rate were estimated per 1,000 people who were ever married, past or present, the figures would be more striking.

From 1970 to 1977 the divorce ratio increased by at least 79%, as compared with an increase of 34% during the decade from 1960 to 1970. Although black people had a higher divorce ratio than white people in 1977, the proportional increase between the two groups during the 17 years from 1960 to 1977 was very similar; the ratio for blacks rose by 160% and that for whites by 136%. In 1977, women had higher divorce ratios (101 per 1,000) than men (66 per 1,000) and persons under age 45, the age of childbearing, had higher ratios (91 per 1,000) than those aged 45 years and over (76 per 1,000). These latter two developments reflect the facts that women have a longer average duration of divorce before remarriage and a lower incidence of remarriage than men and that most of the recent increase in divorce has been among younger couples (U.S. Census, 1978, p. 3).

Children Affected by Divorce

The number of children affected by these divorces nearly tripled between 1960 and 1975. In 1976, over a million children were affected by divorce—1,117,000. In 1965 the mean number of children affected in the decree was 1.32; in 1976 the average number of children per divorce decree was 1.19 for whites, 1.28 for blacks, and 1.36 for others. These figures reflect lower birth rates and the fact that couples with minor children are less likely to divorce than couples with no minor children; they show how the likelihood of divorce declines as the number of such children increases (Illsley & Thompson, 1961). Nevertheless the number of divorces has increased apace.

Hence, differences in divorce exist among racial groups—the mean numbers of affected children are highest for divorcing nonwhite couples other than blacks, lowest of all for whites, with values for black couples falling in between those two groups (Plateris, 1970). It is plain that nonblack, nonwhite children are hit hardest by the divorce rates in the United States. Ease of divorce wipes out the social stigma of divorce even among ethnic minorities but creates the risk of ignoring the hurt children.

Recent data from the U.S. Bureau of the Census (1978) derived from the 1970 census and trend data through 1976 show us that the number of children involved in divorce has increased drastically, yet another way the scourges of both nature and culture—culture especially—are visited upon the youngest members of this society. In 1960, the divorce rate was 18.7 per 1,000 couples with children under 18 years of age. The rate varied between 21.4 for couples with one child and 6.0 for those with four or more children. The divorce registration area (DRA) rate in 1976 was 19.1 per 1,000 couples with one child, 15.1 for those with two children, and 11.3 for those with three or more children. *Divorce rates* are not calculated officially according to divorces per 1,000 married couples, however, but according to the number of divorced persons per 1,000 of the general population. By that standard, the divorce rate in 1981 had shown an increase for the nineteenth consecutive year, reaching 5.3 per 1,000 persons and being 2% higher than the 1970 rate (UPI release in the *Houston Post,* December 27, 1982, p. 3A). From the standpoint of children in America, divorce is a rapidly spreading epidemic for which no cures or prevention appear to be forthcoming.

The Bureau of the Census (1978) reported that small families with one or two children are slightly more prevalent among divorcing white couples than among black or other race couples. Large families with four or more children are proportionally most numerous among nonwhite couples; the percentages for 1976 were 11.1 for the other group, 8.9 for blacks, and 6.4 for the whites. A similar pattern was observed in most of the reporting states. More nonblack, nonwhite children proportionately are ravaged by divorces when they *do* occur.

Factors Contributing to Rise in Divorce

What elements are conducive to this rise in divorces? According to research conducted by the National Institute of Mental Health, *pre marital pregnancy* often leads to *early marriage;* and the earlier the marriage, the higher the rate of marital instability. Other conditions found to be associated with higher rates of separation and divorce are *low SES, husband's occupation* being socially below that of the wife's father, *wife's premarital employment,* and *short engagements* of less than a month. The institute report stated that a larger proportion of black subjects than white are separated or divorced in their *first* marriages. SES might explain this finding (Bumpass, 1978), since frequency of divorce and socioeconomic status are inversely related in the population at large (Carter & Glick, 1970). It may be that the poor are not ready for parenthood, or so it frequently appears to their children.

The lowest rates of marital disruption have been found among women who married farmers. In a highly urban society, the investigators suggested, only farm families may be more traditional in their views on the importance or sanctity of marriage (Bumpass, 1978). Farm children still get a special view of life in the world.

Another circumstance contributing to the rising divorce rates is no-fault divorce legislation. *Newsweek* (May 15, 1978) commented that, after a no-fault divorce law designed to cut divorce red tape and legal fees was enacted in the District of Columbia, divorce cases jumped to 2,392 in the 6 months from May through October 1977, compared to 1,664 in the previous 6 months. This trend has been observed nationwide with the passage of similar legislation (p. 74). When legislators facilitate divorce they seldom think of the children who may be involved.

Schorr and Moen (1979) considered the rise in divorces; besides no-fault divorce laws, they cited the *increased propensity of mothers without husbands to form separate families and women's increased labor-force participation.* They added, however, that society still perceives father to be the wage earner and mother to be caretaker; hence the better father provides for the family, the less likely are mother and father to get divorced. Separation rates are twice as high among families where the husband experiences serious unemployment, suggesting that it is not the amount of income alone but also *income's regularity and stability* that affect a decision to remain married or to separate and, perhaps, divorce (Ross & Sawhill, 1975).

Likewise, Hacker (1979) held that one of the reasons for the increase in the divorce rate is that

most men still expect deference from their wives, an attitude behooving those inherently inferior. Women are the ones who are changing,

> *asking to be seen as equals—a fact they always knew, but saw fit to mask in the past. Men find it difficult, often impossible, to adapt to this new climate. They may say they want wives who are accomplished and independent. But they also want them docile. It is the women, not the men, who are vivid in our present phase of domestic history. They are the force unsettling men, a consequence that can only weaken marriage.* [Hacker, 1979, p. 24]

Others have associated the proclivity to divorce with certain personality factors. Pietropinto and Simenauer (1979) invoked the prevalence of self-centeredness in those who divorce. Loeb (1966) found that marital disruption was associated with some degree of psychological disturbance, and particularly with psychopathic defenses. Peterson (1959) characterized the divorced woman as unrealistic, sex-role conflicted, lacking self-awareness, and blindly propelled by a driving need to marry. That less-than-flattering description seems jaded today. Somehow the easy-divorce ideology has become part and parcel of a "narcissistic society" (Lasch, 1979), for women are not alone in narcissism.

Alimony

Weitzman and Dixon (1978) found that, after the passage of California's first no-fault divorce law in 1969, alimony awards actually declined in California. In 1968, alimony was awarded in 20% of cases. In 1972, this figure was 15%. The sharpest *decline* in alimony awards from 1968 to 1972 was seen among mothers of preschoolers; in 1972, only 11% of preschoolers' mothers were awarded alimony. Judges determine the amount of alimony payments in nonwelfare cases, and when questioned on declining amount of alimony payments, the majority of judges implied that they sought to have the mother of the preschool child go out to work. The payments awarded were intentionally smaller in anticipation of the additional income that would result from maternal employment. The median child-support award in 1972 was $75 per child per month, an amount insufficient to raise a child without additional incomes. The younger children are put at greater risk, as ever.

Census data in 1975 indicated that the average child support from fathers was $2,430 per year for those mothers who received it. For about half of these women the payments amounted to less than 10% of their total income. Only 1 in 20 got more than half of her income from child support. Too, when fathers do not pay child support, courts exert little pressure to force them to do so (Jenkins, 1978).

Two major points are being missed here. One is that most judges are men. That being the case, we would hardly expect their ruling to give economic favor to the female no-fault plaintiff in a divorce case. Second, it is irrational to cut the support payments of a mother of preschool children in anticipation of her working. Even if she can secure employment, the young mother's job is likely to be marginal, low paying, low status, and insecure (Gross, 1968); and she will certainly need additional money for child care, because none is provided by the state in most cases. Justice is blind—to the needs of young children and their mothers.

The scarcity of divorced women who receive alimony payments appears to be a nationwide phenomenon. Only 14% of divorced women who answered a 1975 national poll said that they were awarded such support. However, judges who were asked to guess at the proportion of divorced women receiving alimony estimated 75% on the average, erring by 61 percentage points. The lowest estimates (and probably the most factual) were given by the U.S. Bureau of the Census, which reported that of 4.5 million divorced or separated women in 1975, only 4% received alimony (Reinhold, 1979). According to NIMH (1978) the roots of the alimony myth lie in the high visibility of upper-middle-class and high-income divorce cases (Weitzman & Dixon, 1978). Those are the very families with fewest children.

Emotional Consequences of Divorce for the Mother

Problems of Living and Self-Derogation. What are some of the emotional consequences of divorce for the mother—and, primarily, for the child? Adams (1972a), from his clinical research, drew distinctions between the ravages of the friendly versus those of the angry divorce, also between dirty fighters who respect the child's right to love both parents and those who do not. He described divorce for both spouses as self-perceived failure, carrying the stigma of neurosis and immaturity; and he characterized custody battles as prolongations of the cruel marital ties. He enumerated as the problems of the divorced mother such things as arranging for child care, finding affordable housing and funding the household, obtaining alimony or child support, and overcoming difficulties in parenting when she is the only adult left in the household. The divorced woman is bereft of both material and emotional support and may not have much to give to her child(ren). Schlesinger (1966) advanced a similar stand. Colletta (1979) tabled the matter incisively. She asked: Is the impact of divorce due to father-absence or poverty? Interviewing 72 white working-class families in Buffalo, Colletta controlled for race, number of children, SES, and gender of the target child while studying child-rearing practices—an excellent research plan. When income was held constant, child-rearing practices did not vary significantly between one- and two-parent families. Among poor one-parent families, child rearing was more restrictive and demanding of the child's obedience, especially for divorced mothers of *boys* or of *more than one child*. Stresses mounted therefore in one-parent postdivorce households with these features: low income, two or more children, a male child. The telling difference in child rearing and family functioning had an economic base, not a father base.

Ilgenfritz (1961) characterized the divorced woman as plagued with hostility toward men and fearing for the welfare of the children Specific concerns include provision of male role models, guarding against maternal overindulgence, and educating the children, particularly male children, concerning sexuality and sexual activity Ilgenfritz summarized:

> The problems divorced and widowed mothers face are of two general kinds. There are the objective problems of limited income and the need to find the time and energy for a job to augment it and still be the kind of mother children need in the circumstances—a mother who can maintain a home, discipline and educate young people, and insure their health and safety and their positive emotional growth. Then there are the countless personal problems of guilt, fear, frustration and loneliness, ever-present and always threatening. [p. 41]

The reality and the fantasy, both, can harm the children. Moss and Pleuris (undated) noted that, with single mothers of preschool chil dren, 72% had "a moderate to severe distress problem" compared with only 46% of married mothers. Briscoe et al. (1973) found that 75% of the women and 67% of the men in a sample of 39 divorced probands suffered from psychiatric disease. Those psychiatric disorders seen most frequently in the divorced probands were primary affective disease, antisocial personality, and hysteria.

Social Effectiveness and Social Life. Some observers assert that being a *single* parent may be related to distress problems while multiple marriages are conducive to a kind of "social effectiveness" (Overall, 1971). In Overall's study the never-married tended to evidence more emotional withdrawal and more thinking disturbances. The once-married evidenced more depression. The multiply married tended to have lower levels of all types of symptomatology! Perhaps psychiatrists and movie stars are onto something good.

Speaking of social effectiveness, divorce also tends to erode a woman's effective, good-enough patterns and to necessitate the complete reformation of her social life. When father goes, so go all his work colleagues, friends, and family of origin, in many cases. Often, so goes the mother's social life. Shoicket (1968) reported on these depleted affinal relationships of the divorced mother and noted that, unless she can make some radical readjustments, she may suffer loneliness. Brandwein et al. (1974) reviewed the literature describing the precarious social situation of divorced mothers and their families. Alas, the unhappy mother who heads a household containing young children affects more than her own psyche.

Positive Effects for Mother. Divorce is not always an occasion of failure for the woman, but may in fact be an occasion of success—a new-won freedom, the opportunity to pursue previously denied educational advancements and nontraditional careers, or to seek alternative life styles and embark on heterosexual, celibate, or lesbian sexual practices that earlier had not seemed attainable. While most authors *do* report the destructive and negative sequelae of divorce for the mother, some authors view divorce or separation as a boon for the woman—freedom at last from the bondage of marriage. Tcheng-Laroche and Prince (1979) reported on their survey of 45 French-Canadian middle-class female heads of household who had been separated or divorced from 1 to 3 years:

Interviews showed that, unlike previous reports of divorced women and female heads of families, this group enjoyed relatively good health and normal stress levels, and were generally positive about being head of the family. Among the positive changes, the majority emphasized their great autonomy, freedom, and sense of selfhood. Some mentioned improved relations with their children. On the negative side, loneliness, absence of the father (particularly for their sons), and limited social lives were most often mentioned. It was concluded that the role of head of family is perfectly acceptable for many economically viable women, though not necessarily ideal. [p. 42]

Findings such as these convince the authors that if a woman has the economic wherewithal to make a go of being the head of household, many of the negative concomitants often associated with father-absence need not appear. "What a difference the dough makes" was the way one divorced parent put this. Perhaps the father is not as necessary to the proper functioning of the family unit as many male authors would have us believe.

Emotional Consequences of Divorce for the Child

Research in this area has been criticized for several reasons. According to Jenkins (1978),

the adjustment of children of divorced parents tends to be measured against the norm of children from intact, presumably well-functioning families, rather than against children in homes where there is substantial parental dissention, the pre-divorce norm. In addition, case studies are often done on samples of children seen in treatment, and these may not be representative of all children of divorce. Furthermore, there has been little follow-up study of children after the crisis period is past. [p. 19]

We will, nevertheless, attempt here to summarize some studies that have been published. It is our hope that the reader will be able to get some feeling of what it is like to be a child from a home broken by divorce as well as to get some idea of the need for more accurate and sophisticated research methodology in this field.

What are some of the reported manifestations of divorce in the child? Pollack (May, 1968) wrote, "Family discord and disintegration; resentment toward parents and siblings; jealousy toward friends whose families are still intact—all this falls on the inexperienced shoulders of these children" (p. 179). The child psychiatrist Richard Gardner (1956) described the child from the divorced home as feeling different from other children and as constantly having to explain the absence of a parent to his or her peers. Parents Without Partners expressed concern that often the child who *does* feel deviant or anomalous is the child who becomes self-segregated, declining participation in school social events and extracurricular activities (Schlesinger, 1966). Again the effects of divorce on children probably vary with socioeconomic status. We mentioned before that parents in P.W.P. tend to be from the middle class. The child of divorce living in an inner-city ghetto might not suffer any more from feeling different than from economic deprivation. Furthermore, Condry and Simon (1974) stated that while children from single-parent families do have less adult contact, they tend, in compensation, to increase peer relationships—not to withdraw from them as Schlesinger would have us believe.

Judith Wallerstein (December, 1980) found that, "although designed as a social remedy, divorce has gradually become a source of grave community concern because of its stressful impact on children and adolescents" (p. 455). Only one-third of the children whom she and her associates had studied—at the first 6 weeks following separation, again after 18 months, and finally after 5 years—could be said to have "very good health and [be] content with their lives" (p. 464). Thirty percent of the 131 children studied sensed, at the end of 5 years, that tension and bitterness persisted between their parents. For more than half of the children, neither the divorce nor the 5-year period of cooling down had worked as a remedy for interparental incompatibility.

Pathological Postdivorce Family Patterns. Westman et al. (1970) predicted, on the basis of a sample of 148 consecutive divorce cases passing through a Wisconsin fiscal court, that one-third of all divorces are followed by turbulence and discord that could be pathogenic for the involved children. Pathological postdivorce family patterns have appeared frequently. Wylie and Delgado (1959) drew a clinical picture of such a mother–son relationship: mother hating estranged father and projecting hatred onto son, and son performing poorly in school and acting out hostility toward mother through display of uncontrollable aggression. Heckel (1963) traced the aberrant character development of five Lolita-type preadolescent females to fathers' absence coupled with mothers' inability to function, leaving these children devoid of emotional support and disciplinary control.

Gardner (1956) also depicted pathological patterns of mother-child interaction that could develop following mother–father separation. These patterns may emerge whenever the child becomes an economic, emotional, and social burden to the mother and knows it. Or they may emerge when the child becomes the mother's only love object and is smothered by her affections, solicitations, excessive indulgences, and overprotectiveness.

More recent studies take a closer look at specific mother–child communication patterns in father-absent families. Gooblar (1979) compared communication patterns between mothers and adolescent in one-parent and in two-parent families, finding that more covert patterns of communication existed in one-parent dyads and for dyads with older adolescents. On the basis of this finding he made the following assertions:

> *Withdrawal of the father through divorce was thought to result in ambivalence on the part of the mother regarding her authority in the family and ambivalence on the part of the adolescent regarding perception of his capacity for independence from the family. Consequently these families continually attempt to avoid the task of clearly defining the parameters of their relationships. [p. 4030-B]*

Divorced versus Conjugally Conflicted Homes.   When one views the emotional consequences of divorce for the child as compared with the consequences of living in a conjugally conflicted home, the sequelae of divorce appear to be relatively less damaging (Burchinal, 1964). Landis (1962) wrote that the unhappy marriage is more psychologically disturbing to children than divorce. Many writers cite isolated examples of "good divorces" as seen through the children's eyes. *Look* magazine (1967) reported a case in point, although one seen from the father's perspective:

Everyone knows divorced fatherhood is grim. Some know it needn't be. Like most things, it depends who's doing it. New Yorker Francis J. "Fritz" Shea, for one, is doing it fine. Some of his days with his daughter bog with activities, others are quiet. All seem relaxed. There are treats, but there is discipline. Clearly, the father loves the child and doesn't feel he has to prove it every moment they're together. Clearly, the child knows she is loved by both parents—even though their love is doled out at separate sittings. [p. 28]

Unhappy Home = Broken Home.   Nye (1958) warned against confusing an unhappy home with a broken home. In examining research that correlated delinquency with broken homes, Nye surmised that marital unhappiness was more closely related to delinquency in children than was family composition, whether the child had both parents or only one. He found more delinquent behavior in unhappy unbroken homes than in broken homes. In an earlier study Nye (1957) found that children from broken homes have better adjustment than children from unhappy homes when the gauges used are psychosomatic illness, delinquent behavior, and parent–child adjustment.

Authors who proclaim that divorce has traumatic emotional effects on children cannot distinguish between the effects of the divorce and the concomitants of the discord and turmoil that preceded the divorce although the growing body of evidence indicates that parental conflict, not divorce, is the villain (Luepnitz, 1978). Landis (1960) wrote that divorce is more traumatic for children who perceived their homes as "happy" prior to the divorce than for children who perceived their homes as "unhappy" and torn by conflict. Rutter's (1979) review agrees. Children can discern domestic discord.

Separation and Deprivation.   Howells (1970) dubbed fallacious the view that separation always means deprivation. For Howells, "separation" was physical absence, and deprivation was the loss or lack of love, affection, and security—qualities usually supplied by parents. He alleged that deprivation is the villain in producing childhood psychopathology but that deprivation is independent of separation. Howells further claimed that the most disturbed children suffer emotionally from being *with* their parents and that separation could be used to combat deprivation. Sussman (1978), too, espoused this view, when he wrote: "For a significant number of single-parent families, which result as a consequence of separation and divorce, the removal or absence of a violent parent results in a nurturant and liveable family form" (p. 37).

Specific Immediate Effects on Children.   The situation is complex, multifaceted, and not conducive to facile generalization. McDermott (1968) wrote that, to study the effects of divorce, one must differentiate among the impact of marital strife on the child, the child's immediate reaction to the loss of a parent, the residual impact of the loss of a parental model, and the impact of the divorce on the remaining parent, as that impact reflects onto the child. Hetherington et al. (1979) wrote that single parents show less affection to their children and tend to have less control over them—even 2 years after divorce—than parents in two-parent families, mainly so for mothers with sons.

McDermott himself undertook to trace the effects of divorce on a small number of children seen at the Children's Psychiatric Hospital at the University of Michigan. He characterized disturbed children of divorced couples in the following manner: Some are sad and angry, some lost and detached; some girls are pseudoadult; and some boys have disrupted masculine identification. In a later study, McDermott (1970) associated divorce with *depression* and *acting out in children, excessive identification of male children with the absent father, impaired superego development,* and *delinquent behavior.*

McDermott admonished the legal system that fails to make provisions for families in postdivorce crises, accusing the courts of possibly worsening the trauma for children by providing an arena of brutal custody battles and marital recrimination and by identifying an innocent and guilty party in the divorce proceedings. He stated that although the courts were moving away from passing judgment on the respective spouses with the new trend for no-fault divorce, these polarized attitudes are still held in the minds of the children at risk. Oftentimes, the children think one parent is bad, the other good. Or they may see both their parents as desirable, wanting both and wanting them to be together.

Sometimes children yearn for the restoration of the marriage because object detachment is incomplete. In some instances divorce is harder for the child to accept than death, because decathexis is more incomplete. The process of mourning is prolonged, and repeated contacts with and reminders of the lost parent present themselves as false hopes to which the child reacts with anger and frustration (Grossberg & Crandall, 1978). Ilgenfritz (1961) reported mothers' frustration when children resist accepting divorce and yearn for the restoration of the marital bond, miserable though it may have been.

Several authors have clung to the topic of *disrupted masculine identification in males* from fatherless families. Their assumption is that when father is present the male child models on him. Payne and Mussen (1956), however, reported that the degree of identification is highly influenced by the degree to which the son perceives the father to be a highly rewarding, affectionate person. Thus, the relationship is what counts, and sons who perceive their fathers negatively probably identify with them minimally, present or absent. Donini (1967), too, failed to find significant differences between father-absent and father-present boys in the measure of sex-role identification. This sometimes heatedly discussed aspect of fatherlessness is considered in greater detail in Chapter 5.

Age of Child at Time of Divorce. Several authors have indicated that the age of the child at the time of divorce is a crucial factor in determining the consequences of divorce for that child. Gardner (1956), a Sullivanian, described the effects of parental separation on the child's "concept of self" and "concept of human beings." He wrote that, for the child whose father left during the child's preconscious years, the mother can give no possible explanation of father's absence that will not be harmful to the child. Gardner pointed to the grief reaction of the child whose parents were separated later, after the child had formed attachments to both; such a child has feelings of guilt, ambivalence, and insecurity. Although several authors, including Gardner (1956) and Landis (1960), indicate that the older the child, the more traumatic the divorce for him or her, Thomes (1968) found no significant differences between 9- and 10-year-old children from father-absent one-parent homes and father-mother homes in terms of the children's concept of parental roles, their attitudes and feelings about family members, their peer relationships, and their self-concepts. More recent findings pertinent to the impact of age have been reported by Westman (1970) and Wallerstein and Kelly (1980).

Westman wrote that the worst time for a child to lose a parent is during the Oedipal period. Both boys and girls will be beset by guilt, he opined. Boys fear that their Oedipal wish has been fulfilled. Girls, seeing that mother has been unable to maintain a successful hetero-sexual relationship, may in later years be unable to do so themselves. The school-age child is able to view the loss more realistically, but also suffers the loss more deeply and often becomes severely de-pressed. The adolescent reacts with strong emotions, but emotions that can more easily be resolved than the young child's. The adoles-cent, by tending to seek peer-group support during this time of crisis, may be prompted to early marriage and early divorce. Westman has been criticized for failing to account for evidence contrary to his posi-tion and for drawing his conclusions from a clinic sample, that is, a distressed group (Luepnitz, 1978).

Kelly and Wallerstein (1976), providing evidence from a longitu-dinal study, described the reaction of the preschooler as "regressive, confused and fretful." Early-latency children, they said, were deeply saddened and most poignantly aware of their suffering. Later-latency children and adolescents openly verbalized their sadness and anger. Adolescents were thought to be able to express empathy and compas-sion for their parents. Wallerstein and Kelly have been commended for their efforts to conduct a longitudinal study, but have been criti-cized too for using what appears to be a distressed population, even though they made concerted efforts to control for this shortcoming in their work (Luepnitz, 1978).

According to McDermott (1968), other factors than age come into play when the effects of divorce are reckoned:

> *The child's reactions also depend on such factors as his or her age, sex, . . . each parent's personality and previous relationship with the child, the child's relationships with siblings, as well as the emo-tional availability of all of these important people to him during the divorce period, and his or her own personality strengths and capac-ities to adjust to stresses such as separation in the past. [p. 118]*

Residual Effects of Divorce. The residual effects of divorce take a while to show, some insist. The grown children of the broken home, scrutinized by Frommer and O'Shea (1973), led those authors to surmise that mothers who themselves had been separated from parents and/or siblings during childhood might be more vulnerable to severe postpartum depression and to emotional problems in their adult families than mothers who had not. Gay and Tonge (1967) found marital disharmony in women to be associated with loss of both parents, and mainly with loss through separation or divorce.

Illsley and Thompson (1961) described residual effects on adult women of having experienced broken homes in childhood. These women, they wrote, tended to leave school earlier, take lower-status jobs, and marry semiskilled or unskilled workers more frequently than their counterparts from nonbroken homes. Also, considerably more of them had illegitimate babies; more conceived before marriage; more were delivered in their adolescence. These effects were more severe for women from homes broken by illegitimacy and divorce than by death of a parent. The rate of prenuptial conception was 21% higher among women from broken homes; the illegitimacy rate was 62% higher.

Other authors have attributed adult suicidal behavior to childhood bereavement over the loss of a parent through either death or divorce. Dorpat et al. (1965) compared two populations, one of 121 consecutive psychiatric patients admitted for attempted suicide, the other of 114 successful suicides that occurred during 1 year in the same county. They concluded that there was a higher incidence of broken homes in the original families of the attempted suicides. For completed suicides, there was a higher percentage of parental death in their baby families. Ian Gregory (1966), in a much-publicized study, pointed out that those who attempt suicide tend to be younger than those who complete suicide. Obviously, then, parental desertion and illegitimacy are more likely to be the causes of bereavement among the younger group; and parental death more likely to be the cause of bereavement among the older group. Childhood losses have their harvest seasons of highest incidence in later life.

Gregory collected data on 1,000 native-born white males and females admitted to a psychiatric inpatient unit. He standardized the data according to decade of their birth and to their sex, and used the Minnesota Multiphasic Personality Inventory (MMPI) to indicate depression and suicidal inclination. In contrast to previous studies, he did not find that any form of permanent parental loss during childhood was associated with a vulnerability to depression or with any specific category of neurosis or psychosis in adult life.

Summary of Divorce's Effects on the Child.   Some of the emotional consequences of divorce for the child have been said to be alienation and isolation from agemates or its obverse, excessive involvement by the child with peers. Various psychopathological patterns of mother–child interaction after divorce have been described. The age of the child at the time of the divorce has been tagged as a vital, telling factor in determining the child's emotional adjustment. A dispute appears in the literature concerning the effects of divorce on the child versus the effects of living in a home torn by discord and marital strife. Most of the research, on balance, seems to indicate that divorce is more psychologically beneficial to the child. It is better said, maybe, in this form: Divorce is the lesser evil for a child if the child's choices of his or her evils counted much. Long-term effects of divorce that have been proposed are impaired sexual identification (in males especially), depression, suicidal behavior, problems with marital adjustment, and a tendency to have illegitimate children. These areas must be discussed further in Chapter 5.

Some suggestions of intervention to make divorce less hurtful for children have been provided by Jenkins (1978). Included in these recommendations are: the initiation of innovative strategies for resolving custody disputes, the employment of court-related counseling, the establishment of postdivorce clinics, and the provision of peer-group supports to parents. Luepnitz (1978) recommended Richard Gardner's *The Boys' and Girls' Book about Divorce,* which was published in 1970, to help parents explain their own divorce to children. Kelly and Wallerstein (1976) reported that 80% of the divorcing parents whom they encountered said *nothing* to their children about their divorce.

DEATH

Adams (1972a) described widowhood as the enacting of social ritual; the experiencing of bereavement, laced with grief, ambivalence, and the pain of being the only adult in the household; the questioning of compulsive honor versus respite from mothering; the struggling to make do, to augment income and manage economically through relying on extensions of the family; and sooner or later, perhaps, the seeking of a new mate, remarrying, and encountering associated problems. He noted that the wrenching experience involves the mother much more than the child, but the child does experience the mother's pulling away to confront her own sense of loss and feelings of bereavement.

Langer (1963) wrote some sound information to widowed women that, heeded, would help their children. She noted how often the bereaved woman feels incomplete, amputated, and angry toward the dead husband for dying, for deserting her. Stein and Susser (1969) reported that the transition into widowhood represents a change in status and in role for the mother and as such may precipitate mental illness.

Silverman and Englander (1975) discussed the problems of children faced with the trauma of paternal death. Problems escalate in a culture that is normed to avoid and deny death. Wherever "father is sleeping" or "went away," troubles are worse. The problems of the mothers of these children are great also, since they are called on to meet their children's needs while simultaneously enduring their own grief. For help to these families, the authors described the Widow-to-Widow program, an experiment in preventive intervention. Nonetheless, a high percentage of widows come down within 6 weeks after their husband's death with a crippling illness—physical of psychical.

Peterson et al. (1959) found that a normally healthy family can sustain the effects of father's death. Family strengths rally, bereavement follows its normal course, and individual identities are reestablished. The mental health professional literature is replete with descriptions of the "healthy" way to deal with death and mourning; but this is very different from the literature on divorce. The families who come to the attention of public agencies are those unable to cope with *financial devastation or with mother's unresolved dependency needs.*

Effects of Parental Death on Children

For deepened reading in this area, the reader must consult Erna Furman's (1974) sensitive and thorough review of research on a child's reaction to losing a parent through death. Mother's reaction to father's death will frequently determine the children's reaction (Peterson et al., 1979). Although the healthy family can sustain this trauma, unhealthy reactions can occur. Children may exhibit increased dependency on mother. This bond is one reeking of ambivalence, because the dead parent is fantasized as being perfect while the remaining parent, mother, is imperfect, tainted, or bad; but she is all the child has to comfort him or her in this time of grief.

It is still debated whether children even have the capacity to mourn. If they are able—as Freud described—to achieve a decathexis from the lost object, it is as yet undetermined at what age this potential emerges (Grossberg & Crandall, 1978); Susz and Marberg (1972) described the case of a young Israeli child who lost her father by death at the age of 2 years and subsequently went through all the stages of mourning reported in the literature on adults. Today we generally concede that children can grieve and that they suffer from primary depressions also.

Jacobson (1966), however, wrote that children are unable to go through an actual mourning process and for this reason the dead parent is kept alive and idealized through their fantasies. The parent's loss through death is viewed as a severe narcissistic injury. Freud and Burlingham (1944) wrote that the fantasies of children whose fathers had been killed in the war were "inevitable defenses against the inner feeling of loss and deprivation" (108). Boss (1977), however, indicated that it was dysfunctional to the family unit when Missing In Action (MIA) fathers were kept psychologically present in an expressive role among the surviving family members. In these instances, psychological father-presence was related to a high degree of control, organization, and rigidity in the family environment. The tendency to idealize the dead is so strong that it sometimes grows to the extent of hallucinating a ghostly presence.

Besides fantasy, denial, and depression, two more responses have been observed in children deprived of a parent through death. Depression over a father's death is uncommon in children and often difficult to detect (Keeler, 1954). It is frequently associated with loss through death before the age of 8 years (Caplan & Douglas, 1969). Peterson et al. (1959) provided examples of pathological family adjustment to death. Case studies that are specific for children stressed by traumatic maladaptation to the loss of a parent have been made by Gauthier (1966), Keeler (1954), Nichol (1964), Brown (1966), and Stolorow and Lachmann (1975). Stolorow and Lachmann (1975) described in a psychoanalytic mode the case of a young woman whose father had been killed in a concentration camp when she was 4 years old. Included among the undesirable effects of losing her father during the pre-Oedipal phase was her defensive use of denial in lieu of mourning. The authors elucidated the ways in which the patient's bereavement had influenced her self-image, sexual identity formation, and superego formation, particularly in regard to the role of guilt. Grossberg and Crandall (1978) cited Anna Freud's findings that regression in both instinct and ego development are defenses against parental death.

Other defenses associated with children's reactions to parental death include "reversal of affect" and "loss of recent development gains" (Grossberg & Crandall, 1978). The emergence of delinquent behavior has also been correlated with this phenomenon (Brown, 1966; Keeler, 1954), as have suicidal attempts and preoccupations coupled with anxiety (Keeler, 1954).

According to Grossberg and Crandall (1978), "The developmental phase at which the loss occurs determines to a large extent the nature and severity of the interference" (p. 125). Reportedly, loss of a father during the pre-Oedipal period can result in oral fixations, immature ego structure, and underdeveloped ego controls. A father's death during the child's Oedipal phase is likely to interfere with sex-role identification and or preference. For the little girl, the lost father is idealized, a reaction that "in girls can lead to impaired relationships with men because no 'real' man can compete with the idealized image of the absent father" (p. 126). Little boys who lose their fathers through death may view the deprivation as fulfillment of their Oedipal desires, setting in motion a dynamic that may interfere later with establishing fulfilling and enriching heterosexual relationships. This thinking all harks back to Freud's 1910 treatise on Leonardo da Vinci (see Freud, 1976).

Effects of Parental Death on Adolescents and Adults

Most study of childhood bereavement deals with its residual effects on adolescents and adults. Bartlett and Horrocks (1958) found that adolescents whose parents are deceased show an unsatisfied need for affection, more than adolescents whose parents are still living. They found a significant negative correlation between heterosexual striving and satisfaction from parents, noting that adolescents from homes where one parent was deceased tended to receive less recognition and affection from adults. These adolescents have been observed to overstrive for attention from the opposite sex in an effort to compensate for the emotional deprivation within their families.

Nichol's (1964) review indicated that death of either parent before the age of 15 years is positively associated with depression in later years. Some authors specify that death of the *father,* especially, prior to the youth's fifteenth birthday is significant in this respect (Hill & Price, 1967; Brown, 1961). Others indicate that the crucial period for loss is 10 to 15 years of age (Dennehy, 1966) or 10 to 14 years of age (Brown, 1961; Hill & Price, 1967). Brown specified two crucial periods for loss of the father: 5 to 9 years of age and 10 to 14 years of age. Gay and Tonge (1967) found both adult reactive depression and personality disorder to correlate highly with loss of father between ages 5 and 14 years.

Wilson et al. (1967) analyzed the MMPI profiles of 92 depressed adult inpatients at Dorothea Dix Hospital in North Carolina. The parentally deprived group showed higher scores in the MMPI psychotic tetrad. For the childhood-bereaved group, the MMPI profiles of the *maternally* deprived were more severely disturbed than the profiles of the paternally deprived. Hopkinson and Reed (1966) found no higher incidence of childhood bereavement among hospitalized manic-depressives than among the general population. But, of course, manic-depressive disorder is now considered to be predominantly genetic, or genogenic, in etiology.

Authors who have emphasized loss of cross-sex parent (father of girls, mother of boys) in the etiology of depression include Dennehy (1966), Gay and Tonge (1967), and Birtchnell (1970a). Dennehy (1966) did note, however, that among drug addicts there was an excess of childhood loss by death of the same-sex parent; other types of neurosis have also been associated with loss by death of the same-gendered parent (Gay & Tonge, 1967). Careful epidemiologic studies in large populations are lacking; we cannot say how mother-loss as distinct from father-loss leads to pathology.

Beck, Sethi, and Tuthill (1963) found an overoccurrence of parental death before age 16 among patients who received "high-depressed" scores on the Beck Depression Inventory. Munro (1966) observed that parental loss before age 16 was not significant among depressives as a whole but was significant only among *severe depressives.*

Birtchnell (1970c) noted that the incidence of *early parental death* was significantly higher in a severely depressed group of patients admitted to a Scottish psychiatric hospital when compared to a moderately depressed group and to a nondepressed control group. Watt and Nicholi (1979) reported that premature parental death was distinctively associated with adult schizophrenic disorder—particularly paranoid schizophrenia—in adults. Birtchnell (1970a, b, c) acknowledged the importance to adults of *recent parent death* as a causative factor in *severe depression, suicidal behavior,* and *admission to a psychiatric hospital.* The clinical rule of thumb for adult depressives is that a crisis of mourning lasts 6 to 8 weeks and bereavement endures about 1 year; anything exceeding that should be suspected to be an underlying depression.

Death versus Divorce

Furman (1974) drew a parallel between death and divorce in the respect that both result in the child's experiencing an intense feeling of "longing" for the lost parent. But, in many respects death of a father is considered to be less traumatic for children than is divorce. For one thing, the mother is not faced with the task of deciding to try to make the marriage work. Also, death is something for which the mother cannot be held responsible (unless perchance she murdered father). Therefore, in widowhood there are neither the accusations nor the derogations that often play bedfellow to divorce. A widow may experience guilt, but it lessens as a healthy adjustment occurs. It does not linger on as an unhealed wound, to be reopened frequently with each postdivorce encounter.

Herzog and Sudia (1974) recorded that father-absence due to death is regretted but is usually not attended by the stigma that attends divorce and desertion. In their review on fatherless families, they concluded that family adaptation to father's absence is most facile and productive when his absence is due to honorable causes—death, military service, work—as opposed to divorce, separation, desertion. A family might not adapt so well, then, to father-absence caused by imprisonment, adultery, hospitalization for mental illness and so on. However, as we must reiterate, in such families isolating fatherlessness per se as a major influence is difficult (Rosenfeld et al., 1973). Kogelschatz et al. (1972) found that economic conditions account for most of the variance seen in 105 fatherless children's psychopathology when compared to an intact family group. Most of the widows still were young (1.2 years of fatherlessness) and had good adaptive resources as well as economic security.

We must remember that the widow is usually not so economically devastated as the divorced female head of household. According to Mallan (1975) widows as a group are older: Less than 20% of widows are under age 35 as compared with 55% of divorced and separated female heads of household. Further, widows typically receive inheritances and Social Security benefits and so have higher incomes than divorced or separated women with children.

Adverse repercussions of father-absence have been attributed to three primary conditions: lack of paternal supervision and control, deficit of role model or object of identification for male children, and family disharmony preceding the absence. Because parental death usually occurs when the child is older, and divorce or desertion when the child is younger, the lack of paternal supervision and control, most needed by the younger child, tends to be more highly associated with divorce or desertion than with death. The dead father tends to be more idealized and ennobled than the divorced father, and certainly more than the father who deserted. Hence, odd as it sounds, the dead father tends to be a better role model to surviving sons. Although family disharmony and emotional havoc frequently precede divorce or desertion, no evidence indicates that this hateful turmoil precedes paternal death, except in the case of his prolonged, terminal illness. Also, the family whose father has died is usually not so economically devastated as the family whose father has left through divorce or desertion—or was never there at all. Herzog and Sudia (1974) commented that the child who loses a father due to death is less likely to perceive that loss as abandonment than the child whose father divorces or deserts the mother. Logically, the child of a dead father is less likely to grow to adulthood harboring hatred and re-sentiment toward the lost parent or toward males. Parish and Kappes (1980) found (in 421 college students) confirmation of this: Parental divorce conveyed stigma to the subjects' parents, but paternal death carried a relative halo equal to the high esteem for intact parental couples. Parish (1981) extended these findings to a population of 1,409 college students, but found the students' own concepts of themselves did not vary according to marital status of parents. Francke, et al. (1980) quoted Rabbi Earl Grollman of Temple Beth El in Belmont, Massachusetts who stated that "the big difference between death and divorce is that death has closure, . . . with divorce, it's never over" (p. 198).

Grossberg and Crandall (1978) reported that whether loss of father occurs through death or through divorce, the continuum of the child's normal to pathological adaptation is determined by mother's reaction. So even a widowed mother's responses can be pathogenic for her children. Examples of mother's pathological accommodation include her displacement of unresolved conflicts with her husband onto her child, her libidinal shift from husband to child, entailing maternal seduction, and her overprotection of the child because of her own overpowering fear of another significant object loss.

In such a psychologically unwholesome family climate, "the child's normal intense ambivalence towards the mother, one of love and dependence versus hatred, can turn into an intense fear of being devoured by the omnipotent mother now that the father is not present to act as a buffer in the mother-child relationship" (p. 128).

Summary of Death's Effects

In summary, the child paternally deprived through death is often better off, emotionally and financially, than the child paternally deprived through divorce or desertion. Though it is still unclear whether children do in fact have the capacity to mourn in the way adults do, several psychiatric maladjustments—the most notable being childhood (and adult) depression—have been attributed to childhood bereavement. Much of the child's manner of adaptation depends on mother's methods of coping with father's death. Defensive responses commonly observed in bereaved children are fantasy denial, depression, and regression.

ILLEGITIMACY

Of the types of fatherless families that prevail, the never-completed family headed by the never-married female is likely to experience the most severe financial difficulties and to be lowest in esteem. The mother is also likely to be younger than mothers of other father-absent children. This form of family is on the increase; one birth in six or seven in the United States is now illegitimate (Schorr & Moen, 1979).

One of us (Adams, 1972b) noted that not only lower-class or bo-hemian upper-middle-class but also working-class and petit-bourgeois women increasingly choose to form a family without an adult male. The stereotypes expounded by priests and psychiatrists (usually males) persist as irritants for these women. The special difficulties of the lower-class partial family—never to be completed by the stable presence of a male in the household—include "living with string when rope is called for" and finding ways to cope when no male is around. A child who does not know his or her father, or whose parents never married, often feels disadvantaged. Nobody can glorify a patriarch as much as can a fatherless child.

Leontyne Young (1954) published a 261-page volume of practical casework concerning illegitimate children and their mothers. It is interesting, because it shows what clinical practice was like with un-married mothers some 30 years ago—before liberalized abortion, before liberalized codes concerning illegitimate children, before the shortage of any children for agency adoptions, and before the days when the best adoptions were considered to be agency adoptions. Young viewed the caseworker as an ego support, a more rational substitute mother to the unwed pregnant girl. She declared that the caseworker must be ready to "take the baby, to receive the baby from the unwed mother" since that is all that will satisfy the longings of the unwed mother who wants to give birth but not to rear her child. Times have changed.

Prevalence of Illegitimacy

For a more current view of family life for illegitimate children and their mothers, let us look at some of the recent prevalence statistics and research. Statistics reported here may not be totally accurate, for as Burkart and Whatley (1973) noted, for diverse reasons, current statistics on illegitimacy are unreliable. A number of states do not record illegitimacy rates. Upper- and middle-socioeconomic-level people can afford to buy secrecy for the pregnant unwed daughter. Lower-socioeconomic-class women may claim legitimacy without the benefit of matrimony. Fifty percent of all illegitimate pregnancies are by repeaters. Also, illegitimacy rates never include the illegitimate babies of married women, nor the babies conceived before marriage (25% of all first pregnancies fall into this category), nor the number of pregnant women who get abortions (Godenne, 1977). Despite these flaws, the statistics reported here will serve as crude indices of some general trends.

The number of illegitimate births has continued to rise, even though the total number of live births has reached a plateau. According to Mondale (1977), the rate of illegitimacy more than doubled in the last 3 decades. Indeed, as Osofsky (1970) remarked, there were 87,900 illegitimate births reported in the United States in 1936, which amounted to 3.6% of the total live births for that year. In 1960 they were 5.2% of the total live births for that year, and in 1965, 7.7%. According to *Newsweek* (May 15, 1978), in 1976, 15% of all births were illegitimate. The projected 1980 figure was for an additional 100,000—totaling 403,000—and the largest number of illegitimate children was expected to be born to the 15- to 19-year-old age group.

Reported illegitimacy is high among blacks. Of the 513,000 children who were born to black women in 1976, 50.3% were illegitimate (*Newsweek*, May 15, 1978). Today, white illegitimacy rates are rising much faster than black illegitimacy rates. In the 1950s the black illegitimacy rate was 12 times higher than the white. By the late 1960s, however, the black rate was only 6 times higher than the white (Godenne, 1977). Were the truth known, there might be less race difference in illegitimacy ratios than existing figures indicate. Teele and Schmidt (1970) criticized methods of reporting, and Berkov (1968) stated a well-known condition among demographers: "Less information is available about illegitimate than about total births and it is assumed that concealment of illegitimacy is more frequent for white than for Negro women" (p. 409).

Pope (1969) examined the differences between black and white mothers regarding decisions about their out-of-wedlock pregnancies. We found both that fewer black women than white women marry to legitimize their babies and that more black women actually keep their children after birth. Of course, black women's families and neighbors encourage keeping children. Because race is a major consideration in adoption, mothers of different races do not have equal opportunities in planning for their babies. Black women who offer babies for adoption have to go against the grain. Ninety percent of all children adopted are white (Corrigan, 1970). In 1966, 67% of white illegitimate children were adopted as opposed to 6% of non-white children (Hylton, 1965). This gap may be narrowing, but only slightly.

Pope (1969) also found that a black woman more often than a white woman maintained ties with the putative father after the child's birth; she more often felt that marriage to her sex partner in the future was a viable possibility. Pope proposed tentative explanations of his findings, one being that blacks generally have less of a commitment to the norm of legitimacy than whites, the other that black women have less reason and desire than white women to marry—whether or not they are unwed mothers. Regardless of race, however, as it was observed by *Newsweek* (May 15, 1978), "it is the illegitimate, both black and white, who are most likely to be impoverished, dependent on welfare, deprived of educational opportunities and destined to repeat the cycle with illegitimate children of their own" (pp. 67–68). The outlook for the children is bleaker than that for the fatherless children who are legitimate.

Adolescent Unwed Pregnancy and Births

Recent increases in the age and educational levels of the unwed mother have been noted. Reasons for an older woman to deliver an illegitimate child include premenopausal depression, unfulfilled career expectations, and increased sexual interest (Burkart & Whatley, 1973). Still, adolescents are most highly represented among unwed mothers. In 1965, 45% of all illegitimate children were born to women under 20. In 1973, there were an estimated 2.2 million never-married 15- to 19-year-olds in need of family planning services over a 12-month period (Morris, 1974). In 1976, more than one-half of out-of-wedlock babies were born to teen-agers (*Newsweek,* May 15, 1978). Women under 20 who conceive out of wedlock are likely to have eight additional children during their lifetimes (Osofsky & Osofsky, 1970). Using abortion to terminate an unwanted pregnancy, however, encourages effective contraceptive measures and deters future unwanted pregnancies (Dauber et al., 1972).

One out of every four U.S. births is to a teen-age mother, and although 75% of them are married, 50% of the marriages follow conception. Teen-age marriages formed in order to legitimize the birth of a child end in divorce three or four times as often as marriages formed at a later age (Godenne, 1977). Kellam et al. (1979) indicated that the teen-age mother tends to be and tends to remain the only adult present in the household, has little help with child-rearing activities, and participates in few voluntary organizations. Her child may lack stimulation.

In addition to the sociopsychiatric components, adolescent pregnancy generally is physically dangerous. According to Curtis (1974) unwed adolescent mothers fall into the "high-risk" category due to such factors as late prenatal care, improper nourishment, and inconsistency in following health precautions, leading to such conditions as toxemia, prematurity, and infant morbidity. Godenne (1977) wrote that unmarried adolescent mothers often gain too much weight and are prone to anemia, fetal–pelvic disproportion, prolonged labor, and other obstetrical complications. During labor and delivery, the unmarried mother, generally, is more likely to be heavily sedated and more unlikely to have a companion of her choice present. It has been noted that verbal and physical abuse of the laboring unwed mother occur when she is attended only by the hospital personnel (Scully, 1975).

Personalities of Unwed Adolescent Mothers

Sarrel and Davis (1966) indicated that the adolescent mother is likely to be a repeater. McKay and Richardson (1973) compared M.M.P.I. scores of 21 one-time unwed mothers and 16 recidivist mothers with a control group of "normal girls." Of the two groups, the unwed recidivist mothers deviated most from the norm. Both recidivist and one-time unwed mothers had tendencies such as antisocial attitudes, rebelliousness, and shallow emotional feelings, but these inclinations were distinctly greater in the recidivist mothers. Recidivist mothers also showed more immaturity and emotional instability, more openly conspicuous violation of social regulations, more incorrigibility, and less control of hostility than one-time unwed mothers. Age and education were noted in the study, but socioeconomic status and race were not singled out as telling variables.

Several authors have speculated on the causes of adolescent pregnancy. According to Godenne (1977), "The early adolescent gets pregnant because of lack of information, denial, and knowledge embellished by distortion. The middle adolescent acts out her oedipal conflict and her desire for independence" (p. 345). The unwed mother of 15 to 16 years may be battling acute inner conflicts. She may have lost her identity with her original family group. She may think she is in love with the baby's father and desire to have a child by him (Burkart & Whatley, 1973). The unwed mother of 18 or 19 years may be afraid to be completely independent and may try pregnancy as a lever to marriage. She may use pregnancy as a way to retaliate for pent-up frustrations and belligerent feelings or to escape from an inner change in attitude and reactions to her family. She may be seeking nurture that she has not received in the family group (Burkart & Whatley, 1973). If she does not get that nurturing, one can only pity the often fatherless child who results.

We must point out that these speculations on the causes of adolescent unwed pregnancy may not apply across socioeconomic class and/or racial lines. Some scholars assert that one reason that black adolescent females might become pregnant is as a rite of passage into womanhood; also, whether they marry or not is not of as much importance as it would be to their white counterparts. Probably this variable would also be highly related to social class. Aug and Bright (1970) supported this point of view when they asserted that illegitimacy traditionally has been studied from a middle-class point of view, a standpoint from which the phenomenon is perceived as being deviant, immoral, and indicative of spiraling decadence. Moreover, such attitudes may no longer apply even to the middle class, for today to have children and not to marry is in vogue among some middle-class white women.

According to Burkart and Whatley (1973), unwed pregnancy may be associated with unsuccessful attempts at meaningful work. In some families a cyclic effect may be observed in several generations of women, an effect of cultural factors in addition to socioeconomic status. This same cyclic effect has more recently been associated with communal living.

The unwed teen-age mother presents a unique set of problems. Curtis (1974) stated:

> *These adolescent mothers are frightened, lonely girls caught in a cycle of dependency and deprivation which, without some intervention, will perpetuate itself. They impress me as girls who never developed trust and often use defense mechanisms such as hostility and defiance of authority. [p. 100]*

If the adolescent unwed mother is burdened with psychiatric problems prior to conception, pregnancy merely compounds her problems, adding educational and social dimensions. She may have to discontinue her education. Pregnancy is the largest single cause of female dropouts from high school. The additional emotional and financial needs of pregnancy may not be met if her pregnancy is condemned by parents, educators, boyfriend, and peers. Her self-concept may be drastically altered as she perceives the effects of pregnancy on her young pliable body, still incomplete in its alterations and modifications. The unwed adolescent mother has an inclination to feel fearful and guilty, without hope and without help (Godenne, 1977). Of unwed-female-headed households, teen-age-headed households seem to hold the most suffering—emotional, social, and financial—for the children. According to Adams (1978), "Youthful parents especially can be violent, prone to child battering, child molesting and murder. Older parents are less risky, given our present moral and economic dispensation" (p. 9).

Single Motherhood versus Adoption versus Abortion

Festinger (1971) studied 49 unwed mothers who chose to keep their babies and 49 unwed mothers who surrendered their babies for adoption and found that mothers' decisions to keep their children were associated positively with older age, employment status (not in school), and a nonintact parental home. Other research in the area has found that lower education level, also, is associated with mother's decision to keep the child. There are pressures on unwed women to keep their children; weaker countervailing pressures drive them to let their babies be adopted!

Butts and Sporakowski (1974) compared 74 unwed mothers who chose to have their babies with 38 unwed mothers who chose abortion. They found that "maternity home pregnants were younger, less educated, more regular church attenders, less aware of abortion, less sexually permissive, in poorer relationship with the putative father, and less likely to be satisfied with their pregnancy decision than their abortion choice counterparts" (p. 110). Girls who chose abortion tended to derive economically from the middle class. The maternity home residents' backgrounds, however, tended to be equally divided between middle and lower socioeconomic classes. According to Godenne (1977), "Whatever the reasons, the unwed mothers often come from the low socioeconomic strata of society, are generally poorly educated, and have a history of school truancy and school dropouts" (p. 345).

Advocates of free abortion choice believe that abortion spares women the duty to bear and bring up *unwanted children*.

Of course, abortion is not a panacea. Martin (1973) reported on psychological problems encountered by teen-age women who chose the abortion alternative. The primary distinction between post abortion women who had poor psychological adjustment and those who had good psychological adjustment was the experiencing of intense guilt by the former—possibly a societally dictated response. In any event, recent legislation has made abortion a nonviable option for most poor women in the United States today.

The Role of Personality

Naiman (1966) attributed illegitimacy not to social class or educational background, but to certain personality traits. He examined a total group of 32 subjects and concluded that unmarried mothers were found to have a greater degree of impulsivity and a poorer ability to form stable relationships than a control group of married mothers.

Kravitz et al. (1966) surveyed 83 women referred to an unwed mothers' clinic and found "early deprivation and depression, history of loss or threatened loss as a precipitating factor, unrealistic attitudes to contraception and impulsivity in other areas as well" (p. 463). They wrote: "We are of the opinion that the very fact that a girl finds herself pregnant and unwed in our culture is indicative of underlying emotional problems" (p. 461). Floyd and Viney (1974) found that unwed mothers demonstrated less positive feminine identification and more ambivalence about their ego identities than their married counterparts.

In contrast, Aug and Bright (1970), who interviewed 24 unmarried and 22 married poor mothers 24 to 48 hours after delivery, concluded that

> the "problem" of disturbed interpersonal relationships is well-represented in both wed and unwed groups. Conversely, there are a sizeable number of well-adjusted people in both groups. It therefore seems that it would be wise to take a broad look at the entire subculture if one is to assess the imprint of illegitimacy as a "problem" or as a symptom of "problems" for a particular group. [p. 592]

Services for Unwed Mothers

What services exist to aid the unwed mother? According to Godenne (1977), "The unwed mother who most needs the services of an agency for support and planning for her future is the one who, out of shame, is often the most reluctant to seek help" (p. 345). The mothers may be reluctant, but no doubt excessive prodding does not occur, because programs are insufficient. In the early 1970s, services existed to meet the needs of only 25% of the unwed mother subpopulation (Osofsky, et al., 1973). It has been estimated that the services that do exist to aid unwed mothers (voluntary child welfare agencies, maternity homes, and family service agencies) are used by clients who tend to be white and of higher socioeconomic status and higher educational level than the average unmarried mothers. These recipients also tend to be younger and more likely to place their children for adoption (Herzog, 1969).

Perhaps this differential use of help occurs because existing programs are often staffed by white, middle-class professionals, laden with white, middle-class moral biases. These shortcomings must be overcome if social service agencies can effectively assist the unwed mother (Blair & Pasmore, 1969). Some progress has been made in recent years; that can be observed in various Planned Parenthood clinics. It is feared that such worthy programs will be drastically reduced or annihilated by cutbacks in government spending for social programs.

Programs to help the unmarried mother frequently measure their success by whether the mother conceives *no more* children out of wedlock after participating in the program. According to Aug and Bright (1970),

> *This criterion seems to imply that out-of-wedlock pregnancy is necessarily deleterious in itself, and that if we can but "break the vicious circle" we can do a great service to the unwed mother. This sentiment does not seem to fit with the observations of Barglow et al. (1968), who believed that for certain individuals in their study group, the out-of-wedlock pregnancy, far from being the beginning of a downhill spiral, was an important factor leading to increased depth of understanding between the unwed mother and her family of origin. [p. 593]*

It is to the child's benefit if the mother has healed her outlook and behavior in relation to her family of origin.

It would be less moralistic but more practical to orient programs that assist unwed mothers to fulfill some realistic needs. For example, prenatal medical care is sorely needed among this population, and is less often received by unmarried mothers than by married ones. A program designed to meet prenatal needs of unwed mothers would necessitate the provision of other services as well—transportation, day care, psychological, financial, and others (Herzog, 1969).

Herzog (1969) identified the punitive character of some existing programs. She distinguished between two types of programs. One is designed for adoption of the baby and psychological rehabilitation of the mother. These programs are usually supported by the community to serve the middle-class, frequently white, unwed mother. Still other programs are geared to socioeconomic rehabilitation and damned by the community for using their tax dollars. These programs, whose apparent aim is "keeping the mother off relief rolls," most often serve the lower-class, usually nonwhite mother. Herzog recommended that sufficient public funds provide necessary programs for lower-class unwed mothers; she cited the example of Denmark where the unmarried mother is expected to receive help in establishing adequate living quarters, adequate day care for her child, and adequate training for herself, sometimes for several years. In the wake of such a program, illegitimacy rates are reported to have *decreased* in Denmark.

Problems of the Illegitimate Child

What are some of the problems encountered specifically by the illegitimate child? The mother may feel ambivalent toward the child and may vacillate in her approach to her or him. Thus, the child may suffer from overprotection or from rejection or from both sporadically (Wimperis, 1960). Peterson (1959) thought that illegitimate children represent to the mother her failure to find gratification for herself. The mother who feels strongly ambivalent toward her illegitimate child may keep him or her in an effort to force the father to meet her dependency needs—or she may leave him or her with the maternal grandmother as a type of revenge for her own neglected upbringing. When the child learns of his or her origin, he or she may feel stigmatized and initiate the experience of mutual ambivalence in relation to the mother. Around the matter of a child's illegitimacy, many sadomasochistic struggles arise.

Corrigan (1970), however, compared child-rearing practices of 181 unwed mothers with two control groups and found that children born out of wedlock were not for the most part victims of inadequate child rearing. The unwed mothers tended to be warmer than control mothers and less permissive. The unwed fathers tended to be less warm than wed fathers, but they did not discriminate in their treatment of male and female children. Unwed mothers tended to emphasize school performance more than the controls. From these findings, unwed mothers do not appear to be either more permissive or more rejecting than wed mothers. The extent of the child's psychiatric disturbance tends to be directly and positively correlated with the extent of mother's psychiatric disturbance and inversely correlated with income. The most prevailing and most devastating characteristic noted among these families was their extreme poverty. The author noted, "Poverty has a cumulative eroding influence. It erodes the individual's spirit and mind, but mostly it erodes family relationships" (p. 67).

DESERTION

An illegitimate child is usually not considered to have been deserted. Yet technically, the child has been deserted by the father before birth (Lerner, 1954); assuredly, both mother and child could be said to have been deserted before marriage.

Little scientific study has been done on the impact of desertion per se, since few statistics exist in this area, and those are likely to be unreliable. Some authors have written generally on its effects, however. According to Lerner (1954), desertion is much like other types of father-absence in that children's reactions often depend largely upon mothers' reactions. The attitude of mother, the only present parent, can make a tremendous difference in the emotional health or ill health of the child(ren). Lerner noted that because childhood is an extremely dependent state, fears of desertion and abandonment commonly arise in children. When this catastrophe does in fact occur, confirming the child's worst premonitions, the child feels rejected, guilty, insecure, anxious, and full of dread about the future, to a greater or lesser degree depending upon the child's age and other extenuating circumstances. It is thought that the younger the child is, the more severe are the effects of desertion by a parent. Nevertheless, a 6-year-old too can be distressed by father's desertion of the family.

Once more it becomes obvious that the primary problem facing the father-absent family is financial. The law deals with this problem, in cases of desertion, by attempting to locate the errant father and to extract from him payments for child support. In many cases the attempt is unsuccessful. Skarsten (1974) suggested:

> *In view of the fact that the administrative costs of collecting monies from the deserting spouses exceed the amount of monies collected, why not use this public money to pay the deserted spouse to provide adequate care for the children as well as educational and up-grading courses to enable the person to become more self-sufficient? [pp. 24–25]*

This quotation appeared in an article dealing with family desertion in Canada, but the same situation might be thought to apply in the United States. Canadians usually tend to take a more active approach to solving problems rooted in social needs than do we of the United States; perhaps we could take a lesson from Canadians. There was no discussion available in our search for what it means to be a deserted child, or a child whose absconded father is punished and forced to pay up. The literature is seldom written with an eye on the child.

TEMPORARY FATHER-ABSENCE

Temporary father-absence occurs when father's work demands it or when state intervention removes him from the family. His work may keep father away from home in another city, as may state intervention that occurs when the father is imprisoned, or, as another example, when the father is drafted into military service. Herzog and Sudia (1968) found that, of the 59 studies they reviewed, when grouped on the criterion of continuing or temporary father-absence, more studies indicated deleterious effects for temporary than for continuing absence. However, when studies with gross defects in methodology were eliminated, there was the same number of studies in each category. Nevertheless, they stated that temporary father-absence could not be equated with continuing father-absence; it is too difficult to compare or to assume that studies are equatable that use different definitions of the term *broken home*. But the temporarily absent father may have serious impact on the temporarily fatherless children.

Absence Due to Work Demands

Wylie (1942) calculated that of 168 hours in a week, the average man spends 40 hours working, 15 hours traveling, and 56 hours sleeping. This leaves 57 hours of free time. Three hundred boys in seventh and eighth grade reported that of 57 free hours, their fathers spent approximately 7½ minutes with them during a week. James Turnbull, a psychiatrist, reported that fathers spend no more than 25 minutes per week involved in one-to-one interaction with their sons (Roche Report, 1980). As a result of this scant interaction time, Turnbull said, boys do not model their fathers' behaviors, but rather they model the behaviors of mothers, peers, and male instructors at school. Still, clinicians see workaholic fathers who wonder why their sons do not feel close to them.

Lynn (1974) viewed father-absence on account of work as a consequence of the growing complexity of our society, particularly among executive-professional fathers. Lynn remarked that the executive-professional father may leave for work before the children are awake and return after the younger ones are asleep; his paltry leisure hours are devoted to tennis, golf, or civic activities with other adults, not his children. The number of hours devoted to work and to travel declines as the status of the job declines. Elliot (1978) characterized temporary father-absence due to excessive work demands as primarily a middle-class phenomenon. However, working-class fathers tend to see children more as within the purview and orbit of the mother, in some cases as belonging solely to the mother. Consequently, working-class men may have more time to spend with their children but they rarely use their leisure time for that purpose; rather, they spend more time "out with the boys." Lynn (1974) stated that father absence due to work demands is so taken for granted in our society that "the absence of the father through death or divorce can be considered simply an extreme on the prevailing continuum of father absence" (p. 6).

Levine (1977) commented on father's temporary absence due to work-related travel as it affected wives and children in what appears to be middle-class society. The mother remaining at home may show bellwether signs of depression and/or boredom for the whole household. These mild problems usually can be overcome easily with adjustment to father's absence if underlying pathology is not great. Fagen et al. (1967) described effective and ineffective patterns of maternal coping with temporary father-absence. Cohen (1977) depicted the situation of a group of British middle-class wives, residing on a housing estate, who suffered the effects of their husbands' temporary absence due to work demands. These wives and mothers, wisely and expediently, established instrumental relationships with one another, forming what became a peer-group support system and enabling themselves to deal more effectively with the problems of daily living and the temporarily solitary rearing of small children. McCubbin et al. (1976) described six patterns of coping behavior exhibited by wives coping with war-induced separations from their husbands during the Vietnam War. They determined that the choice of coping patterns depends on background variables related to the wife, the husband, the family, and the marriage. The authors did not examine in detail the functional or dysfunctional nature of the six coping patterns. Tiller (1958) made a classic contribution concerning Norwegian sailor fathers whose prolonged recurrent separations from their children were a requirement of their work.

Effects on Children. A child's reactions are in large part predicted and colored by mother's adaptation or maladaptation to father's absence. Elliot (1978) wrote of mothers who attributed behavior problems of their children to "paternal work-absorption":

> *But even where a mother is correct in thinking that there is a link between her child's behavior problems and paternal work-absorption, the child's reaction may be a response to the atmosphere of tension and stress created by her frustration rather than to paternal deprivation per se . . . a child may be affected not simply by his own experience of parental deprivation but by his mother's reaction to her husband's work-absorption and by the way in which she presents it to him. [p. 312]*

Sauer (1979) described the effects of temporary father-absence due to work demands on the male children in a small coal region in Pennsylvania—where the "absentee father syndrome" had become tradition. Of the typical referral to the county mental health center, he wrote:

> *The common ingredient in most of these referrals is that the budding autonomy of the child is thwarted by his utilization in his parents' relationships as a buffer. He protects his mother from loneliness and despair by his availability to her and he serves as a stand-in for his father, thereby reducing the father's anxiety about his non-commitment to the family. [p. 248]*

The child's reaction depends on the child's age. Young children may cry and fear desertion, may be unduly anxious, and may need additional comfort and reassurance for the duration of father's absence. "Older children may be demanding and rebellious or quiet and withdrawn" (Levine, 1977, p. 75). Of detriment to the children is to have inconsistent standards of discipline; standards that vary when the father is at home and when he is away breed insecurity in the children and sometimes result in their being more upset by father's return than by his absence.

Absence Due to Military Service

By far the majority of the literature on temporary father-absence concerns itself with fathers away in military service. Authors of these studies rarely note that research conducted with military personnel examines only the reactions of a population that tends to be authoritarian, patriarchal, politically conservative on the whole. It is the opinion of the present authors that results gleaned from such studies cannot be justifiably applied to other segments of society.

An early study reported by Freud and Burlingham (1944) explored the effects not only of temporary father-absence, but also of temporary total-family-absence, on children placed in residential nurseries during World War II. It was observed that children deprived of parents in this manner tended to model after, imitate, and identify with residential nursery staff members as they would have related to their parents in a home situation. Nevertheless, the children invented and clung to exorbitant fantasy figures of their absent parents, for whose return they lived in longing anticipation. McDermott (1970) observed the tendency in emotionally disturbed children from father-absent families to exhibit the same symptoms. An identification with a part of (or a fantasized part of) the absent father was employed as a way of dealing with the loss and conflict surrounding the father's absence.

Crain and Stamm (1965) investigated whether intermittent absence of Navy personnel fathers affected 30 second-grade children's perceptions of both parents. Comparison with 22 father-present second-grade children of civilian employees revealed little difference between the two groups with regard to perceptions of mother and father as sources of love and authority. These results conflicted with previous findings in the area, and the authors speculated that a possible reason might be that their study measured only attitude and not performance. Moreover, other later studies did support the findings of earlier studies.

Effects on Children, Male or Female

Studies of temporary father-absence have concentrated primarily on changes manifested by male children. Research findings have indicated that father-absent boys show increased immaturity, compensatory masculinity, elevated masculine striving, and poorer peer adjustment (Lynn & Sawrey, 1964; Baker et al., 1967). Reports that father-absent boys generally become more feminine, less aggressive, and more dependent, and experience more Oedipal fantasies, however, have not been borne out in the research on temporary father-absence (Baker et al., 1967, 1968; Seplin, 1952).

Pedersen (1966) also failed to demonstrate that temporary father-absence is related to emotional disturbance in male children. He did, however, show that the *extent* of father-absence *is* related to degree of emotional disturbance. Other studies report that father-absent males show increases in conduct problems, hostility, and rivalry toward siblings (Baker et al., 1967) as well as in independent-mature behavior and in feelings of relative rejection, sadness, and inferiority (Baker et al., 1968). Changes observed in temporarily father-absent girls have included increased dependency on the mother (Lynn & Sawrey, 1964) and decreased quantitative ability (Hillenbrand, 1976).

Age at time of father-absence and sex, number, and age of siblings appear to be important variables to be considered when assessing the effects of temporary father-absence. Hillenbrand (1976), who looked for the effect of temporary father-absence on sixth-grade military dependents, found that in firstborn male children cumulative father-absence related significantly to enhanced quantitative ability and to perception of the mother as the dominant parent. The author hypothesized that the explanation for this beneficial effect of father-absence might be found in Talcott Parsons' role theory, which would predict that the older son adopts the instrumental role in father's absence and likewise sharpens his "masculine" skills. More detrimental effects were observed for younger firstborn sons—as with Adams and Horovitz's (1980b) study. In older firstborn boys, early-beginning father-absence related to increased aggression and dependency, but absence did not relate to quantitative ability or maternal dominance.

Crisis of Father's Return

Rosenfeld et al. (1973) examined family reactions to father-absence among Israeli sailors. Length of father-absence was sporadic among the 10 families interviewed. As in other studies (Baker et al., 1967, 1968) mothers reported difficulties in child rearing, and particular concern about the male children. Specifics were not given. Overall, however, it appeared that most of the upset was caused by father's visits home, rather than by his absences. Mother and children adapted and made do in his absence. In his presence, adaptations had to be suspended to make way for the reentry of the ordained household head. In some cases it appeared that father's brief visits were analogous to entertaining a dear guest who received the red carpet.

Crumley and Blumenthal (1973) explored the effects of father's absence for military service on 100 children, primarily white, male, and middle class, ranging in age from 3 to 18. They found that it was impossible to distinguish the effects of father's absence from the effects of the crisis of his return. They concluded that the entire cycle of departure, absence, and return resulted in detriment to the children's development in the areas of superego formation, the capacity to tolerate depressive affect, and object relations.

Father's return has been thought to have negative effects on both mother and children. According to Marsella et al. (1974), who examined the differential effects of father's presence and absence on maternal attitudes, fathers do not have a gentling influence on the wife-mother:

> There is more breaking the will, strictness, intrusiveness, and acceleration of development (all maternal domination) and more martyrdom, rejection of homemaking role, marital conflict (all marital discord) when father is present. The increased maternal control under conditions of father presence may be accounted for by modeling of the husband's behavior, complementary authoritarian role behavior,

control of husband's attention, and changes in children's behavior. [*p. 257*]

Crumley and Blumenthal (1973) explored deficient father–son relationships as a function of military life. They stated that sometimes the remiss father–son alliance could be traced back through three generations. Deficient interrelationships were merely exacerbated by father's repeated absences:

> *The fathers seemed to have re-created with their sons the poor relationship they themselves had experienced as children. Their own deficient masculine self-image was bolstered by assuming a super-soldier role and by an attempt to mold their sons in this image. Often the son felt completely unable to live up to this ideal expectation and felt rejected by the father. The child's anger at his parent was then turned inward against himself or outward toward others as acting out. Sexual identifications were inadequately developed.* [*p. 781*]

LINING UP A (NEW) MATE

Realistically speaking, what are the odds that the female head-of-household will marry or remarry? The odds are overwhelmingly toward no marriage in most cases, particularly as the woman grows older. For women aged 40 to 44, there are in the United States 137 unattached women for every 100 unattached men, a figure that varies according to the category of "unattached." For women who are divorced and currently single, there are 141 women per 100 men. For those who are separated, there are 213 women for every 100 men. For those bereaved, there are 644 widows to every 100 widowers. If the group of never-married men, who are unlikely ever to marry, are eliminated from the totals, there are 233 unattached women for every 100 unattached men. Nine out of every 10 women have been married at least once by the time they reach 30 years of age. The presence of children, too, decreases a woman's odds. There is a 73% chance of remarriage for a divorced woman with no children; 63% chance for a divorced woman with two children; 56% chance for a divorced woman with three children (Hacker, 1979).

But suppose the mother does remarry. What of the children in the reconstituted family? NIMH (1978) estimated that close to 15 million children under the age of 18 live in reconstituted families. Psychoanalysts say this situation promotes the Phaedra complex, the sexual attraction between stepparent and stepchild, often more lethal than either the Oedipal or the Electra triangles, especially when it results in consummation—the incest taboo having been diluted—through sexual molestation, usually of the female child under 10. The dangers of incest in such a family are not so much biological as they are emotional (the Medico-Legal Society, 1969). Messer (1969) advised that family romance—not incest—is not only a healthy and natural process, but that it is in fact necessary for the teaching of appropriate courtship behavior to adolescents. Thus he recommended that the phenomenon be dealt with in an open and forthright manner, in the natural family as well as in the reconstituted family. Denial, he said, leads to incestuous preoccupation and guilt. Bringing the issue to the fore allows it to be bypassed and repressed ultimately.

NIMH has issued two publications to help stepparents deal with some of the turmoil their tenuous liaisons with their newly formed families inevitably bring. Children tend to resent stepparents as intruders, unworthy replacements of their beloved lost ones. It is recommended that the stepparent try not to replace the lost parent, but to use time to befriend the child gradually. Remarriage is traumatic for children; it finalizes the departure of the absent parent. The child may feel increasingly guilty for the absent parent's egress—may hate the "replacement" and most hate the "betrayer" (mother) for intensifying his or her suffering. Kellam's (1979) study in the Chicago ghetto showed that the mother-only and mother-and-grandmother families led to better adjustments than did mother-and-stepfather families, nudging us to recall that economic class matters a great deal in family matters and notably so, for example, in stepfamilies.

Stepparents must be sensitive to these feelings in the child and be aware that the child who feels most isolated and alone and most needs love and protection may often assume a guise of hostility as a defense (NIMH, 1978).

In the words of Dennis Wilkes, a former stepchild, now stepfather:

I think it's difficult for children to accept someone who is not really their father as their father. It puts them in an awkward situation.

They think, "How should I treat my stepfather? Shall I treat him as a father or shall I treat him as an outsider?" [Ward, 1980]

Some authors extol the beneficial effects of the presence of a step-father or father surrogate on the development of children, particularly male children. Oshman and Manosevitz (1976) found male college students, both those who had had stepfathers and those who had never experienced father-absence, did not differ from each other on measures of psychosocial functioning. But both groups scored higher than subjects from father-absent families in which no father surrogate was present. Jenkins (1978) indicated that some of the negative connotations attributed to stepparents may be the effect of sociocultural conditioning—wicked stepparent syndrome—and she cited authors such as Maurice W. Levine and Margaret Mead to support this supposition. Indeed, only one short novel known to the authors portrays a stepparent lovingly, and that is a stepmother; see Peter Taylor, *A Woman of Means* (1950).

Other authors report that stepfathering may have detrimental effects on children. For example, Douglas (1970) observed that the greatest excess of enuresis is recorded for the children who were fostered or in institutions, and the least amount for those who remained with their mothers and did not have a stepfather. Waldron (1979) described some of the effects of the "intrusion" of the stepparent into the family system and the role conflict experienced by that person. Waldron made recommendations for therapeutic intervention in reconstituted families, but Visher and Visher (1979) have given the most complete treatment of the topic.

Whether stepparenting generally and stepfathering specifically have positive or negative effects on children in reconstituted families is a question that can be resolved only when variables such as age of child at time of reconstitution, length of time spent in a mother-only family, income, and other factors are controlled. Jessie Bernard (1971) asserted that very young and very old (adult) offspring suffer fewer negative effects from the assimilation of a stepparent into the family unit than do adolescents. That is in agreement with clinical practice.

In summary, it appears that the number of children growing up in father-absent families is increasing dramatically, and the likelihood is poor that the mother will be married eventually. The main problems besetting these families seem to be financial problems, problems that we fear will escalate with the present trend toward cutbacks in social spending. The type of fatherlessness tells everything in the individual case and in the mass also. When financial strains are relieved, as is sometimes the case when father-absence is due to death or work demands, rather than to divorce, desertion, or illegitimacy, we are able to look more closely at some of the strictly emotional or mental sequelae of father-absence. Then again, the children's adjustment seems to be determined largely by mother's reaction to father's absence, so it is difficult to establish specific cause–effect relationships between father-absence and children's development. This problem will be examined in greater detail in the following chapters.

Effects on Offspring: School and Sex Role

Many authors have speculated on the consequences for children of living in a female-headed household. Ironically, as Hetherington et al. (1979) pointed out, these writings are referred to as "father-absent" literature: "This rubric reflects a bias that when differences are found between children in single-parent and in intact families, they are attributable to the absence of the father rather than to differences in family functioning, stresses, and support systems in the two types of families" (p. 118). Not all children who live in households without a father suffer directly and exclusively from father-absence. Nevertheless, in this chapter we consider some of the presumed effects of father-absence on children. In this and the following chapter, we shall go into the areas of academic accomplishment, sexual identity and sex-role preference, psychopathology, and delinquent behavior. We shall try to determine whether the variable of father-absence is in fact the telling factor in a world inhabited by members of a single-parent, female-headed household, or whether that world is shaped by other forces, for example, by the economic deprivation that often accompanies fatherlessness.

SCHOOL PROGRESS

No evidence shows that fatherlessness rather than poverty or another variable causes poor school performance, but many researchers have tried to prove that it does:

> There appears to be some relation between retarded school progress and the lack of a parent in the home. The lack of one or both parents seems to affect every phase of school work unfavorably. Even if the difference between the groups is not large, the results always favor the group with parents. [Risen, 1939, p. 531]

Research into the influence of father-absence on educational performance and adjustment has grown rapidly. The pertinent studies deal generally either with academic performance, including measures of IQ or ability and achievement, or with general academic social adjustment, including motivation orientation. Specifically, in the first studies father-absence is often associated with an erosion of mathe-

128

matical skills and giftedness, and in the second it is associated with inferior adjustment to peers and teachers. A third group of studies deals with academic performance and adjustment of poor and minority children. Only a small percentage of these studies use appropriate methods; they frequently fail to control for the following variables: *race, socioeconomic status, type of father-absence, length of father-absence, age of child at time of father-absence, ordinal position, and number of siblings.* Because each of these variables affects children's academic functioning, we are skeptical of studies that omit them.

Socioeconomic Status (SES)

Differential academic achievement among socioeconomic classes has been well documented. Lewin (1969) noted a positive association among housing conditions, self-concept, and academic achievement. The different measurements of cognitive functioning among races is an issue more clouded and complex. Social or behavioral scientists do not falter in putting down poor people—nowadays, however, they seem more cautious about putting down nonwhites.

Even clinicians who stress "intrapsychic" matters have come, over the past 2 decades, to accept the view that extrapsychic factors, for example, poverty, impinge heavily on the real lives and fantasies of children in school. School breakfasts, free lunches, and early "compensatory" education such as Head Start are among the realistic steps taken to lessen poverty's blight on schoolchildren. More and more, although they are in the style of Karl Marx, radical therapists are joined by neoconservatives in seeing the family as the arena in which economic class confronts values and fantasies.

Black and Poor. Deutsch (1960) recounted differential indices of scholastic achievement for white children and black children, even when social class was controlled. Henderson and Long (1973) suggested that racism among teachers may affect the poorer academic achievement often found among black children, that teachers get what they expect from black pupils.

Mischel (1961) found, with 112 Trinidadian subjects 11 to 14 years old, a significant relationship between preference for immediate smaller rewards and acquiescence and, conversely, between preference for delayed larger reinforcement and school achievement. Although Mischel hedges, his later studies suggest that a people who for centuries have not been given equal opportunity to achieve will opt for the immediate, smaller reward, so that their measured achievements, even at a very young age, will be significantly lower than those of a people who have been in power and have not had to acquiesce for small prizes. Herzog's (1974) more sophisticated and imaginative conclusions about West Indian children are presented later.

Bronfenbrenner (1967), having reviewed the research on poor children, wrote that serious inadequacies of disadvantaged schoolchildren, primarily black males, result from prenatal damage, father-absence, impoverished home environments, and dysfunctional patterns of child rearing. He called for a counterstrategy of more active involvement with disadvantaged children, asking middle-class children and adults of both races to help, a plea that now may look patronizing. Egalitarians no longer endorse George Bernard Shaw's wish to make everyone as socialistic and middle class as himself; rather they wish to grant more equality irrespective of subculture, dialect, or life style.

Controversy surrounds discussion of the effects of racism and poverty on cognitive functioning. Jensen (1969) has made an unusual contribution to this controversy—to the science and politics of IQ and race—with his conclusion that blackness is associated with lowered IQ. However, Burnes (1970), for example, analyzed the WISC scores of middle- and lower-class black and white preschool children and found differences between social classes, but not between races. (See Chapter 7 for descriptions of tests.) In general, Burnes' ideas have held more securely than Jensen's. Burnes' report scrutinized Deutsch's (1960) and Stodolsky and Lesser's (1967) studies, which indicated disparate scores both between socioeconomic classes and between black and white children even when socioeconomic status was controlled. Since this contradiction remains unresolved, and since fatherless children are disproportionately black and poor, researchers must control for both race and socioeconomic status when assessing the effects of fatherlessness on cognitive functioning, and clinicians must remember that an apparent decrement of 15 IQ points may need to be added for a more accurate appraisal of a black child's IQ or potential IQ.

Father-Absence Variables

The type of father-absence is an important qualitative variable, as noted by Santrock (1973) and Herzog (1974) as well as by others considered in the preceding chapter. Landy et al. (1969) confirmed the importance of both length of father-absence and the child's age during the father-absence for girls' cognitive development. Herzog (1974) noted the importance of age at time of father-absence on boys' cognitive development and school adjustment.

Lifshitz (1976) reported that especially those children who lost their fathers before the age of 7 "tended to show significant constriction in awareness and differentiation of their broader social milieu, and tightening of diverse psychological indices; the smaller the perceived difference between self and parents, the more changeable and restless their behavior appeared to be" (p. 196). Lifshitz suggested that children who lost their fathers early may have been more preoccupied with internal organization than with situations at large. Other authors remarked the apparent effects of father-absence on perceptual differentiation in children (Goldstein & Peck, 1973; Goldstein & Gershansky, 1976; Gershansky, Hainline, & Goldstein, 1978), although Roach (1980) did not find such effects in sixth-grade Jamaican children. Lifshitz's findings would indicate that age at the time of father-loss is a consequential variable in the larger picture of a child's perceptual and learning style.

Even in infants, father-absence is differentially correlated with cognitive development at different ages, according to the findings of Miller (1977), who tested infants at 12, 15, 19, and 24 months with a battery of seven tests of competency. The need to have a developmental perspective, and to control for the fatherless child's age, has been confirmed by Maxwell (1961), Sutton-Smith et al. (1968), and Santrock (1973).

Family Composition. Sutherland (1930) compared two groups of fatherless children with controls and found that measured IQ was less for children from fatherless families than from fathered and that

IQ correlated with size of family. Thus, the number of siblings in the fatherless family should be controlled in studies of the effects of fatherlessness, a point also made by Sutton-Smith et al. (1968), Sutton-Smith (1969), and Soloman et al. (1972). Rosenberg and Sutton-Smith (1968) noted that in two-child families, particularly, siblings have systematic effects on each other and on their parents. Rouman (1956) found that the oldest-born and youngest-born children were more often referred for counseling than children in other ordinal positions. Herzog (1974) stated that controlling for birth order wipes out paternal residence effects, but that the reverse is not true. Hence, ordinal position or birth order may strongly influence how well a fatherless child does in school. The same is true for sibling group size since a mother-only family of two or three children seems to more than double or triple the demands imposed on the mother and the unmet needs of her children (Colletta, 1979).

Gender of Child. That the sex of the child as well as the gender of siblings is important has also been noted by Sutton-Smith et al. (1968), who recounted the widespread belief that the school effects of father-absence are more pervasive for male than for female children. In contrast to other research, they found that a same-sex sibling modified the effects of father-absence for females as well as males. They also observed that an only girl is affected by father-absence but an only boy is not, theorizing that in single-child families the child identifies more with the opposite-gender parent and that is to boys' advantage, relatively. The only sensible conclusion we see is that, while a fatherless boy reacts differently than a fatherless girl, we don't know why fatherlessness affects boys' and girls' academic achievement differently. We may even suspect that the cause, whatever it is, is mediated by the mother's differential care for male and female child when father is away.

School Ability and Achievement Studies

Authors who have studied general academic performance are Risen (1939), Maxwell (1961), Lessing (1970), Collier et al. (1973), Santrock (1973), Mackie et al. (1974), Shinn (1978), and Moffitt (1981).

In an early study Risen (1939) found that lacking one or both parents negatively affects junior-high-schoolers in the following areas:

1. IQ
2. Overageness for the grade
3. Cooperation
4. Subject failure
5. Scholastic honors
6. Referral for counseling
7. Election to student council
8. Physical defects

Unfortunately, the gender of the absent parent was not controlled in this pioneer study by Risen. The control group of high-school students selected was matched only for educational level, IQ, and gender.

Later studies show finer methodology, but still have obvious flaws. Maxwell (1961) attempted to correlate WISC subtest scores of British child psychiatric patients, aged 8 to 13, with father-absence, finding that children who experienced father-absence after the age of 5 years, more often than those fatherless before 5, scored below the median of WISC Comprehension, Vocabulary, Picture Completion, Picture Arrangement, and Coding subtests. (See Chapter 7.) He used no control group of psychiatrically normal patients, and although age at time of father-absence was noted, uncontrolled variables included sex, race, and socioeconomic status. Later studies suggest that differential performance on some of the WISC subjects may be a function of gender rather than fatherlessness (Bayley, 1968), which could not be verified from Maxwell's data (Lessing et al., 1970).

Lessing et al. (1970), too, examined a population of psychiatrically disturbed children, aged 9 to 15:11 years, to ascertain the effect of father-absence on their cognitive abilities. They too, failed to use a control group of psychiatrically normal children and neglected to control for race, although they did control for social class, sex, and the availability of a surrogate father. The 138 subjects, who had experienced prolonged father-absence, showed lower WISC Performance IQs and lower scores on Block Design and Object Assembly, regardless of sex or social class. (See Chapter 7.) Lower scores on Arithmetic were noted for father-absent boys only. Working-class father-absent children earned a lower mean Verbal and Full Scale IQ. There were no significant differences in IQ between father-present children and father-absent children who lived with a step-father in the household. Kellam et al. (1977), however, found the adaptation of poor black children with stepfathers to be no better than that of children with mother only.

Collier et al. (1973) tested 31 black lower-class ninth-grade students, 15 father-present and 16 father-absent, to find which of the following were most affected by father-absence: IQ, achievement, self-concept, or personality. The two groups did not differ significantly on any of these variables. Race, socioeconomic status, and educational level were held constant but sex, type of father-absence, length of father-absence, age at father-absence, ordinal position, and number of siblings were not controlled in this small sample. Santrock (1973) studied white lower-class boys and girls and went further than Collier in his attempts to exert proper methodological controls. He found that on measures of achievement father-absent boys consistently performed more poorly than father-absent girls or father-present boys. Duke and Lancaster (1976) theorized that father-absent boys performed poorly because they had developed an external locus control, as opposed to the internal locus of control of father-present boys.

When we compare Collier's and Santrock's findings we are again left wondering whether father-absence exerts its deleterious influences only among the white middle class or the white lower class aspiring to become white middle class—groups who tenaciously cling to the normative concept of the patriarch-headed nuclear family. In any individual case, of course, a clinician has to study the perceptions, meanings, and values of the given child.

Mackie et al. (1974) studied 220 kindergarten children in a black ghetto neighborhood, controlling educational level, race, and social class. Using information from the parents, the authors divided the children into three groups: one with father in residence, one with father absent and one with surrogate father in residence. The three groups were administered the Test of Primary Mental Abilities (see Chapter 7), and the resulting data were analyzed according to sex.

Intellectual differences were found only among the boys and appeared to be due to the amount of preschool education, not to father-absence. Type of father-absence, length of father-absence, age at time of father-absence, number of siblings, and ordinal position were not controlled, nor were subjects matched on these variables as displayed in the tables of Chapter 7.

Shinn (1978) reviewed 54 studies of the effects of father-absence on cognitive development, measured by standardized IQ and achievement tests, and observed differential effects according to cause, duration, and onset of father absence; age, sex, race, and socioeconomic status of the child; and the skill tested, whether quantitative or verbal. Noting methodological defects from inadequate controls, she concluded that financial hardship, high level of anxiety, and low levels of parent–child interaction cause poor academic performance among children in one-parent families and that sex-role identification is insignificant. Her belief that the mother's ability to compensate for the loss of the husband-father helps children to adapt makes sense but does not lessen such a mother's burdens.

Arithmetic and Gender. Some authors, including Carlsmith (1969), Nelsen and Maccoby (1966), Collins (1969), Herzog (1974), and Chapman (1977), contend that father-absence diminishes mathematical performance, specifically in male children. This puzzle may be like the high positive correlation, in Sweden, between storks and birth rate: More storks are correlated with more babies in rural areas.

Females often score higher in verbal skills than in mathematical skills on standardized tests, while the reverse is true for males. Cultural conditioning may account for this discrepancy, and the present trend toward androgyny may change it. Nevertheless, research indicating that males from father-absent families tend to have cross-sex identities does correlate with the finding that boys from father-absent families tend to exhibit a more feminine pattern on standardized tests. Bernstein (1976) reported that children who experience early father-absence have weaker mathematical than verbal skills and the effect, which appears as early as age 11, is more pronounced among girls. Such research cannot distinguish between the effects of father-absence and the effects of other conditioning.

Carlsmith (1964), observing male middle-class college freshmen and high-school seniors whose fathers had served in World War II, found that early and long separation from the father resulted in higher verbal than math (Vm) scores on the Scholastic Aptitude Test (SAT). (See Chapter 7.) Late, brief separation causes slightly higher math scores (vM).

In response to the hypothesis that early separation from father increases anxiety and that anxiety affects math achievement more than verbal, Richards and McCandless (1972) implied that it is not anxiety but how children cope with anxiety that influences verbal ability. Gathering data from over 300 4- and 5-year-olds, both black and white, they found that coping with anxiety by withdrawal interfered with verbal facility while coping by aggression did not necessarily interfere; girls with high verbal ability found nonverbal ways to cope with anxiety. Koch (1961) found that preschool children of divorced parents had higher anxiety scores on Amen's Projective Test of Anxiety (see Chapter 7) than did control children from intact families, matched for IQ and age, but what looks like an effect of father-absence may result from bickering and animosity that preceded the divorce.

Nelsen and Maccoby (1966), expanding Carlsmith's findings by including additional variables of family dynamics associated with patterns of math or verbal achievement, found that the Vm pattern in males is associated not only with father-absence but also with being punished exclusively by the mother, fearing the father, and reportedly having been a "mamma's boy" or "daddy's boy." The vM pattern in males is associated with punishment exclusively by the father and with sharing personal problems with the father, while the Vm pattern in females is associated with fear of the mother and "only sometimes" sharing personal problems with the father.

Chapman (1977), on the other hand, found verbal SAT scores lower among father-absent males than father-present males, but *not* significantly lower quantitative scores. (See Chapter 7.) Sciara and Jantz (1974) found that both male and female father-absent fourth-graders achieved lower reading scores on IQ tests than their father-present counterparts. Michael Chapman suggested that his own findings together with those of Blanchard and Biller (1971) and Landy et al. (1969) point to the general rather than differential impact of a mother on verbal abilities of her children.

The studies of Carlsmith (1964) and Nelsen and Maccoby (1966) deal primarily with effects of father-absence in the middle and upper-middle classes, although only the second study specifically says so. Broken families are far more common in the lower class, where alternative life styles become more socially acceptable as financial need outweighs the desire for an intact family unit. In a social climate where fathering is not expected, perhaps children are less traumatized by living in a partial family. Research findings on this point are ambiguous. Collins (1969) compared the reading and arithmetic scores of 150 third-grade, black, lower-class students from broken homes with the scores of 150 controls from intact families and found no significant differences in performance on standardized tests—contradicting Sciara (1975), who found lower test scores in both math and reading for father-absent, black, lower-class fourth-grade boys and girls, particularly for students with IQs greater than 100. Collins (1969) did report, however, that on teacher-rated achievement, the sixth-grade, father-absent group performed significantly worse in arithmetic. Of course, the term *broken home* was vague, the specifics of father-absence were not controlled, and teacher ratings tend to be negatively biased against father-absent children (Santrock & Tracy, 1978)—but Collins' study is suggestive. A later and more methodologically sound study of black lower-class children, conducted by Fowler and Richards (1978), indicated that father-presence facilitates the mathematical achievement of girls more than boys. But Fowler and Richards—like Sciara—decried the presumed negative effects of father's absence on boys and girls alike.

Moffitt (1981) had this comment on the supposed "reversal" to a feminine pattern by fatherless boys (Vm):

One interesting aspect of the math–verbal pattern reversal has been left unanswered to date. That is whether the math–verbal pattern reversal results from depression of boys' mathematics scores or from elevation of their verbal scores. . . . If growing up without a father impairs a boy's mathematics aptitude, the pattern reversal is a detrimental effect of father separation. On the other hand, if growing up without a father leaves a boy just as good in mathematics, and better than could be expected in verbal skills, then it would be clear that father separation can have at least one beneficial consequence.

Moffitt did not find the Vm phenomenon in either fathered or father-less boys from S. A. Mednick's control sample of 60 Danish boys with nonschizophrenic parents. The high-SES boys from this nonclinical group numbered 28, only 4 of whom had experienced "father separa-tion," while 32 were low-SES with 22 showing separation from an adult male as father or father surrogate. The boys averaged 15.1 years in age (ranging from 10 to 20) and took a Danish translation of the Vocabulary and Arithmetic subtests of the Wechsler Intelli-gence Scale for Children. (See Chapter 7.) Among the four high-SES boys father-absence was associated with increases in both vocabulary and mathematical scores, the vocabulary being higher; for the 22 fatherless, low-SES boys both vocabulary and mathematics scores were slightly decreased. Moffitt sagely averred that if she had ignored SES (as done in several studies showing the Vm reversal) she might have concluded that fatherlessness per se had been associated with lowered scores, simply because there were 22 low- and 4 high-SES children studied. Across economic levels the fathered boys showed nearly identical ability scores, leading Moffitt to ask to what degree differences in intellectual ability, supposedly related to race or pov-erty, have been influenced by the intervening variable of the high prevalence of father-absence among poor and minority populations.

Herzog (1974) controlled for socioeconomic status, race, and cul-tural attitudes toward paternal residence, with some attention to the reasons for and the timing of the father's absence. She investigated the effects of father-absence on the school performance of 119 black Barbados boys between the ages of 6½ and 15½ years. Father-present boys "do better in conforming to the school's expectations; absorbing the specific arithmetic taught, trying hard to do their work, and be-ing quiet and cooperative" (p. 80). Father-absent boys do better on novel tasks and are often called "troublesome" by their teachers. In-terestingly, boys with early (B-1:12, or birth to 2 years) or complete (B-4:12) father-absence during their first 5 years did better on the Chicago IQ Test (see Chapter 7) and the Graded Arithmetic Test (see Chapter 7) than boys whose fathers were present during all 5 years. Herzog concluded that, in Barbados, it is academically better for a male child to live with no father during his early years, allow-ing him to enhance his relationship with his mother, and then to live with a father after age 2 or 3 because the father can provide the economic support and discipline that assist the child in adapting to school. Herzog's study, controlled and cautious, lets us see that the father's absence and presence affect children of different ages in different ways.

Studying 418 sixth graders in Jamaica with a conceptual style test and a questionnaire, Roach (1980) found a positive correlation between poverty and depressed analytic style scores for girls only. Low-SES boys scored as high as more affluent children. Roach found no significant patterns of variation for conceptual style and father-absence, conceptual style and family size, or conceptual style and birth order. The study of almost anything in 418 children is worth pondering. One speculation prompted in us by Roach's study is this: Could the oft-found relationship between girlish cognitive style and the tangle of poverty/father absence/large families be due to the investigators' tendency to study samples in which poverty-stricken girls are overrepresented? And at all events is it not the pattern of maternal care (punishment or encouragement of autonomy, high verbal interaction and discussion versus low verbal behavior, etc.) that should alter and shape cognitive practices among young children?

Giftedness and Creativity

To confuse the issue still further, we must mention the work of Albert (1971), who noted the frequent occurrence of early parental loss among historically famous, highly intelligent people: "Among persons designated as 'eminent' or 'historical geniuses' there appears a rate of parental loss at least three times that of the average college population (gifted), with the ratio of father-loss to mother-loss being 2 to 1, and, occurring proportionately among Ss in the arts, the humanities, the sciences and the military" (p. 25). Eisenstadt (1978) found early orphanhood and bereavement to be characteristic of a group of 699 eminent people whose biographies he examined. Drawing on Freud's examples, many "tele-analyses" (Adams, 1972c) of literary authors and characters have been done—of Leonardo, Judge Schreber, the Brontes, Poe, Swift, Hawthorne, Beaudelaire, and others, even Little Black Sambo. See Kanzer (1953) for a typical essay, ending on this note: "Early loss of a parent was a factor that predisposed them to lifelong morbidity and excessive development of the imagination, traits that revolved about identification with the dead parents" (p. 151).

Woodward (1974) noted also that among eminent scientists, two out of five have lost a parent during their formative years. Becker (1974) observed that father-absent subjects are significantly more creative than father-present subjects, especially that mother-influenced subjects, regardless of father-absence or -presence, were superior to father-influenced subjects in all three aspects of creativity—fluency, flexibility, and originality. Martindale (1972) related father-absence not only to creativity, but also to an increase in psychopathology and cross-sex identity among poets. In all respects, father-absent children see things in a nonstandard, deviant way; they are less conventional and less conforming and may be more original and inventive, especially if not economically disadvantaged.

Some evidence suggests that creativity in father-absent children corresponds to the child-care attitudes of the mother. Heilbrun (1971) found a deficit in creativity in sons of mothers who were high in controlling and low in nurturing (HC-LN) behaviors. In an earlier paper, Heilbrun (1970) postulated that LN subjects base their performance on visual–motor tasks more than on environmental cues while HN subjects base theirs more on their own self-expectations. The creative person and the pathfinder must be motivated more by their own inner expectations than by environmental cues; the guideposts of others usually point to the well-trodden path of conventional thought. In some ways fatherless children supply their own cues and they may, especially with good input from the mother, be creative.

School Adjustment Studies

More mundane studies of children's social adjustment to school suggest that, although fatherless children adjust less well than others, fatherlessness alone does not cause poor adjustment. We begin our look at school adjustment by noting that adjustment and maladjustment have preschool precursors. Pedersen et al. (1979) reported on the early development of cognitive skills and motivational characteristics, as well as social responsiveness, in black lower-class infants, 5 to 6 months old. Comparing father-absent to father-present infants, they found no significant relationship between these qualities and the father variable for *female* infants, but for *male* infants, the father-present group scored significantly higher on the Bayley Mental Development Index (see Chapter 7), their scores varying with the amount of father interaction. The authors commented, "We do not believe that single-parent families are without important strengths, but perhaps it is because of the generally disadvantaged circumstances of the families in this study that the infants were particularly vulnerable to the effects of father absence" (p. 59). In reality, of course, these authors studied not father-absence but a complex network of noxious conditions that cluster around father-absence during infancy.

Elementary School Adjustment. Rouman (1956) studied 48 father-absent students in kindergarten through twelfth grade who had been referred to the school counselor, primarily for *academic failure*. Elementary-school-age children were referred more frequently than older children, and more youngest-born and firstborn children were referred than those in other ordinal positions. Consistent with this, Adams and Horovitz (1980b) found more aggressive behavior problems among younger than older firstborn black and Cuban fatherless males and suggested maternal sensitivity was higher when the son was young.

The greatest problem in social adjustment in Rouman's group was a lack of self-esteem or a diminished sense of personal worth. These children appeared deficient in motivation and internalization of societal standards. Rouman indicated that the father serves as a role model for these qualities—a widely held assumption. However, in this early study, race and socioeconomic status were not controlled. Racism and poverty probably contributed mightily to the low self-esteem of father-absent children almost 3 decades ago.

Later School Adjustment. Studying junior-high students with one or no parents, Risen (1939) found overageness compared to their classmates, less chance of becoming school leaders, and increased chance of being referred to the school counselor. Kopf's (1970) findings, based on a new awareness of societal facts, differed from Risen's. Looking at the demographic traits that vary with the negative effects of father-absence in 52 urban, eighth-grade boys and their mothers, she concluded that school adjustment was *not* related to degree of father-absence, age of child at separation, son's ordinal position, sex of siblings, amount of extended family interaction, or prior father–son relationship. Instead, the mother's attitudes and behavior toward sons were crucial to the son's adjustment. Kopf did not control for race or socioeconomic status and did not study a comparison group of father-present boys.

Economic Disadvantage

Deutsch (1960), in a classic study of how economic disadvantage relates to the school achievement and adjustment of fatherless children, compared the academic achievement of lower-class black and white children in fourth, fifth, and sixth grades; they all scored lower than the middle-class norm on standardized tests. The black children, victims of racism and poverty, performed even worse than white children at the same socioeconomic level. Both black and white children from broken homes did less well scholastically than children from intact families, though the white control group was very small ($n = 15$), and *broken home* was undefined. Black students differed from white students in verbal-to-math ability ratio, with girls outperforming boys in both reading and arithmetic, as well as on the standard test total score.

Standardized tests of mental ability have been criticized for being normed on white middle-class children, so when these tests show differential abilities among races or socioeconomic classes, one must be skeptical (Stodolsky & Lesser, 1967). Authors like Mumbauer and Miller (1970), who stated that intellectual performance suffers among culturally disadvantaged preschool children, should be faulted on this count and also for using the term *culturally disadvantaged*.

Summary

Research on the measurement of IQ, academic ability, and achievement in fatherless children yields muddled and contradictory results. Early studies flatly attributed retarded school progress to parental absence, but later studies, considering variables such as race, SES, and age of child at time of father-absence, raise important questions:

1. Is differential performance on the WISC a function of father-absence or of sex-role conditioning?
2. Are differential cognitive abilities functions of father-absence or of previous educational training?
3. Is the performance differential on standardized tests a function of father-absence or of anxiety in children from father-absent homes?
4. Are the effects of father-absence general *or* differential and specific on math and verbal abilities?
5. In measuring cognitive abilities, are teacher's ratings or standardized tests more accurate predictors?

Again, we return to the perpetually recurring question in this endeavor: *Do detelerious effects so often attributed to fatherlessness really result from fatherlessness or from the poverty, exploitation, and prejudice so often experienced by children living in fatherless homes?* We do not know, but the evidence suggests that fatherlessness counts less than social inequity does.

SEX-ROLE IDENTIFICATION

The cliché that fatherless children, especially boys, lack a role model for masculine identity (Colley, 1959) is a political cop-out, in the very first instance. Emphasizing the individual's identity problems rather than the total social world of fatherless children allows one to disregard the socioeconomic conditions associated with fatherlessness, resulting in a psychologism that suits the prevalent ideology of a nonwelfare society, a society turning to the right. Fatherless families have more than their sexual attitudes to get set straight.

Many writers claim that father-absence interferes with the boy's development as a healthy male but less with the girl's development as a sound female: "A boy really needs a father." Freudians paradoxically contend that fatherlessness makes boys sissies and, if they overreact to being sissified, makes them become tough and violent, macho. The girl's story has received less attention.

Conventional wisdom is echoed by the psychiatric dogma that a boy is harmed when he does not interact with an adult male, not only seeing the adult's penis but also developing the appropriate envy, fright, tolerance of rough-housing, and domination of others that the father as bearer of the phallus can exemplify for him and that he can "mirror" and copy. Ultimately, by this paradoxical logic, castration anxiety initially will be mobilized and intensified within the boy by the father and thereupon reassuringly quelled. The little boy will identify with his fantasied aggressor, the father, castration anxiety will be dissipated, and a more or less strong father identification will occur in the boy's mind. That is the analytic viewpoint that interpenetrates and interrelates with conventional wisdom, each adopting parts of the other, but the common-sense attitudes do not go quite so far.

Edgar E. Stern (1980), a psychiatric social worker, studied the attitudes of "single mothers" (i.e., divorced, widowed, and separated women who were the parents of boys) compared to "nonsingle mothers." The ideology prevalent within his entire study group was that a father was more important than a mother; that attitude reigned most forcefully among singles, especially regarding a father's importance to a boy in play activity and sex role. Single mothers also rated higher a mother's importance to a child than did nonsingles, an indication of the former's feeling that any and all parenting—though needed—might be in hurtfully short supply when a child has lost one parent.

One sensible way to study the problem of whether and how being fatherless ties with sex-role identification problems is to do a cross-sectional study of fatherless children of the same gender who are similar to one another socially but different in age, taking samples of fatherless boys at different ages and studying them during one brief period of time, as Adams and Horovitz (1980b) did. Another good approach is to study the boys longitudinally, selecting a large number who come from similar social and economic backgrounds and following them from infancy through childhood, adolescence, and adulthood. This second approach is costly and difficult in a fast-moving capitalistic society where sound planning based on firm data has not really caught on. A third approach may leave more to be desired but is less costly. Most of the studies surveyed by Herzog and Sudia (1970) took the third way: They selected one particular age group for intense study, drawing on child development theories and facts to predict the trajectory of the individual's life, inferring rather than studying development during later ages. In this section, we examine particular researches on sex-role development in this way, age by age, finally combining information about children of different ages into a general theory. Some major theories of sex-role learning are status envy, identification, imitation, and complementation. We review theories and then turn to the various age groups of children.

Roger V. Burton and John W. M. Whiting's (1961) cross-sectional study of 64 different cultures looked at 11- and 12-year-old boys in several cultures from the standpoint of status-envy theory. Although their views lack high scientific merit, they represent the hypotheses that reigned during the 1950s in the whole field of sex-role development, concepts that linger even now, such as primary identification with the mother, initiation rites as a masculinizing turning point, status envy, and compulsive masculinity.

According to Burton and Whiting's status-envy hypothesis, only scarcity of resource leads people to envy the status of others, positing an economy of scarcity even in parent–child interactions, making (in a manner reminiscent of Alfred Adler's view of children as the dispossessed, have-not people) learning of gender role into a matter of the weaklings envying and copying the strongest, most resourceful member of the family. Copying may occur in fantasy or in practice, but the weak always envy the powerful:

> *If there is a status that has privileged access to a desired resource, the incumbent or occupant of such a status will be envied by anyone whose status does not permit him the control of, the right to use, the resource. Status envy is then a motivational component of status disability, and such motivation leads to learning by identification. [Burton & Whiting, 1961, p. 86]*

Other authors who have similarly explained sex-role development with status envy are D'Andrade (1973) and Carlsmith (1973). Burton and Whiting wrote with an eye to mental health practitioners:

A completely satisfying complementary relation between two people will not lead to identification. By this hypothesis [of status envy], a child maximally identifies with people who consume resources in his presence but do not give him any. He does not identify with the people he loves unless they withhold from him something he wants. Love alone will not produce identification. Thus, the status envy hypothesis advanced here makes identification with the aggressor just a special case, and the Oedipal situation is also simply a special case. [pp. 86–87]

Burton and Whiting paid particular attention to the father's presence or absence in the maternal and infantile bed for the first 2 years of the child's life, a concrete measure of whether father and infant are close. An axiom of human nature for these authors is that familiarity breeds envy. In 36 of the societies studied, the infant slept exclusively with the mother; in 28 the infant slept with mother and father in the bed, or else slept alone.

Burton and Whiting's traditional answer to the question of how little boys can identify with mothers, yet later perceive themselves as male and masculine, restates Freudian theory but sidesteps Freudian contradiction about the emergency and resolution of the Oedipus complex, grandly treating Freud's views as narrow and special instances of the status-envy phenomenon. Maccoby and Jacklin (1974) may rightly call this legerdemain "stumbling over" rather than "sidestepping":

If the mother is the nurturant figure, children of both sexes should imitate her for this reason; if the father is the dominant figure, children of both sexes should imitate him for this reason. Freud, in his discussions of the psychosexual development of the two sexes, stumbled over this issue and attempted to solve it by simply saying that the boy identifies with the aggressor, whereas the girl's identification with her mother is "anaclitic"—that is, based upon nurturance and dependency. This "solution" is merely a restatement of the problem. . . . It simply asserts that this is the case. [p. 286]

Studying a polygynous Mormon group from which fathers were often away and in hiding, Seymour Parker et al. (1975) took exception to Whiting's views; they found no differences between father-absent and father-present boys' strong sexual identification as males, adding that "the Whiting theory of puberty rites is not acceptable as it stands, and its credibility should no longer be automatically perpetuated." Without fathers and without puberty rites the Mormon boys became masculine.

Psychologists (like Whiting, an anthropologist) usually focus on the learned aspects of sex-role development and (save for Money & Erhardt, 1970) minimize the endocrine and cerebral physiologic conditions that influence sex-typed behavior (see Mischel's lead-off chapter in volume 2 of Mussen, 1970). Psychologists who are anything but Freudians often take up Freud's bias that sex-typing comes about from modeling of children on the same-sex parent; as such, most psychologists study identification, imitation, and observational learning. Only Money and Erhardt have attended as well to complementation: "The fact is that children differentiate a gender role and identity by way of complementation to members of the opposite sex, and identification with members of the same sex" (p. 13). The theoretical addition of the opposite gender to sex-role learning is indispensable for understanding how a mother can enhance the masculine self-concept of her son when no male is on the horizon.

Nancy Chodorow (1978) also applies the complementation concept to how mothers influence not only their sons but also their daughters in *The Reproduction of Mothering*: "Her son's maleness and oppositeness as a sexual other become important, even while his being an infant remains important as well" (p. 107). Chodorow recommends that fathers must do their half of child care in America so that daughters too will have counterpart caretakers not so closely similar to them as are their mothers. She thinks that caretaking fathers will make for stronger females and reduce the muting and blurring that girls feel after having been parented so exclusively by their mothers. Chodorow makes the fascinating switch from good Freudian doctrines to a rather radical feminism in phraseology disarmingly gentle:

> *Mothers tend to experience their daughters as more like, and continuous with, themselves. Correspondingly, girls tend to remain part of the dyadic mother–child relationship itself. This means that a girl continues to experience herself as involved in issues of merging and*

*separation, and in an attachment characterized by primary identifica-
tion and the fusion of identification and object choice. By contrast,
mothers experience their sons as a male opposite. Boys are more likely
to have been pushed out of the preoedipal relationship, and to have
had to curtail their primary love and sense of empathic tie with their
mother. [p. 166]*

Infants

The science of infant watching, although with us since Charles Darwin, has come into prominence only recently. Studies of infants have
examined prenatal and perinatal influences, temperamental and
other individual differences, sensory capacities, learning abilities, activity levels, and innate behavioral repertoires. The few studies comparing male and female infants (see Birns, 1977) have exaggerated
their differences.

At the time of birth, boys tend to be heavier, particularly in
muscle mass, and a little longer than girls; their basal metabolism is
higher than that of girls. But development quickly tilts the balance
in the girl's favor by virtue of her earlier teething, walking, talking,
and bone growth. Birth defects are unquestionably more common
among males as are all forms of "reproductive casualty" (Pasamanick
& Knobloch, 1959), adding one more reed of evidence that the female
possesses a natural biological superiority (Montagu, 1968). Birns observed that results of studies of sex differences in newborn to 2-year-
old infants are confusing and at times fit no theory about infancy.
The Scottish verdict of "nothing proven" summarizes what separates
boys and girls during infancy. Only the genital and related differences hold as true differences. Infant boys have penile erections at
birth or soon afterwards; little girls show vaginal lubrication in a
rhythmic cycle shortly after birth. Infant boys as a group can be
made more active and restless than baby girls only if they are circum-
cised—but that is hardly a way to bring out deep, innate gender differences. Birns (1977) said accurately for boy and girl infants that
"behavioral sex differences, like beauty, might exist primarily in the
eye of the beholder."

John and Sandra Condry (1977) studied the eye of the beholder by
designing research to elicit the effects of labeling an infant as male

for some observers, as female for others. Extremely interesting were their findings that when the infant was in an ambiguous situation, the observers' sex stereotypes came to the fore most strongly; male observers beheld greater sex differences in the responses of the infants (more stereotyping by attributed sex); male observers who had had more experience with infants saw the greater differences between the attributed male and female; female observers who were more experienced with infants saw the infant labeled female as feeling with greater intensity than the infant said to be male; less experienced female observers perceived the putative male more as did the male observers. Condry and Condry concluded that "a lot more than 'beauty' resides in the eye of the beholder."

Fagot (1974) and Smith and Lloyd (1978) found a differential treatment of very young infants according to the gender-based expectations of their child-care givers. Graves (1978) dealt with an Indian group of mothers playing with 1- and 2-year-olds: In that patriarchal culture too the mothers were more vigorous in their interaction with boys, more attentive and responsive as well. Considering the effective masculinization done by mother, there is not much need for a hypothesis covering father-absence or -presence in infant sex-role learning.

Age 2 to 5 Years

For toddlers and preschoolers the works by Maccoby and Jacklin (1974) and Beverly Birns (1977) provide the best reviews of the conflicting findings about sex differences. It will suffice here to provide only the sketchiest summary and leave it to the reader to learn the welter of pro and con arguments by consulting those two reviews.

Preschool boys appear to be more active motorically than girls, less passive and quiet than girls, but that may be a function of the situation in which the boys and girls are observed. Aggression, likewise, can be influenced by the situation, but strong evidence indicates an intrinsic male penchant for aggression greater than for overall activity. Maccoby and Jacklin concluded that males are, after all is said and done, more aggressive, but they hastened to add that that did not mean that girls are more *passive* than boys or that boys show their aggression more frequently to girls than to other boys. Maccoby and Jacklin found furthermore that sex differences in preschoolers' behavior are situation-specific and dynamic. For example, boys may be more impulsive than girls only as preschoolers; girls may become more nurturant than boys but only as elementary students. Aggression (meaning biting, hitting, physical violence against persons or things) is considered by Maccoby and Jacklin as a fairly well-established sex difference, one associated with maleness in the preschool era. Boys and girls, despite Erikson (1963) and much subsequent folklore to the contrary, do not choose notably different play materials; as cited by Birns, preschool boys choose to play more often with trucks while girls choose blocks and dolls more frequently, but one does not find boys choosing phallic objects nor girls choosing "incorporative, inner space" toys. A truck or van can have more inner space than a doll or a solid block.

True sex differences begin to appear in the behavior of boys and girls in late nursery-school and kindergarten years:

> *Preschool boys engage in more aggressive play, manipulate toys more, and are more exploratory. Girls are more sedentary, imitative, persistent, and attentive. Cognitive difference in coding and memory are not observed, but differences in field independence, characteristic of males in adolescence and adulthood, favor females in the preschool years. The hypothesis that sex differences begin to emerge only in the preschool years appears supported. [Birns, 1977, p. 276]*

Few reports exist on the uniquely male characteristics of fatherless preschool boys, but those of Meiss (1952), Mussen and Distler (1960), Kohlberg (1968), Biller (1968), Houston (1973), and Reis and Gold (1977) merit some attention. Meiss favored a psychoanalytic approach, discussing only one case, a boy whose father had died when the son was about 39 months old. Meiss interpreted the child's obsessive and fearful symptoms at age 5 as directly caused by his "loss of the rival parent early in the phallic phase"; she observed that no other instances of such developments were reported in the psychoanalytic literature of that era (1952). She attributed little Peter's strong avoidances to his belief that he—having been angry at father—had been responsible for his father's sudden death on a train.

Mussen and Distler (1960), from the tradition of academic psychology, used a learning-theory rationale in their study of kindergarten children who were fathered, and who were more masculine when their fathers were more nurturant and warm. A population of 5-year-olds made an isosexual identification with the father, when the father was in essence nonmasculinely affectionate and warm. The mother's warmth, in contrast, did not correlate with greater masculinity, and may provide a corollary principle for fatherless children. Zunich (1971) reminds us that lower-class mothers of boys may not be as warm to boys as they are to girls, so class position really matters when we look at any kind of parental influence.

Lawrence Kohlberg (1968) and Kohlberg and Ziegler (1967) took up a Piaget-Werner hypothesis in their cognitive–developmental analysis of sex typing and gender preferences of bright young children. Roughly, they found that the stage of cognitive development measured by IQ showed precocious sex typing by gifted children, so that 4-year-olds made choices and typings that average older children make. More precisely,

> the bright boys are preferentially oriented to the adult male at age four, at a time when the average boys are preferentially oriented to the adult female. As they grow older, the bright boys seem to shift to a preferential orientation to females, and then from seven to ten, to shift once more to a neutral orientation. . . . From age five–seven, the average boys begin to become more female-oriented, as the bright boys had done two years earlier. [Kohlberg, 1968, p. 150]

Hence, while he introduced thinking about cognitive structure, Kohlberg showed that these dynamic and fluid structures depend on the child's overall cognitive level. Kohlberg put cognitive development first, indicating that children learn attitudes about their gender consistent with their developmental stage and then seek models to inspire them while they perfect their role learning.

Henry Biller (1968, 1969) deserves a prominent place in the study of sex-role learning by fatherless boys. The 1968 study of 29 lower-class, black (15) and white (14), fathered (18) and fatherless (11) boys aged 5:10 to 6:11 years showed that white boys with father present scored higher on the IT scale (see Chapter 7) than black father-present boys; too, white father-absent boys had higher masculine IT scores than black father-absent boys. Race differences in masculinity were not a function of father's presence or absence, Biller concluded, nor were differences in masculinity between father-absent and father-present boys a function of the boys' race. Moreover, what the boys scored on the IT test did not correlate with a rating scale of masculinity. Hence, Biller believed that the IT test taps sex-role orientation (almost equivalent to "core gender identity") more than masculinity.

In subsequent work, some of it carefully detailed and methodologically astute, Biller refined his beginning views (coauthored with Borstelmann, 1967) on sex-role orientation, preference, and adoption. Most recently, he held that sex-role orientation is influenced most by father-absence, and that sex-role preference and adoption result from other forces but have more to do with masculinity. The male's masculinity when father is absent, furthermore, has been influenced strongly by the mother. Oddly, then, for a writer who devised a Father Power bloc, Biller came to hold that the mother orchestrated the son's masculinity when a father was not present, encouraging her son in masculine activities, showing her positive attitudes toward men (especially toward the absent father), eschewing overprotectiveness, and promoting the boy's stereotyped masculine assertiveness and aggression.

Stewart Houston (1973), indebted to Biller, studied the sex-role orientation, preference, and adoption of Australians, eight of whom were boys 5 to 6 years old. Boys with no father and those with sisters were less masculine, Houston reported. However, at 5 to 6 years, boys who were singletons and who had fathers were also less masculine, even less than the father-absent boys of that age. Boys with either brothers or sisters, younger or older than they, were more masculine than either father-absent or singleton boys. Houston could not account for these findings using his rather pro-father bias; that the differences in masculinity did not hold for older groups of boys he accounted for by invoking the familiar doctrine of compensatory masculinity.

Late in the 1970s there came the work of Reis and Gold (1977), Reyes (1978), Lowery (1978), Kramer and Prall (1978), and Galenson and Roiphe (1980). Reis and Gold (1977) looked at sex-role orientation of 30 4-year-old American boys whose fathers varied in their availability to the boys. The hypothesis was that boys with low-available fathers would resemble father-absent boys in their sex-role orientation and be less masculine. While the boys who had a lot of friendly contact with their fathers did better on problem-solving tasks, they did not show greater masculinity than the relatively father-deprived boys. In the spectrum of fathering, slight fathering does not produce low-masculinity preschool boys as expected.

Reyes (1978) gathered a sample of 127 children between 3½ and 5 years old from day-care centers of southern Michigan, comparing the affective and social involvement of those without fathers to that of those with fathers. Data were collected on the child's age, ethnicity, ordinal position, playmates, number of years of father-absence, number and relationship of father surrogates, type of dwelling, number of females in the home, and day-care experience. Reyes found that father-absence did not affect the social behavior of preschool children; length of father-absence did not affect development of social behaviors; neither father-absent, father-present, nor father-surrogate families differed significantly from one another. Reyes noted a homogeneity among the *mothers* of all children he studied, which may have evaporated father differences.

Lowery (1978) reported for a doctoral dissertation at Temple University his findings on 16 black boys from ages of 3:7 to 4:11 years. Neither dependency nor father-absence made the boys more prone to model their behavior on male teachers, contradicting those who think little boys, particularly ones from father-absent backgrounds, are overexposed to women and need male models. In fact, in Lowery's sample, boys with father present tended to be more receptive to male teachers, to depend on them more, and to model after them. Father-hunger is not a sequel of father deprivation in Lowery's study group.

The American Psychoanalytic Association panel, chaired and reported by Selma Kramer and Robert Prall (1978) respectively, brought together some of the newer trends in psychoanalytic meta-theories on sex-role identification of young children, especially in the pre-Oedipal years. E. Abelin's (1977) paper entitled "The Role of the Father in Core Gender Identity and in Psychosexual Differentiation" echoes some of the work of Galenson and Roiphe (1980) with preschoolers; Robert Stoller presented a paper on fathers of children who as adults underwent sex change. Discussion of the panel centered on how fathers (if not aloof) could help little girls to separate

and individuate from mothers; if fathers would do it they could become breaths of fresh air and knights in shining armor to their children in the second and third years of life. Abelin along with others
postulated an "early triangulation" at 18 months of age that heralds
later Oedipal developments, perhaps with even greater castration
fear than in the later period; a dominant mother "therefore interferes
with early triangulation and has the same effect as absence of the
father." Old-fashioned and patriarchal as much of it appeared, the
analysts leaned toward a prescription that fathers are needed, and
when they are present they should be both nurturant and punitive,
dominant but not sadomasochistic.

Early School-Aged Boys

Two noteworthy studies of young elementary-school boys by Bach
(1946) and Keller and Murray (1973) show considerable change in
psychologic thinking about fathers over 3 decades. Bach studied 40
lower-middle-class children 6 to 10 years old, 20 of whom were fatherless because of the war and 20 of whom had fathers present, de-
ferred from military service. He found that the "European psychoanalytic" view of father as "a punishment-threatening, tyrant–giant"
was not apt among U.S. children then, regardless of father's presence
or absence. The absent father was highly idealized as an enjoyable
person who likes his family, giving and receiving much affection but
alien to any family strife or discord: "This fantasy-father shows very
little hostility and does not exert his authority. The children of the
control group, however, living as they do in daily contact with their
fathers, elaborate significantly more upon the punitive function of
the father and his contribution to intra-family hostility" (Bach, 1946,
p. 71). That was plausible but unexpected in the forties.

Keller and Murray (1973) selected a larger group ($n = 57$), all 6
years old, black and poor, 28 of whom were fatherless for at least the
most recent 3 years of their lives: "It was expected that the boys from
the father-absent home(s) would show relatively less imitation of the
adult male model's aggressive behavior although both groups of boys
would show more imitation of the male than the female model."
However, they found no significant difference in overt aggression between father-absent and father-present boys and no difference in their

choice of a male as a person they would like to be. Witnessing an aggressive female inhibited the males' aggression, for they showed less aggression than after seeing a male model or no model at all. Keller and Murray's concluding words were, "Thus, aggressive behavior in young Negro boys may be more directly related to the role of the mother than the presence or absence of the father."

Their views were reiterated by Trachtman (1978). Trachtman found that early-latency-aged boys, 16 fatherless and 10 fathered, none of them patients, showed no difference in psychopathology or in health adaptation; the mother played a crucial role in that outcome. If anything, boys with father present showed greater castration anxiety. Studying nonclinical populations means surprises, disconfirmations of many of the generalizations from clinical samples. Father-absence in the population at large does not have the effects it does in *patients* who are fatherless.

The overall situation is not much different with school-aged boys a year older. With 58 Canadian second-grade boys, Drake and Mc-Doughall (1977) found that their chosen instruments did not distinguish between the 29 with fathers absent and the 20 with fathers present. Levels of .01 significance were found but not in sex-role preference or adoption. Not the IT test but Draw a Person and Drawing Completion tests (see Chapter 7) were used to elicit data on sex-role orientation; again the primordial parameters of masculine sex typing (orientation and core gender identity) did differ according to father's presence. Multivariate analysis of covariance showed no significant association between the measures of sex role and father's absence or presence, early versus late father-absence, availability of male siblings, and availability of father substitutes.

Joel Badaines (1976) also studied 7-year-olds, Chicano and black (26 of each), from Dallas. Blacks chose to imitate black male models more exclusively than Chicanos chose Chicanos; Chicanos often preferred Chicanos and whites. Badaines believed that blacks have stronger ethnic pride than Chicanos at 7 years, and about sex-role orientation, he found "that by age seven boys tend to show a preference for the masculine role, but that paternal absence has a detrimental effect on its development; or, conversely, that father presence enhances it."

Walter Mischel (1958) deserves mention for some work that throws an oblique light on conscience development in fatherless boys of early elementary-school age. He found that fatherless black Trinidadians from 7 to 9 years old showed a significant predilection for immediate reinforcement. They were what anthropologists and social scientists would later call "action oriented" and psychiatrists would call "acter-outers" but as boys may be termed only masculine. Impulsive antisociality may be a special risk for fatherless, lower-class boyish boys in many Western cultures, as psychoanalysts often claim.

Later School-Aged Boys

E. Mavis Hetherington (1966) told of her work with 32 black and 32 white firstborn males when they were 9 to 12 years old. She found no variance attributable to race difference but did find that father-absence beginning before the boy became 5 years old was associated with fewer sex-typed behaviors by the time the boys were 9 to 12 years of age. If fathers left after their sons were 5 years old the sons were just as masculine as when the fathers were present. Hetherington's design was an excellent one; controls were set in place against bias because of race, sex, economic status, age of child when father-absence occurred, and whether father was present. Left out were such variables as ordinal position of child, mother's images of the absent father, and so on. Nonetheless, Hetherington's work is solidly respected and often quoted.

It is readily apparent that Santrock (1977) and many others have done their investigative work with an eye to what Hetherington did so soundly in 1966. Santrock studied 45 lower-class white boys from West Virginia, 30 of them fatherless. From the father-absent group he paired one whose parents were divorced with one whose father had died; the pair was matched to a control boy with a father present. Matching was based on IQ, age, and attendance at the same school in the fifth grade. As an added and important refinement, a third of the fatherless boys had experienced separation from fathers during the first 3 years of life, a third between 3 and 6 years of age, and the remaining third at 6 through 9 years of age.

The findings included the following: Boys from father-absent homes were as a group more masculine, more physically aggressive, and more disobedient, and showed more plucky initiative; "the problem, however, becomes one of determining whether the father-absent boy's behavior is too masculine, to the extent it encompasses anti-social behavior such as disobedience and excessive fighting" (Santrock, 1977, p. 8). Little emerged from comparing divorced and widowed homes except the "divorced" boys' greater aggression on the doll-play interview. Looking at child's age when father became absent, Santrock found that the older the child when separation commenced, the more aggression shown, but the earlier the separation the greater the child's disobedience at ages 10:1 to 11:11 years.

Joining Santrock during the past 2 or 3 decades is a growing list of investigators who find that preadolescents from divorced, father-absent families have a real penchant for disobedience, violence, and other behaviors that their mothers alone apparently cannot curb or modify, as if, for control purposes, two parents are better than one. The elementary-school years are hardly quiescent times for these macho youths, nor do they comprise an epoch of conscience development along a straight line of progression. Hoffman (1973) reviewed the literature and reported a study of father-absence and conscience development in seventh graders. The father-absent group, matched for age, sex, IQ, and social class (the four perennially vital sociobiologic distinctions), were rated by teachers as more aggressive and scored lower than the father-present comparison group ($p < .01$) on "internal moral judgment, acceptance of blame and conformity to rules." Hetherington et al. (1979) wisely surveyed such studies under the rubric "The Development of Self-Control." Some categories employed in studies of self-control are antisocial, rebellious, impulsive, acting out, unable to delay gratification, weak conscience, disobedient, destructive, showing conduct disorders, delinquent, aggressive—perhaps it is the macho package. Interestingly, the girls in fatherless homes do not show these leanings. Even the boys show fewer of them when the father has died and more of them following father's exit by divorce.

The link between fatherlessness and sex role among boys beyond primary grades of elementary school has been the subject of works by Rabin (1958), Stephens (1961), Phelan (1964), and Vroegh (1972). Phelan's father-absent sixth-grade boys drew more other-sex figures on the Draw a Person test (see Chapter 7) than did fathered boys from middle-class schools; Rabin's father-absent fourth graders who were aged from 9:3 to 11:3 and lived in kibbutzim showed, on the Blacky cartoons (see Chapter 7) IV, VII, and VIII, lower "Oedipal intensity, more diffuse positive identification with father and less intense sibling rivalry." Stephens' early, faulty investigation showed that social workers regarded fatherless boys as both more effeminate and belonging to gangs more frequently. Vroegh (1972), as reported earlier, debunked the idea that male teachers are highly salient to fatherless boys. Joining Rabin in studying latency-aged boys from varied ethnic backgrounds were LeCorgne and Laosa (1976), who studied Mexican-Americans, Longarbaugh (1975), who studied 51 black boys derived from both North American and Barbadian stock, and Rubin (1974), who found that Philadelphia blacks at this age had good self-esteem, better than might have been hypothesized. LeCorgne and Laosa found that poverty-ridden Mexican-American boys drew females in a more masculine way than fathered boys and cautiously suggested that this "could be interpreted as indicative of a less differentiated concept of female sex-role attributes among the father-absent children." That odd reasoning does not account for the fact that, having no fathers, the boys saw the female as less feminine, more masculine. Why not see the male as more feminine, instead? When there is only one parent, most writers agree that that parent becomes the focal, salient adult figure in the life of the child. A husbandless woman may take on attributes that violate stereotyped feminine demeanor; she may find herself with more things she has to organize decisively and expeditiously if her family is to endure.

Adolescents

Developmentalists typically assume that the unhealthy effects of early fatherlessness on sex role may not appear until adolescence. Available studies variously suggest that as older boys become emancipated from the strictly familial pressures of the formative years, the marks from earlier father-absence drop in importance; that early father-absence deeply and directly affects later behavior; and that we do not know enough to name the latter effects of fatherlessness: a spectrum of conclusions.

Discussions of how growing up with no father affects adolescents are relatively rare, possibly because by adolescence most differences in gender identity and sex-role performance have leveled out so that fatherless adolescents are not distinguishably different. In a naive study, Leichty (1960) reports examining "Oedipal intensity" in father-absent boys, using the Blacky test cartoon IV (see Chapter 7) as the index of that variable. Leichty found greater Oedipal intensity (as defined) in boys whose fathers had been away at war, later returned, but the probability that this result could not happen by chance alone is only .02. Hetherington (1965) then concluded that a nondominant father damaged the sex-role identification of both boys and girls, but fortunately she has since become more skeptical.

Most adolescent boys prefer and practice the male role; even more feminine boys may hold a firm idea of male identity and role. Helper (1955), Hetherington (1965), and Moulton et al. (1966) all looked at what adolescents are like when their fathers are or are not dominant over mother, affectionate to offspring, and free in dispensing praise (or punishment). Without questioning sex-role stereotyping much, they concluded that a traditional father is the best father, an intact family the best family.

Other writers, however, discovered few adolescent and adult consequences of fatherlessness. Altus (1958) found that 25 college males from divorced families did not differ significantly from 25 males from intact families, although he believed that the males from divorced families were more feminine in personal attributes, a surprising opinion from Altus, who in 1943 reported that a group of illiterate black recruits from broken families adjusted better to military life than their compeers from intact families.

Barclay and Cusmano (1967) contributed the finding that adolescents from broken homes did not differ on the usual manifestations of masculinity, but father-absent boys (mean age 15.43 years) did show more field-dependence on the Rod and Frame Test (see Chapter 7), often interpreted as a feminine attribute. They did not stress clinical application or policy ramifications of that finding. Domini (1967) gave 300 black males between 13 and 19 years of age the Draw a Person test (see Chapter 7); the 30 who had lived without fathers did not differ significantly in sex role from the others. Carlsmith (1964) studied Harvard freshmen (all males then) whose fathers had been absent during the war, from a date prior to the infant's reaching 6 months of age and extending thereafter 22 to 36 months. He found that the father-absent youths had a more feminine cognitive style and outlook but seemed to do all right among their fellow Harvard students and also in their rather intellectual families. Kellam et al. (1977) found that teen-agers from mother-only families were not more disposed to seek psychiatric help when offered it and that the overall adjustment of people from mother-only families, although worse than that of persons from mother-and-father families or mother-and-grandmother families, was better than that from reconstituted mother-and-stepfather families. Kellam and associates did not (perhaps wisely in view of that state of the art) give special attention to sex-role development of the teen-agers in the Woodlawn area of Chicago.

Hunt and Hunt (1977), studying black and white youths, found the mixed message that fatherlessness meant "gains for blacks" but "losses for whites." The critical issue was ethnic: the kinds of intimate family cultures in which the boys had been nurtured and the structuring of status and power in a racist culture.

Delinquents, often regarded as proof positive that fatherless males become overly and compulsively masculine to compensate for their earlier lack of fathers, often come from fatherless families; since so many lower-class families are fatherless, we should perhaps expect a high incidence of all things relating to poverty and fatherlessness among delinquents. Two studies since the much-cited one by Mac-Donald (1938) have aimed pointedly at the masculinity of delinquents: Greenstein (1966) and Mitchell and Wilson (1967). Greenstein found, with 75 delinquents in New Jersey, ages averaging 15.5 years, no significant differences in sex-role identification of those without fathers and those with fathers. Mitchell and Wilson, looking at the masculinity of 34 delinquents aged 12 to 19, found neither increased femininity on the MMPI (see Chapter 7) nor indications of compulsive masculinity. Despite these studies, clinicians are fond of saying with conviction that delinquents are hypermasculine in order to compensate for feeling insufficiently masculine. Clinical lore dies very hard.

The TAT stories of 28 father-absent and 103 father-present college males—in response to Cards 4, 6BM, 7BM, 8BM, and 13MF—were scored and analyzed comparatively by Merton Shill (1981), operating on Freudian views (as modified by Stoller) that are vividly spelled out: "Castration anxiety is, therefore, the hallmark of masculine gender identity. . . . This fear of castration is based on the intimate sense of one's identity being dependent upon having a penis . . ." (p. 137–138). (Cards 6BM, 7BM, and 8BM were the cards to which the father-absent males responded with by far the greatest castration anxiety.) Shill's finding that father-absent college males had significantly *more* castration anxiety than those with fathers present led him, however, to doubt his original Stollerian hypothesis that male gender identity can be defined operationally as castration anxiety. To a Freudian, fatherless males should have little castration anxiety, so finding they have more made Shill backtrack as follows:

Although there was a significant difference in castration anxiety between father-absent and father-present subjects, no significant differences were found between father-absent subjects who had lost their fathers before the age of (five) versus subjects who lost their fathers thereafter. [p. 143]

The failure of this study to find significant differences in castration anxiety between the three groups of father-present subjects is disappointing. . . . It is conceivable that the experience of the father as a mirroring object during the second and third years provides the son with sufficient gender consolidation which even subsequent adverse father–son interactions do not reverse. [p. 144]

Adults

One could measure influences of father-absence on sex-role identification and behavior by testing feminine males who grew to adulthood to determine what part fatherlessness played in their development. Homosexual males would not do to test the effect of fatherlessness because feminine core gender identity goes a lot deeper than a choice, exclusive or partial, of male sex partners by an adult male.

Males who as adults seek sex changes may be an instructive group; male-to-female transsexuals, although chromosomally male, feel that they *are* female and seek to right the state of affairs that makes them seem male. Person and Ovesey (1974) described the "primary transsexual" (male to female) as someone whose separation from mother did not occur in infancy and someone whose femininity was assured. In that view Robert Stoller (1978) concurred, but Stoller differentiated the *feminine* boy from the *effeminate* one, considering effeminacy a mimicry whose hostility shows that some separation from mother took place. Stoller asserted that an inverted Oedipal situation may occur in the effeminate male but never in the feminine-identified boy. Though they need serious questioning, Stoller's words deserve attention: "Most feminine boys result from a mother who, whether with benign or malignant intent, is too protective, and a father who is either brutal or absent (literally or psychologically)" (Stoller, 1974, p. 545; italics deleted).

Bieber (1962) and Kardiner and Ovesey (1962), reporting that adult homosexual males show diminished fathering in their early lives, wished to connect paternal deprivation and later homosexuality. Richard Green (1978), studying the later fate of effeminate or girlish boys, found that the more feminine of them do become transsexual or homosexual, the intermediately masculine or feminine may become homosexual or heterosexual, and the more masculine may wind up as heterosexual but episodically transvestite. Of course, both homosexuals and transvestites may have highly masculine tastes and manners, but not the truly feminine-identified transsexual person, whose self-concept dictates that plastic surgeon and psychiatrist help to establish a correspondence between self-concept and sex role: The compulsion is to undo the wrong body. The homosexual male's self-concept is more varied—it may be masculine, feminine, bisexual, or "ambisexual" in Masters and Johnson's terminology (1979), "amphimixous" in Ferenczi's (1968, original 1923)—and the homosexual male's sex role may be masculine, feminine, unisex, or other. A longitudinal study of transsexuals requires tracking of fewer variables than does a study of homosexuals. Such research on fatherless transsexuals would be very illuminating.

On other matters of psychiatric relevance the picture is not much clearer than with sexuality, sex role, and gender identity of males. Father-absence during childhood is written vividly on the life histories of adults who are neurotic, psychotic, depressed, schizophrenic, suicidal, and geniuses. What gets faint recognition is that most fatherless children may turn out to be quite normal, ordinary people. A statistically significant increase of their numbers among the deviant is similar to the swallow that does not index a summer; most deviants still come from intact nuclear families, after all is said and done.

The reports of the dozen or more authors who have pointed to psychopathologic sequels of childhood fatherlessness will be considered in the next chapter.

Methodologic and Clinical Comments

Valid research in this area needs to control for several variables, including the following: age of child at time of father-absence; socioeconomic status; race; presence or absence of father surrogate; ordinal position; number, age, and sex of siblings; and type and length of the separation from father. To these variables we add the following: gender of the child studied; family educational level; geographic locale; and possibly mother's attitude about the absent father. Few studies control for all these variables. Behavioral science is hagridden by elegant designs for clinically uninteresting questions and poor designs for interesting matters. Some examples will follow.

Age at Time of Father-Absence; Type and Length of Absence.
The importance of controlling for the child's age at the time of father absence has been considered by Ucko and Moore (1963), Herzog (1974), and Biller (1975). Ucko and Moore (1963), using doll-play techniques, operated on the theory that both boys and girls tend to identify with the mother initially: they indicated that 4-year-old boys are squarely in process of shifting from identification with the mother to identification with the father. Boys at 4 years tend to attach equal importance to both parental figures, but at 6 they tend to bring father into their fantasy play more than mother. On the other hand, girls at 4 years tend to perceive the mother as the dominant figure in all aspects of parental function, but at 6, while they still perceive mother as the most positive parental figure, girls recognize father as the primary authority figure. Children's perceptions change with age more than the adult-focused world admits. A child is not only a child, but a unique person who changes at different ages, in different circumstances.

Biller (1975) commented that the father's presence is highly important in the child's early years for sex-role differentiation and touted Father Power. The older child with a strong relationship with the father is less likely to be negatively affected by temporary absence of the father, Biller observed. Herzog (1974), however, as we noted earlier, suggested that among lower-class boys from Barbados, it was most beneficial for the father to be absent during the child's early years in order to enhance the child's relationship with the mother, and then to return after the first or second years in order to provide economic support and assistance in socialization.

Holman (1953) long ago stated that it is imperative that type and length of father-absence be controlled; she concluded that temporary parental absence has little etiological significance in child maladjustment but that permanent separation does. Holman thought that early (before age 4) separation from the father is more deleterious than late (after 4 years) separation. It must be noted that Holman was comparing two mentally ill groups. However, her methodological admonitions were well taken and her clinical commentary apt. The Canadian child psychiatrist David R. Offord wrote with a colleague (Offord & Abrams, 1978) focusing on the child's interests and paid more heed to children than to the person of either of the parents. In that way, total parenting was what was measured, not mother's or father's absence or presence. Their approach was clinically and logically sound because all who work attentively with fatherless children, of any level below middle class, know that such children become relatively motherless as well as fatherless as soon as the father is gone. The overburdened mother also gives less time to the children and her children derive diminished security from a smaller dosage of parenting that they both crave and *objectively* need for healthy growth.

Socioeconomic Status (SES).   Biller (1975) has noted the importance of socioeconomic status on sex-role identification and on sexual behavior when children grow up. Sigusch and Schmidt (1971) observed the effects of SES and nationality on human sexuality—certainly *a crucial* stance when one considers interaction between the sex roles. The results of their study implied that European attitudes toward sexuality are more healthy than U.S. attitudes. The two European samples, more than the U.S., regarded sex as a social activity with mutuality, fidelity, and romantic love. The double standard, the desexualization of women, and the brutalizing of sexuality were not observed with the same frequency in Europe as in the United States. The authors concluded by writing:

What we have described as the Scandinavian pattern of lower-class sexuality is actually the pattern of the "stable working class" of affluent workers; what we have described as the American pattern is the pattern of the "unstable working class" or nonaffluent workers. . . . The differences between the Scandinavian and the American pattern, on the one hand, and Swedish and West German workers, on the other hand, are ultimately class differences. [p. 43]

Comparing Scandinavian "stable working class" or affluent workers with American "unstable working class" or nonaffluent workers adds an unwarranted support to their hypothesis. Economic stratification drastically affects the outcome of all research on sexuality and sex roles. The size of sibling groups and the size of the households also vary according to economic status and all of these must be considered.

Age and Sex of Siblings. Among many authors who have dealt with the importance of siblings and surrogate role models are Brim (1958), Santrock (1970), and Wohlford et al. (1971). Brim (1958), using Koch's (1954, 1955 and 1956) data, found that having cross-sex siblings, especially older siblings, yields more traits appropriate to the cross-sex role. A girl with an older brother has a boy for a model or at least for a reference. The older sibling, more powerful, can better distinguish his or her role from his or her sibling's role. These effects are more potent for siblings closer in age.

Seegmiller (1980) designed a study of sex-role differentiation in 398 preschoolers, comparing the sex-role differentiation (SRD) of those whose mothers worked with those whose mothers did not work and examining the relation between sex-role differentiation and maternal employment with variations in child's gender, presence of father, and sibling characteristics. Maternal employment, it turned out, had no correlation with SRD, regardless of the mother's job level, regardless of the child's gender, and whether the father was present or absent. However, the reference child's siblings did carry some significant traits that accounted for variations in sex-role differentiation. Everybody omits much consideration of the role of a preschooler's siblings but they are highly salient to SRD.

Singletons and children with brothers only gave the greatest number of sex-typed responses (most masculine choices for boys, most femi-

nine for girls), whereas children with sisters or siblings of both sexes were least sex-typed. . . . Taken together, these results suggest that young children may not be as dependent on their parents for sex-role learning as most theorists have suggested. Nor are they uninfluenced by factors in their environment as cognitive development theory has postulated. . . . Maternal employment probably does not exert a very strong influence on SRD until after the age of five or six. Before this time, siblings play an especially important role. [p. 188]

Presence of Father Surrogate. Regarding father surrogates, Santrock (1970) concluded that preschool father-absent black boys were significantly more feminine, less aggressive, and more dependent than their father-present counterparts. These boys, however, were significantly less dependent when a father surrogate was present. Santrock found no differences between father-absent and father-present females; he did find that father-absent females with older female siblings only were more dependent than father-present females with older male siblings only. In addition, father-absent females with only older male siblings were significantly more masculine than father-absent females with older female siblings only. An older brother may be adopted as a kind of substitute father, as we see repeatedly in clinical work with fatherless children.

Ordinal Position. Wohlford et al. (1971) assessed the variables of masculinity–femininity, aggression, and dependence in 66 impoverished black preschool father-absent boys and girls. Children with older male siblings were significantly more aggressive and less dependent than children with no older male siblings. The presence or absence of older female siblings did not offset the older brother's influence. Ordinal position appeared secondary to the presence of an older brother in establishing assertiveness and independence. The presence of an older male sibling, however, did not affect the masculinity–femininity variables, only aggression and independence.

On Cultural Definition of Sex Roles

Culture and social structure define male and female roles in U.S. society, but we question whether it is negative for children to acquire cross-sex traits. We do not attribute society's ills to the blurring of sex roles in today's society, as did Voth (1977). In much research, the masculine role, including the role of the father, is associated with power, control, and success or status. The male, particularly the white male, has the edge on prestigious jobs, the receiving of professional training, and the making of earth-shattering decisions—literally.

Why should we try to make only masculine boys and feminine girls? Why should we denigrate males who are passive, dependent, and timid? Why cannot women be equally represented in government and men equally represented by the hearth? We could do with more egalitarianism in the nursery, less compulsive assigning of "appropriate" sex-role identities to our male and female children.

Giele (1971) discounted the father's crucial role in appropriate sex-role identification, asserting that either parent can perform any function as long as the children's needs and interests are met. In the future family, male and female roles will be more alike than they are now, so sex-role modeling might as well begin to train for individuality among social equals. Boss (1980) found that mothers whose husbands were missing in action fared better when they were *more masculine,* not only androgynous.

Research on both boys and girls has generally shown males to be more affected by father-absence than females, although less than expected; however, vague and contradictory research results make attribution of specific effects difficult. Some authors suggested that father-absence affects a child's display of aggression. Sears (1951) examined 150 preschool children of working mothers, one-half with fathers absent, matched for sex and age with the father-present group. She found that father-absent boys show more aggression in doll-play according to their sibling status and length of father-absence. Santrock (1970), however, using doll-play with 60 economically disadvantaged black preschool children, one-half of whom had fathers absent, found that father-absent boys were significantly less aggressive, more feminine, and more dependent than their father-present counterparts. The expression of aggression was significantly influenced by the sex of older siblings and the presence or absence of a father surrogate.

Doll-play with preschool girls indicated no differences in their display of aggression whether they are father-absent or father-present. Father-absent girls with only older brothers, however, were significantly more aggressive than father-absent girls with only older sisters. Aggression can be learned from brothers as well as from parents present or absent. Andrews and Christensen (1951), who studied college freshmen, showed that among both males and females, father-absent adolescents' courtship was precocious and accelerated and engagements were broken more often than among father-present adolescents. The authors hypothesized that young people who experience father-loss may form affectional relationships to compensate for their loss, and in their haste, they choose poorly.

Female Sex-Role Identification

Little research has explored the impact of father-absence on female sex-role identification, and the rare papers are often case studies (Hetherington, 1973; Neubauer, 1960; Kestenbaum & Stone, 1976; Deaton, 1979) rather than methodologically sharp, empirical studies of larger groups of children. Biller and Weiss (1970) and Biller (1971b, 1974) have reviewed the literature, while Neubauer (1964), Pollack and Friedman (1969), Adams-Tucker and Adams (1980) have suggested implications of father-absence on the sexual development of women.

The theoretical formulations that precede scientific study are often no more than clinical hunches prompted by one case. Neubauer (1960) wrote that when a parent leaves during the Oedipal period, Oedipal conflicts are intensified. When the child loses the parent of the opposite gender, the child's Oedipal longing remains unsatisfied, and increased longing leads to a fantastic idealization of the missing parent. Father-absent Oedipal females may evade Oedipal conflict through "phallic fixation" and an arrest of development at the primary homosexual level. Such pathological Oedipal development appears in Neubauer's case of Rita, a 3-year-old only child whose father had been absent (almost totally) from the date of Rita's birth. Pincus and Dare (1978) cited many examples of secrets and myths that grow up about absent fathers. Adams (1980b) dealt with a case of a female-to-male transsexual whose father had been delusionally erased from consciousness in infancy.

Pollack and Friedman (1969) indicated that female sex-role identification varies with class boundaries and family structures, and father-absence varies in its imprint on sexual development according to the type of father-absence. Pollack and Friedman differentiated the once-intact, middle-class family broken by death, divorce, or desertion from the family that is lower-class, female-headed, three-generational, and incomplete from day one. They proposed that, in the broken family, pathologic Oedipal fantasies are more likely to come into play since a phantom father fills the role of the absent father. A lost father is missed far more than a father who has never been there. In the incomplete family, where no father has ever been present, there is no paternal screen on whom to project the child's ideas of a father's desirable and undesirable traits, nobody to cherish or to dread, no image to venerate. The middle class, Pollack and Friedman maintained, is anxiety prone, unable to enjoy sexuality, and inclined to sacrifice the present for an overinvestment in the future. Middle-class females are the guardians of morality because they must bear any physiological sequels of premarital sex. This is probably less true today than when Pollack and Friedman wrote. Thanks to the availability of contraceptive techniques, premarital sexuality has lost much of its seriousness, moral or otherwise, today. The burdens of conception, contraception, and abortion, however, still impinge mainly on the female.

On the other hand, Pollack and Friedman described the lower-class three-generation family as operating on the pleasure principle, advocating promiscuity in the young, obesity in the middle-aged, and physical aggressiveness at all levels. In that three-generation family without father, girls learn their sexual identities and their perceptions of men by borrowing from the sometimes freewheeling grandmother and mother, and by associating with male siblings or peers:

> *They will gain very negative and devaluative impressions of men, because they will have encountered them mostly as fleeting contacts of their biological mother—exchangeable, unreliable, and possibly not the exclusive partners of their mother, even for the period of their appearance. They may also have encountered them as brothers, who, surrounded by women of three generations while themselves confined to the formative years, will appear to be drowning insignificantly in an ocean of femininity, truly the material of which the paramours of mother seem to be made. [pp. 27–28]*

Although Pollack and Friedman recounted a rather stereotyped view of the poor as promiscuous and irresponsible, their insistence on the need to control for type of father-absence and socioeconomic status is commendable.

Hunt and Hunt (1977) also underscored the need to control for race of girls studied when they revealed that, among white females whom they studied, father-absence appeared to weaken sex-role identification, but it "released" girls for higher achievement. Among black females the effects of father-absence were less dramatic, possibly because black females do not value males very highly, fitting with the high status of white males and the low status of black males in the United States.

Kestenbaum and Stone (1976) considered other important factors—race, religious and ethnic affiliations, the presence or absence of preexisting psychiatric disorders, age at the time of absence, the quality of mothering, and the number of siblings. Age is of particular importance in loss by father's death—if, as Wolfenstein (1966) argued, true mourning is not possible before adolescence. Prior to adolescence, any loss of a love object, particularly through death, is so traumatic and painful that it must be denied. Kestenbaum and Stone gave a judicious summary:

> The impact of paternal loss upon daughter appears varied and not easily predictable. One cannot assume that absence of the father need be pathogenic, although through interaction with other negative factors, it may become so. [p. 186]

Kestenbaum and Stone presented 13 case studies of father-absent girls ranging in age from 10 to 13 years. All the girls had lost their fathers between infancy and adolescence. All 13 failed to complete Oedipal resolution and suffered impaired feminine identification.

We reported earlier that Andrews and Christensen (1951) observed precocious courtship among both males and females from father-absent families, accompanied by a higher percentage of broken engagements. When seeking a mate, the father-absent female has a less sufficient reference person than her father-present cohort. Hetherington (1972) unearthed more heterosexual activity among female adolescents who had lost their fathers by divorce than among those who had lost their fathers by death. But Hainline and Feig (1978) failed to replicate those findings among college women. Fleck et al. (1980) found a greater frequency and extent of "heterosexual behaviors," along with greater state and trait anxiety in 160 father-deprived female college students. Thus, the effects of father absence may diminish with age (among other variables)—or they may change from sexual ones to depression or pessimism and so on.

We hear of adolescent promiscuity in regard to females only. Males are not considered to be promiscuous. They "sow wild oats" and "learn to be men." Teen-age girls, however, who become impregnated by boys "sowing their wild oats" have "gotten themselves into trouble." Behavioral scientists often refer to the "promiscuous" behavior of father-absent adolescent females. Hetherington (1973) observed that teen-age females who had lost their father through divorce tended to be "clumsily erotic" with men, while girls who had lost their fathers through death tended to be scared of men. A *Time* (1970) reporter who interviewed some 35 female strippers wrote that approximately 60% of them came from broken homes in which the father, if present, was unreliable, or from otherwise unstable homes. *Time*'s journalist concluded that these women bared their bodies to strangers in an attempt to obtain that male love and attention they had never received from their fathers. We often run into a similar explanation for female prostitution—a seeking for male attention and patronage, accompanied and underlined by deep-seated hatred for men.

Biller (1971b), having surveyed the literature regarding female sexual development, concluded that females who had suffered a lack of fathering or inadequate fathering had more difficulties in feminine development and interpersonal relations than girls who had experienced adequate fathering. Shaw (1977), too, described psychosexual and psychosocial problems encountered by young women—victims of inadequate fathering—as she outlined the implications for psychotherapy of such women. Biller wrote that females who endured inadequate fathering were more likely to become homosexual and to develop severe psychological problems than those who had had warm affectionate relationships with their fathers. He conceded, however, that "other facets of family functioning and the child's constitutional and sociocultural background must be considered if a thorough understanding of the influence of the father–daughter relationship is to be achieved" (p. 137).

Schrut and Michels (1974) dsecribed impaired sex-role identification in nine suicidal women with nonstandard father–daughter relations. In these women they found "a lifelong history of an insufficiently organized and frustrated ego structure based upon an inadequately fulfilling parent–child relationship, punctuated by mother's intolerance of feminine sexuality and of men, and by father's indifference, hostility, or absence" (p. 345). Most of the women had been unable to work out satisfactory relations with their fathers. Their mothers' allegations of feminine inferiority and sexual uncleanliness were confirmed by father's absence, hostility, passivity, or indifference, so the daughters developed an unconscious need to be accepted by the idealized male. Death by suicide was viewed as the prototype of union with the father in the unconscious. "To death is attributed not only elements of the protective mother, but also the omnipotent power and insuperable strength she feels is necessary for her redemption. If accepted by death, she will be forever enshrined in the sorrow of those who lost her or she will be reborn pure and virginal" (p. 334). Mead and Rekers (1979) have provided a complete—if not fully consistent—review of psychological literature concerning female sexual development.

Adams-Tucker and Adams (1980) outlined the father's role as it contributes to sex-role identification in the female. They distinguished between benevolent and noxious father influences and between healthy families and "hotbox" or incestuous families. At no point, however, did those authors hang such heavy consequences onto the father's role at any one stage in the daughter's development. They felt that father, present or not, could be salient or not and, when salient, healthy or not.

Again, we meet with a scientific void—theories unconfirmed by facts and disjointed facts that do not generate fresh new theory. A multitude of variables enter into female sexual development, including, in addition to those previously mentioned, the mother–father, intersibling, and mother–daughter relationships. With this host of extenuating circumstances surrounding father absence, we cannot attribute specific sexual maladaptations of female persons to fatherlessness per se. We agree with Popplewell and Sheikh (1978) that more and better research would help us achieve some basic understanding of these topics.

CHAPTER SIX

Effects on Offspring: Delinquency and Mental Disorders

A topical index of the literature on fatherless children always shows four big substantive issues to be well represented:

Academic performance
Sex-role behavior
Juvenile delinquency
Mental illness

In the preceding chapter we surveyed research literature devoted to academic achievement and sex role; in this chapter we shall consider theory about and researches into the delinquency and mental illness effects of fatherlessness.

Behind the reviewing of this literature is our desire to determine some data base that makes enough clinical and theoretical sense to serve as a guide for mental health workers. It is apparent, we believe, that some important matters for clinicians are clarified when the entirety of the literature is surveyed (and judged). While we are not more interested in the deviance or pathology than in schools or sex roles of fatherless children, we do find a literature that seems more solid, more pertinent to mental health disciplines, when we take up the topics of this chapter—delinquency and mental illness.

DELINQUENCY

Traditional common sense holds that a child without a father is more likely to have conflict with the law. The absent father has been implicated in the etiology of delinquent behavior, particularly among male children. Classic examples of this theory are provided in psychoanalytic writings that have been produced in an attempt to explain, if not justify, the delinquent careers of such renowned criminals as Sirhan Sirhan and Lee Harvey Oswald. Although popular misconceptions are still widely accepted by many academicians as well as by social strategists, the research in this area is becoming gradually more sophisticated. Additional and perhaps more important variables causative of delinquency are being unearthed. An emerging concept is that perhaps fatherlessness and delinquency are both resultants of underlying economic deprivation rather than themselves being associated in a cause–effect relationship.

Let us examine some of the work that has been accomplished in this area, beginning with the early studies and moving to a more modern perspective. There is a trend from the general and speculative to the specific and empirical. Early studies rarely controlled for many of the salient variables on which later studies themselves are based. Early research looked at the "broken home" as a variable. No distinction was made for the type of break, the sex of the missing parent, the age of the child at the time of the break, the number of siblings, the ordinal position, the socioeconomic status, the sex, or the race of the child, among other variables. Early studies looked at "delinquent behavior" without taking into account the seriousness, nature, or frequency of the delinquent behavior, the degree of recidivism, or the specific personality type of the delinquent child.

Early Studies—Broken versus Unbroken Homes

Early studies acknowledged that children from conflicted families, which went on to see the parents separated, had problems. Most series of cases showed broken homes to lie prominently on the histories. Thus the broken home was to be studied often, but not always well.

Russell (1957) wrote concerning early studies conducted in this field:

> A thorough search of the literature related to behavior problems of children coming from broken homes reveals that the few significant studies available were conducted in the first quarter of the present century. These studies were conducted without controls, and a cause and effect relationship implied variables which influence behavior. [p. 124]

Russell's own research was designed to discern whether certain behavioral characteristics were associated with children from broken homes. His experimental and control groups were matched for age, sex, race, and intelligence; he did not distinguish among types of broken homes. He concluded nonetheless that children from broken homes exhibit significantly more behavior problems than children from intact homes. He followed in his predecessors' footsteps. Three authors cited by Shaw and McKay (1932) as ones who early implicated the broken home as a causative factor in delinquency are Shideler, Slawson, and Burt. Although Slawson considered his control and experimental groups to be matched, there was a paucity of variables actually held constant between these two groups. Imputations to broken homes were made in the early days of this century even when rigorous definitions and controls had been omitted. Slawson and Shideler examined boys only, but Cyril Burt examined both boys and girls. Shaw and McKay themselves did not indicate whether these authors controlled for race.

Elliott and Merrill (1950), the authors of *Social Disorganization,* did examine a group of white girls who were committed to Sleighton Farms, Pennsylvania, during the years 1913 to 1915, mostly for sex offenses. These authors found that for delinquent girls too there was a higher percentage of broken homes within the experimental group than within the control group. Although "broken home" itself was employed as a variable, when type of break was specified, it was found that in cases of parental death, the death of the mother was significantly higher among those delinquent girls than was death of the father.

One of the classic longitudinal studies in this area is the Gluecks' 1950 study, followed by a more global wrap-up in 1968. Their study concluded, as one might expect, that there are multiple family traits that spawn delinquency in certain children. Of the five familial characteristics, three had reference to the father in particular—paternal discipline, paternal affection, and family cohesiveness. As did Lee Robins (1966), the Gluecks often stressed the noxious impact of delinquents' fathers who were *present,* or present but deserted later. The Gluecks have been criticized often but bettered seldom for their summary statement that

> the main impact of the external societal environment, or the general culture, is less significant in generating delinquency and extending it into criminal recidivism than are the biological endowments of the individual and the parental influences of the formative years of early childhood. [1968, pp. 171–173]

Boys who are delinquent, and thereby also delinquency prone, showed as a group a father–son relationship that was cold and distant, a mother–son relationship that was overprotective, and a lack of effective communication within the family. Presumably, these criteria could be met easily in the father-absent family. A less likely prospect is that these criteria could be met in many intact and complete families that do not spawn delinquents. But the biggest protest against the Gluecks' criminology came out against their contention that their delinquent boys were *mesomorphs* to a significant extent, and not *ectomorphs,* and that the boys who were delinquent showed delayed maturation. As seems to be inevitable, the social scientists raise up an attack on any hypotheses that bend in the direction of a psychobiologic predisposition, as does the Glueck hypothesis. It is probably salutary that social scientists do attack views that propound biological determinism since our era has had to be disabused over and over about the overdrawn emphasis on race, breed, stock, temperament, physique, gender, and IQ.

Two other results of the Gluecks' research worthy of mention are:

1. The break in the home of delinquent children occurs at an earlier age for the child than does the break in the home of nondelinquents.
2. At the time of the first court appearance, a delinquent child is likely to have a broken home history of several years and a string of preceding offenses that were not detected and prosecuted.

These findings were thought to have preventive implications; they were issues to be considered in greater depth by later research.

Studies that denied that delinquency was associated with the broken home followed the work of Shaw and McKay (1932). Shaw and McKay themselves found no significant relationship between broken homes and rates of delinquency. Their methodology has been criticized by several writers, including Colcord, Lenroot, Shulman, and Maller (1932), Monahan (1960), and others. Hodgkiss published a 1933 study that emulated the Shaw and McKay methods of research, but used girls rather than boys as the experimental group. Hodgkiss's girls were not like the Shaw and McKay boys; the girls who were delinquent *were* from broken homes. Shaw speculated that these findings were the result of intervention by social agencies in broken homes to a greater degree than in unbroken homes. Early case findings more often channeled the delinquent daughters in such family settings to the court system. Sterne (1964) gives a review of delinquency research prior to 1964 that we heavily recommend and rely on.

Weeks and Smith were cited by Sterne (1964) as having attempted to replicate the findings of Shaw and McKay, using a population of 326 male delinquents in Spokane. They arrived at a correlation of $.61 \pm .12$ between broken homes and delinquency; so another attempted replication wound up negating the original findings of Shaw and McKay.

Sterne concluded his excellent review of the research in 1964 by calling the results of early studies "ambiguous" due to "unresolved uncertainties in sources of data and some shortcomings in the methods of analysis used" (p. 47). He specifically criticized past studies for their failure to: (1) employ adequate controls; (2) note whether one family rupture followed another; (3) note the type of break and time of break; and (4) state with whom the child lived following the family rupture. In his own research, Sterne attempted to remedy some of these gross methodological errors, although he was skeptical of his own findings as well:

> There is differential reporting, prosecuting, and committing of delinquent children for legal transgressions according to race, socioeconomic level, and intelligence level. Delinquent children with high or higher than average intelligence levels are often more skillful at hiding or evading the consequences of their delinquent acts. [pp. 94, 95]

Still, research techniques being what they were in the early 1960s, Sterne's results contributed in an important way to future explorations. Only 31% of the 1,050 white delinquent boys he examined were from broken homes. That finding of an incidence below one-third precludes the broken home from being the major cause of delinquency. Having looked also at the seriousness of offense as a function of broken or unbroken homes, Sterne concluded that there was no support for the preexisting hypothesis that boys from broken homes commit more minor offenses than boys from unbroken homes.

With regard to social planning, Sterne wrote, "Delinquency cannot be fruitfully controlled through broad programs to prevent divorce or other breaks in family life. The prevention of these would certainly decrease unhappiness, but it would not help to relieve the problem of delinquency" (p. 96).

These remarks were in direct contradiction to those of Monahan (1957) a few years earlier. In speaking of the correlation between the "broken home" and delinquency, Monahan wrote with assurance:

The relationship is so strong that, if ways could be found to do it, a strengthening and preserving of family life, among the groups which need it most, could probably accomplish more in the amelioration and prevention of delinquency and other problems than any other single program yet devised. [*p. 258*]

Herzog and Sudia (1968, 1970) carefully reviewed early studies of fatherless families. We need to remind ourselves that prior to 1965, widows (not divorcées) were the most frequent female heads of households. Those articles that correlated juvenile delinquency with broken homes contained seven that upheld the classic view, "although five of these did so with strong qualifications or reservations . . ." (Herzog & Sudia, 1968, p. 178). Of these seven, they rated only four as being reasonably sound in method. They identified six studies that opposed the classic view, but of these they rated only one as being reasonably sound in method! A further point they made was that,

although the differences reported are statistically significant, they are not necessarily practically significant. For example, with regard to juvenile delinquency, one state-wide study reports that about 2 percent of the boys in two-parent homes and about 3.5 percent of the boys in one-parent homes were classified as delinquents. . . . Even without the appropriate qualifications, these figures do not suggest that most boys in fatherless homes are likely to be delinquent. [*Herzog & Sudia, 1968, p. 179*]

In their later review, Herzog and Sudia (1970) noted that other factors are more important in the emergence of juvenile delinquency than is the presence or absence of father per se. They wrote that the overrepresentation of fatherless boys among delinquents

> *could not be attributed primarily to father's absence but rather to stress and conflict within the home, inability of the mother to exercise adequate supervision, depressed income and living conditions (including exposure to unfavorable neighborhood influences), the mother's psychological and behavioral reaction to separation from her spouse as well as to the social and economic difficulties of her situation as a sole parent, and community attitudes toward the boy and the family.* [Herzog & Sudia, 1970, p. 154]

Later Studies—Methodological Issues

Later studies designed to find the causes of delinquency have taken on a more empirical air. Methodological issues have come to the forefront and individual variables have assumed a higher priority than general notions with an a priori base. Hetherington, et al. (1971) wrote:

> *Early studies of juvenile delinquency frequently involved a simple comparison of characteristics of delinquents and nondelinquents. Such an approach was based upon an implicit assumption that delinquency was a homogeneous form of psychopathology and as such should have identifiable patterns of behavior and etiology associated with it. However, recent investigations have indicated that delinquency should be viewed as a legal classification which subsumes a variety of psychological dimensions, each associated with unique characteristics, motivational factors, and experiential antecedents which have contributed to the development of the delinquent behavior.* [p. 160]

As one reads scientific literature in this area, two distinct approaches to the study of delinquency emerge. One is a psychoanalytic or theoretical approach; another is a strictly phenomenal–research approach. Usually some attempt has been made to combine the two. From the psychoanalytic approach, theories have emerged regarding delinquent personality types. Nonanalytic theories consider the role of the mother, the role of the father, the self-concept of the delinquent, the child's conscience development, the family climate in which the delinquent lives, institutionalization, and religious and ethnic affiliations. Methodological issues that emerge give consideration to race, socioeconomic status, age of child at time of break in home, type of break, differential reporting of delinquent acts for different races, classes, and family types, sex of delinquent, ordinal position, number of siblings, recidivism, and type and seriousness of offense.

Delinquent Types

Albert Reiss (1952) identified three types of delinquents: the relatively integrated delinquent, the delinquent with markedly weak ego controls, and the delinquent with relatively defective superego controls. A more sociological stance was originated by Jenkins and Boyer (1967), who proposed the three types of the *unsocialized aggressive* delinquent, the *unsocialized runaway* delinquent, and the *socialized cooperative* delinquent. A still later model designed by Hetherington et al. (1971) offered these classifications as alternatives: the neurotic, the psychopathic, and the social delinquent. The *DSM-III* (*Diagnostic and Statistical Manual,* Third Edition, American Psychiatric Association, 1980) made an atheoretical, phenomenologic stab at classifying delinquent behavior that may embody the best practice available for the contemporary clinician. *DSM-III* wound up with four classes of "conduct disorders" in children: (1) undersocialized, aggressive; (2) undersocialized, nonaggressive; (3) socialized, aggressive; and (4) socialized, nonaggressive. The authors of *DSM-III* claimed that these classes are "controversial" as, indeed, was most of the work on *DSM-III,* but at least there were ways to make some reasonable differentiations between the children who are unsocialized and those who belong to gangs and seem to be participants in group norms. Likewise, the children who are aggressive are sorted out from the ones who are nonaggressive, a very telling distinction for the children's neighbors. *DSM-III* agreed that the unsocialized or undersocialized children set up their patterns in the prepubertal era and the socialized ones only in the pubertal or postpubertal years.

The Socialized Delinquent. Jenkins' and Boyer's socialized cooperative delinquent seems to approximate Reiss's delinquent with relatively defective superego controls and Hetherington et al.'s.

(1971) *social delinquent.* The socialized delinquent is distinguished by gang activities, cooperative stealing, habitual school truancy, running away from home, and staying out late at night. Usually, the socialized delinquent hails from a poor residential area, a zone invaded by commerce and industry and having high rates of delinquency. Often the prime candidate to become a socialized delinquent is the young child from a large family with delinquent siblings. Delinquency represents a typical form of group participation in an urban lower-class neighborhood, as opposed to a suburban middle-class neighborhood, where delinquency, or at least gang activity, is atypical (or so it is said to be).

Of the three delinquent categories defined by Jenkins and Boyer, the socialized cooperative delinquent appears to have the most normal personality and to come from the most normal home situation. His (or her) delinquent activity is representative of conforming to peer-group pressure. From some authors, father-absence comes to play in the etiology of the socialized delinquent. Walter Miller (1958), writing of the boy in the lower-class street gang, stated, "In many cases it is the most stable and solidary primary group he has ever belonged to; for boys reared in female-based households the corner group provides the first real opportunity to learn essential aspects of the male role in the context of peers facing similar problems of sex-role identification" (p. 14). This observation seems to be based on a presumption that most lower-class families are fatherless.

Miller also chided so-called scholars for lumping gang delinquency with other forms of delinquency and incorrectly defining it as a form of rebellion against middle-class values. He wrote that although lower-class street gang activity often violates the middle-class norm, this transgression is not the primary motivational component of such behavior. Departure from middle-class values is instead "a by-product of action primarily oriented to the lower class system" (p. 19). Furthermore: "No cultural pattern as well-established as the practice of illegal acts by members of lower class corner groups could persist if buttressed primarily by negative, hostile, or rejective motives" (p. 19).

The Unsocialized Runaway Delinquent.

Jenkins and Boyer claimed that the unsocialized runaway delinquent appears to have the most poorly organized personality. Delinquency in this case is a form of psychopathology associated with parental rejection. Hetherington et al. (1971) asserted that parental rejection, particularly maternal rejection, is associated with the "unsocialized psychopathic factor"; "psychopathic delinquents describe their mothers as rejecting, autonomous, non-enforcing, and hostilely detached" (p. 161). That jibes well with the clinical appearance of runaways who feel they have "been run off" by the remaining family members.

The Unsocialized Aggressive Delinquent. The unsocialized aggressive delinquent is characterized by starting fights, cruelty, defiance of authority, malicious mischief, and inadequate guilt feelings. Jenkins and Boyer described this category of offender as occupying an intermediate position with respect to both parental rejection and degree of personality organization. They predicted that this type of behavior is most likely to emerge in a child who experiences child rearing that consists of parental rejection combined with parental overprotection and shielding from the authorities. "Such a combination might be expected to give him both hostility and the courage to act on it" (p. 76).

Certainly the three types described by Jenkins and Boyer are recognizable by the clinician involved in work with delinquent families and individuals. The typology rings very true.

Two of the most used and confused terms in all the psychologic and psychiatric literature on delinquency are *aggression* and *conscience*. The unsocialized child is supposed to be high in aggression and low in conscience and, as we discussed earlier, the male child is supposed to be superior in both aggression and conscience, but the fatherless child is supposed to be both lower in aggression unless overcompensating and lower in conscience. The *DSM-III* way of categorizing seems to us to promise a construction facilitating research that can be helpful in this mixed-up state of conceptualization. For, in reality, the *DSM-III* subtypes are simply ways of ordering the varied pairings of violent, aggressive behavior or its obverse, with socialization (rule observance) and its obverse. The aggressive delinquent is not well understood at the present time.

Psychiatry in its psychodynamic schools has added to unclarity: aggression is equated with initiative, increased motor and intellectual activity, increased and active fantasies and imaginations, hitting, pulling hair, mugging and destroying property, and sometimes unconscious motivation by a death drive, Thanatos. Nondynamic psychiatrists often mean overt behavior that is destructive or assaultive of things, animals, and persons—easier to define and research, often a matter of court record or among the troubles known to a child's parent, school personnel, and peers.

There are a few recent studies of aggression as a delinquent trait that we present now. Children who kill have not been notably fatherless despite the fact that Lee Harvey Oswald and some other notorious ones have grown up to be killers. Killing is one of the prime causes of death among adolescents today in the United States. Our figures on murder and violence consider, of course, only that violence that is not condoned by the state and excludes killings by police and soldiers at war. Psychologists often attempt to devise questionnaires and tests that will ferret out a trait of aggression or proneness to aggression. Using a questionnaire and a three-dimensional puzzle game, Montare and Boone (1980) matched Puerto Rican, native black, and native white impoverished male children in Newark with examiners of their same ethnicity and derived information about the relation between aggression scores and fatherlessness, concluding from videotape analyses that fatherless children as a group did not differ significantly from the fathered ones, but that when ethnicity was considered Puerto Rican boys were more highly aggressive than either black or white, and that while black fatherless boys were less aggressive than black fathered boys, white fatherless boys were more aggressive than their fathered counterparts. Hence, race or ethnic background becomes critical for discerning aggression in fathered/ fatherless boys. Montare and Boone had the impression that Puerto Rican boys were the newcomers to inner-city Newark, and that fact combined with their culturogenic positive valuation of machismo accounted for their greater aggression scores. White boys, being the local minority group, showed completely different relations between aggression and fatherlessness than did the local majority black boys of the inner city. Oddly, this was not true of Miami's Cuban newcomer poor boys (Adams & Horovitz, 1980b).

Arthur M. Horne (1981) studied Oregonians, 24 families, 9 of these mother-only families, all seeking help for an aggressive child.

Matched to these were 25 normal families with a target child of the same age as the clinical target child, and 9 of the nonclinical families were also mother headed. All mother-only families were postdivorce. Families were observed and codings were made by two observers who had high interrater agreement. Rates of aggressive behavior (overt and observed, not deduced from a paper-and-pencil test) appeared in this order, moving from highest to lowest:

Mother-only clinic children
Clinic children from two-parent families
Mother-only nonclinic children
Two-parent nonclinic children

Furthermore, the siblings from families with a clinically referred child had higher rates of aggression than the siblings of nonclinic children. Siblings from nonclinic two-parent families surpassed in aggression the nonclinic mother-only ones, too. Horne surmised that in clinic families the father might have been needed as a stabilizing influence, curbing the aggression of the children, but that in non-clinic "normal" families "this stabilizing factor may not be necessary." Horne's work supported the research of Barry (1979) with single-parent families: The well-being of the parent who was present became the model that stamped other family members into appropriate behavior. Once more, the mother in the mother-headed family exposes her neck because she is alone, and as mother-headed households grow in number mothers may once again be singled out as "schizophrenogenic," or other kinds of culprits—made more likely by our tendency to blame victims whenever possible.

Cynthia Pfeffer and colleagues (1983) examined a clinical population of 103 children to see what characteristics predicted their being assaultive. They found boys of all racial heritages to be more assaultive than girls and to have predictably greater assaultiveness when parents are assaultive and the child has a record of past aggression and currently shows less anxiety or depression. Impulsive acting out does not accompany the kind of anxiety and depressive insight found in child psychiatry patients as a group. Of interest to us was the finding by Pfeffer et al. that mother's assaultive behavior was significantly correlated with child assaultiveness but father's assaultiveness did *not* reach statistically significant correlation. The mother as a model for young males appears strongly again.

One more report may be of interest to clinicians who work with diverse ethnic groups: the 1981 study by Castellano and Dembo of the University of Southern California. Eighty Mexican-American females 13 to 17 years were divided into four groups (all were from families with annual income between $4,000 and $6,000) with the following scores of egocentrism:

High antisocial, father absent—highest egocentrism

High antisocial, father present—next highest egocentrism

Low antisocial, father present—third highest egocentrism.

Low antisocial, father absent—lowest egocentrism

Even in the Mexican-American family, where the father is reputed to be a central person, there was no significance found for his presence or absence in respect to egocentrism. Antisocial behavior was what made for the important differences among the groups studied. There were no special considerations given for IQ or surrogating by other males, or for the type of father-absence.

Castellano and Dembo did give support to an old clinical maxim, namely that people who have some empathy for others and are not totally egocentric, or who may even have some occasions to be altruistic and care for others, do not as often violate the rights of others by antisocial acts. It may be, we speculate, that they will also show more moral development or conscience even before they reach the final Piagetan stage of formal operations after 12 to 14 years of age.

The describing and specifying of the psychosocial conditions in which altruism and conscience develop most reliably remain a task of the future; we do not know enough at present. However, it seems plausible that writers such as Thomas S. Parish are on the right track in their suggestion that a child with more basic needs unmet is not a good candidate for smooth, precocious, or even normal moral development. See Parish and Parish (1977) and Parish (1978) for their Maslovian comments that "advances in moral development are tied to the fulfillment of various physiological and psychological needs."

Role of the Mother in Delinquent Behavior

Here we review the writings of proponents of the theory that gives mother alone the responsibility for the child's character formation, as well as the writings of some of the opponents of this theory and some of the research relating specific delinquent behaviors to mother–child interaction. Naturally, we are most interested in mothers who head up their households, whose homes do not have an adult male cohabiting there.

Bowlby (1951) in the *World Health Organization Bulletin* declared that separation from the mother or mother surrogate during the first 5 years of life was among one of the foremost causes of delinquency—at least delinquency of the psychopathic or affectionless type. Others have since refuted this theory. Notable among these is Andry (1962), who questioned whether Bowlby and the maternal deprivation theorists could certify that their concept was both sound and useful, since it did not evolve from rigorously controlled experiments. Andry criticized Bowlby and others for not presenting their evidence in factor-analysis terms, thereby failing to rule out other variables as causing the results Bowlby and company had specifically attributed to maternal deprivation. He pled for recognition of the role of the father as well as the mother in child development, and appealed to analytically oriented psychologists for a greater recognition and appreciation of the usefulness of the learning theory model. Andry certainly did not belong in the Bowlby camp.

Grygier et al. (1969) also attempted to dispel the traditional psychiatric view that character development is primarily the result of the mother's role in child rearing. They attributed mutual or joint responsibility to the father's role, and espoused the view that "separation from either parent does not seem to be a single factor in delinquency; rather it is part of the entire family situation of the pathology inherent in unstable families" (p. 247).

Koller (1971) wrote that it is the presence of the mother, rather than her absence, that contributes to children's delinquency. Koller's remarks seem applicable to fatherless families only, although his position assumes that when father leaves, any preexisting psychopathology in mother is intensified.

In sociopsychiatric literature there are several patterns of pathological mother–child interactions thought to be contributory to delinquency. Martha MacDonald (1938) recounted her observations of a group of eight boys who showed both criminally aggressive and passive effeminate behavior. None of these boys had had an early gratifying relationship with a father or a father surrogate. All had been raised by their mothers and/or grandmothers, women described by MacDonald as being "aggressive, dominant, rejecting, punitive women. They are women who more or less despise the adult males they have known and feel themselves capable, superior and in control" (p. 71). MacDonald hypothesized that because the boys had had no male role models with whom to identify, all opportunities for parental identification were overbalanced toward the maternal side. The boys behaved like "perfect little gentlemen" when among women or girls, feeling secure in exhibiting the passive effeminate behaviors they had learned. By contrast, the criminally aggressive behaviors exhibited by these boys when around men or their male agemates were thought to be attempts to "overcome strong passive homosexual drives in which they would play a masochistic role with resulting projection of the aggressive, sadistic role to the exterior and identification with the fantasied aggressor" (p. 78).

Later literature is less psychoanalytic and paradox laden than that presented by MacDonald. Hetherington et al. (1971) described a family system dominated by the mother, that is, the neurotic delinquent family. Jenkins (1968) wrote that overanxious children are likely to have an anxious, infantilizing mother, while unsocialized aggressive children are likely to have a critical, depreciative, punitive, inconsistent mother or stepmother. This mother tends to have a character disturbance or psychoneurosis. According to Jenkins, the unsocialized aggressive child is more likely than the socialized delinquent to be an only child, to have a stepmother or a punitive mother, and to experience much parental inconsistency. Jenkins and Boyer (1967) described unsocialized aggressive delinquents as children who had experienced "a gross lack of a normal experience of being mothered" (p. 65).

On the other hand, the socialized delinquent was described by Jenkins as having a more normal relationship with a mothering person, but as having grown up in a delinquency area, usually a deteriorated urban slum. If one highlights the effects of an absent or inadequate father figure, race and socioeconomic class must be considered at every step along the way. Rosen (1969) noted that the absence of a father figure was of little importance in deriving the etiology of lower-class black male delinquency; other forces were at work in that determination.

Role of Father in Delinquent Behavior

Research that implicates the father in the etiology of delinquency is not so abundant but it ranges from general accusations to specific condemnations of paternal behavior. Andry (1962) wrote that when he compared 80 delinquent boys with nondelinquents, the delinquents implied that they felt rejected by their fathers (but felt loved by their mothers). The nondelinquents indicated with much greater constancy that they felt loved equally by both parents. Nondelinquents had a marked tendency to obey the father and recognize the father as the head of the family. Delinquents, on the other hand, while recognizing their fathers as heads of household, did tend to obey them the least. Hetherington et al. (1971) noted that although parents of delinquents generally are more hostile and rigid in disciplining their children, they are less effective disciplinarians. Lang et al. (1976) indicated that delinquent girls also feel rejected by their fathers.

Grygier et al. (1969) indicated that an inadequate father image is more likely to contribute to delinquency than a faulty mother image. Permanent parental separation is generally significant, and it is more frequent on the part of fathers than of mothers. Temporary separation is less frequent and less pathogenic. Faulty parental image appears in their research to be at least as important as permanent separation, and it more often involves fathers. Again, it is a matter of negative or pathogenic fathers who are present in the household but outstrip absent fathers as noxious influences on child and family. See Robins (1966) on the father, alcoholic or sociopathic, as predictor of the children's delinquency and adult sociopathy.

Jenkins (1968) stated that socialized delinquents frequently come from large families and suffer from neglect. Parental pathology is typically more paternal than maternal and frequently involves the alcoholic father or stepfather. Hetherington et al. (1971) wrote that the family of the socialized delinquent is dominated by the father, as opposed to the maternally dominated family of the neurotic delinquent. They described a socialized delinquent's family as patriarchal in nature, with a passive, resistant, inactive, and quiet mother whose son is negative and rigid, who feels free to talk, but whose talk is rarely considered or implemented. Talk is cheap, after all.

By contrast, Hetherington et al. (1971) described the family of the psychopathic delinquent as one in which the father appears to be dominant; but the mother plays a more active role than the father in the family of the socialized delinquent. The psychopathic delinquent son seems to participate minimally in decision-making processes in the intact family. Fathers of both neurotic delinquents and psychopathic delinquents set stricter limits on their children's activities and are less permissive than the fathers of either socialized delinquents or nondelinquents.

No clear and invariant pattern of parental dominance is shown in the nondelinquent's family, and the children have a more active role in decision making. The father of the nondelinquent is less anxiously involved with his son than the father of any delinquent subgroup.

Self-Concept

One of the classic effects thought to be associated with children, particularly male children, in father-absent families is the modeling of a negative self-concept (Rosenberg, 1965; Biller, 1970). This was discussed in Chapter 3. When Song (1969), however, compared delinquent boys from broken homes with delinquent boys from unbroken homes, he found no difference in self-concept between the two groups. Moerk (1973) compared two groups of father-absent male children—a group of male children whose fathers were imprisoned and a group of male children whose parents were divorced. Both groups scored below the norm on the self-concept scale, and there were no significant differences between the groups. The author did note, however, that profiles of the children with imprisoned fathers were more similar to the profiles of juvenile delinquents and less similar to the norm than the profiles of the children from divorced families. Moerk speculated that these findings may have been attributable to discordant family relationships that existed in the home prior to father's imprisonment. Family discord has frequently accompanied both delinquency and father's temporary absence. Of course, discord has also been associated strongly with divorce.

Moerk suggested that low socioeconomic standing may be responsible for both groups' scoring below the norm on the self-concept scale. Malone (1963) described a group of skid row children from highly pathologic families. In terms of their ego development and self-concept, he wrote, "The experience of the self as active and capable of self-direction has been thwarted" (p. 35). In psychoanalytic terms, he described the condition of these children as having "a relatively weak cathexis of objects, both human and inanimate, and also a relatively poor concept of the belief in the permanence of people and things" (p. 35). Malone described the tendency to act upon impulse, observed in these children, "as an outgrowth of certain developmental deficiencies arising from disturbances in the mother–child relationship" (p. 41). "The areas of developmental lag stressed were the dominant use of action rather than words for expression, delays in certain aspects of cognitive development, and the children's difficulties in forming integrated identifications and a firm sense of identity" (p. 41). Thus, Malone saw the problem in poor self-concept formation as lying with the mother and not the father. But, just as important, he saw a negative self-concept as a function of social class and pathological conditions inherent in impoverished living conditions.

Other authors claim that the absent father is not a factor in poor self-concept formation, but rather that self-concept formation is a function of the child's qualitative interaction with whichever parent he or she has present or of the total parenting available to the child from any source (Offord & Abrams, 1978). Parish and Copeland (1979) reported that in father-absent families college students' self-concepts tended to be closely correlated with their evaluations of their mothers and stepfathers (if present) but not with their evaluations of their absent fathers. Also, if father is present, but inadequate, the effects of the poor father–child interaction may be more devastating to the child than having the father absent. Millen and Roll (1977) indicated that there was a positive relationship between the son's feeling of being understood by the father and the son's self-concept. They also found a negative relationship between the son's feeling of being understood by the father and his reported somatic complaints. So the child's perception of the quality of interaction with father is important to many areas of the child's development.

Some of the discrepancy among research findings in the area of self-concept can be explained by the inaccurate and imprecise research methodology that has been employed. Kaplan (1970) reported that significant correlations existed between adult self-derogation, a manifestation of negative self-concept, and (odd or even) number of siblings, ordinal position, and sex distribution of children. Kaplan indicated that these variables, at the very least, need to be controlled in studies attempting to examine the dynamics of self-concept formation and maintenance.

Conscience Development

A notion that we discussed earlier is that the father provides a model for superego formation or conscience development in the young child, particularly the young male. That was the notion of Freud and of Aichhorn (1935). As a corollary, impaired conscience development is thought to follow father-absence. But would that apply to girls and boys alike? Hoffman (1973) compared two groups of seventh-grade white boys and girls, controlled for sex, IQ, and social class. He found that father-absent *boys* attained lower scores for all moral indices; they also exhibited more aggressive behavior, according to teacher ratings. However, there were no differences shown between father-absent and father-present *girls*. Father-absence means more for conscience development of male children than for females. Hoffman replicated the findings of several other studies (Glueck & Glueck, 1950; Gregory, 1966; Miller, 1958; Siegman, 1966).

Hoffman supposed that his findings could be the consequence of changes in mother's child-rearing practices subsequent to father's departure. Some experts believe that in father's absence the mother becomes more affectionate to her female children and less affectionate to her male children. Atkinson and Ogston (1974) found that the behavior of children without fathers is not significantly different from the behavior of children with fathers. They stated that what may change as a function of father's absence is parental behavior. In the end, their speculations would concur with those of Hoffman.

Other authors suggest that father's absence may not affect internal controls, or conscience development per se, but rather that it affects external controls or the administration of punishment. Goldstein (1972) compared black father-present preschool boys with a father-absent group and found that father-present male children had no more internal controls than father-absent children. But, Goldstein reported that the father-present boys were more frequently punished for aggressive behavior. Both groups, surprisingly, if one believes in father-as-disciplinarian, were punished more frequently by mother than by father even when a father was present.

Adams and Horovitz (1980a) studied 108 fatherless firstborns through their mothers' reports on problems with their aggressive behavior. They compared them with 93 fathered, poor firstborns, and found that only *younger* lower-class boys showed more such problems, as perceived by the mothers. As firstborn boys grew older the mothers had less to complain about. That agreed with child clinicians' experiences that *young* sons present mothers with their gravest conduct and discipline problems; the mothers see their older sons as actually helpful and benign figures.

Family Climate

In research endeavors conducted following the era of Shaw and McKay, the concept of the *inadequate home* began to replace that of the *broken home* (Sterne, 1964).

Different types of inadequate families have accompanied different types of delinquent behavior. Tuckman and Regan (1966) found that the type of home that is high in aggressive behavior tends to be the home that is also high in antisocial behavior but low in anxiety, neurotic symptoms, and problems of habit formation. Conversely, the type of home that is high in anxiety tends to be the type that is also high in problems of habit formation, but low in aggressive and antisocial behavior. Peterson, Quay, and Cameron (1959) suggested that conduct disorders and neurotic disorders were found in different types of home climate. The primary variable for discriminating between these two types of homes was the amount and kind of parent supervision. Aggressive behavior, antisocial behavior, and conduct disorders may be associated with absence or laxity of supervision: do not supervise and you get a delinquent.

Hetherington et al. (1971) credited parental *rejection* with the unsocialized–psychopathic factor in delinquency; *overcontrol* with the neurotic–disturbed factor in delinquency; and *neglect,* with exposure to delinquent norms, with the socialized–subcultural factor in delinquency. So refraining from supervision may spoil some children, rejection and harshness others, and overcontrol still others.

Religion

Much so-called religion is rather nondescript and pallid, so American religion has not been studied often in regard to delinquency. Nye (1958) wrote that less delinquency was found in families where the parents and children attended church regularly. In the southern United States, juvenile court judges often mandate church attendance for delinquent children and make religious observance (of either a parent's or the judge's religion) a condition of the child's staying out of a correctional institution. Regarding extent of piety, Sterne (1964) stated that among Protestant boys, a significantly high proportion of serious criminal offenses was found among the devout. Baptists are people of the Book, it is said; they may also be "people of the booking." Among the nondevout of all faiths the proportion of serious offenses committed by Protestants was generally highest. These relations did not hold for Catholics or Jews. That exactly parallels the situation with suicide—higher for Protestants than Catholics or Jews.

Sterne (1964) described "the renegade son of the minister" as a distinct delinquent type unlike either the gang delinquent or the "middle-class boy who revolts against the domination masked in his 'good' mother's affection" (p. 26).

Foreign-Born Parents

Nye (1958) wrote that foreign birth, which formerly was the focus of Americanization and delinquency reduction efforts, did not appear by the fifties to be associated with delinquent behavior. Sterne (1964), however, claimed that delinquent children of foreign-born parents still tended to commit more serious offenses than delinquent children of native-born parents. There has been some speculation that foreign-born parents try to exercise more rigid controls over their children than native-born parents. When the children do revolt, it is in a more serious manner, because the restrictions against which they are rebelling are more stringent.

Not enough is known about delinquency among the foreign-born here in the melting pot becoming pluralistic. However, in a study of fatherless, firstborn sons of poor Cubans in Miami, Adams and Horovitz (1980a) found surprisingly little delinquency or aggression among either the Cuban fatherless children or the black fatherless children with whom they compared the Cuban refugee group, both groups of nonpatients.

Race

Shaw and McKay (1932) insisted more than 50 years ago that the rate of broken homes for a group of boys in the general population is of little or no value if the nationality and racial composition of the group are not known. They did *not* mean that the genes governing skin color also governed delinquency, but they discerned that, in a racist society, disadvantage and deviancy are bound up with color and the latter's evaluation in the society. Of all racial categories, Shaw and McKay also found the highest proportion of broken homes to be among blacks and the lowest proportion of broken homes among Jews. Some write that the broken home gives little input to delinquent behavior among black youth who are poor (Eisner, 1966)— among black males, particularly, (Rosen, 1969; Adams & Horovitz, 1980a). However, Monahan (1957) found the highest correlation between delinquency and broken homes for black girls and the lowest for white boys, with black boys and white girls falling in between, showing that close inspection of class, ethnos, and gender is always called for before sweeping general statements are uttered.

Willie (1967) remarked that delinquency rates were similar for members of white and nonwhite populations who live in the most disadvantaged environments, of broken homes and low income. Although delinquency rates may be the same, other authors indicate that children from broken homes and black youths are more likely (than are children from unbroken homes and white youths) to be committed to institutions following their delinquent acts, a measure leading to much greater recidivism (Herzog & Sudia, 1968). Axelrad (1952) indicated that black children "are committed to a state institution as delinquents younger, with fewer court appearances, less previous institutionalization, and for fewer and less serious offenses than white children" (p. 571).

Regarding the type of offense they committed, Axelrad wrote that white children were institutionalized for more serious offenses than black children. White children were also committed more often for truancy than black children. "It is probable that the community, or at least the school system, considers truancy in the white child as something about which it is willing to be active. Seemingly, it did not care so much in the case of the Negro child" (Axelrad, p. 571).

Bartollas (1976) wrote an interesting study of an Ohio correctional facility thoroughly dominated by its majority, delinquent black males. Studies of imprisoned youth in America always find the poor and minority members overly represented.

Socioeconomic Status (SES)

Delinquency has long been associated with the lower socioeconomic strata. There is doubt that statistics on delinquency are accurate indicators of the incidence or prevalence of delinquency because middle- and upper-class delinquents are less frequently found, reported, prosecuted, and committed than lower-class delinquents (Nye, 1958; Herzog & Sudia, 1968). Nevertheless, we will attempt to review such literature as exists here.

Shaw and McKay (1932) were among the earliest who found a high correlation between rates of delinquency and socioeconomic status, although they did not find a relationship between broken homes and delinquency. Fleisher (1966) wrote that the effect of income on delinquency is remarkable: A rise in income is followed by a much larger drop in delinquency than is a corresponding drop in unemployment. Perhaps it is not surprising that delinquents respond better to money (a result) than to work (a means). Willie (1967) suggested that community programs designed to prevent juvenile delinquency will have maximum success if they focus first upon increasing the economic status of the target population. Raising the economic status is real; it provides more jobs and elevates the general standard of living, rather than just providing more welfare payments. Besides, Sterne (1964) found that those receiving relief or "welfare" were prone to serious, not minor, offenses. Minor relief is very minor and its small payments give little help to its recipients. Lower-class impoverishment is associated with the emergence of gang delinquency, too (Miller, 1958). Miller described the features of lower-class culture that exacerbate the formation and maintenance of gangs: trouble, toughness, smartness, excitement, and autonomy. Malone (1963) enumerated a series of psychosocial maladies, including crime and delinquency, which arise from a sociocultural climate of economic deprivation. Other detrimental effects included alcoholism, neglect, brutality, and illegitimacy.

Generally, a much stronger relationship has been established between low socioeconomic status and delinquency than is the case between broken homes, or father-absence specifically, and delinquency. The only methodological shortcoming that prevents our being able to state this categorically is the differential reporting of delinquent acts between social classes that we remarked on earlier. The poor in general may be "hidden America" but their crimes are put on public display.

Age of Child at Time of Family Disruption

The early years are reportedly the most crucial years during which a child can lose a parent. Whiting, Kluckhohn, and Anthony (1958) predicted that the probability of a boy's becoming delinquent is highest when the separation of the mother and father occurs during the boy's early infancy and the mother remarries when her son is 2 or 3 years old. Sterne's 1964 data supported this theory somewhat. Newman and Denman (1971) wrote that white adult males who had lost their fathers prior to the age of 18 are more likley to be involved in criminal behavior categorized as "felonious." More specifically, they provided support for the hypothesis that the *early* years, 0 to 6, are the most important for personality formation. The Gluecks (1950) found that in addition to the proportion of broken homes being higher among delinquents than among nondelinquents, the break in the home also occurred *earlier* for delinquents. Other authors disagree that the age of the child at the time of the break is of unvarying significance (Koller & Castanos, 1970).

Shaw and McKay (1932) found an increase in the number of broken homes with the increasing age of the delinquent. That is logical, since greater total numbers of homes are broken with each new year. Monahan (1960), however, wrote that most breaks occur under 7 years of age, but most delinquency occurs between 10 and 17 years of age. This finding implies that a residual effect of early parental absence is expressed in later years. It has been hypothesized, however, that by the time delinquency is detected and the child actually appears in court, he or she may have a long series of delinquent acts behind him or her, that have been committed but have not actually been detected, reported, or prosecuted (Glueck & Glueck, 1950).

Type of Break

Unfortunately, most of the large group studies we examined do not specify which parent leaves or the type of break that occurs. Rather, much of the research done in this area employs merely the broad category of "broken home" when assessing influences on delinquent behavior. To some researchers, this omission makes precious little difference. For example, Andry's (1962) results failed to support the maternal deprivation theory, the paternal deprivation theory, or the dual deprivation theory. Were his results accepted fact, the sex of parent or type of break would not be worth investigating.

Other authors, however, have found significant relationships between specific types of break and delinquent behavior. The Gluecks' (1950) study indicated that illegitimacy and desertion were types of fatherlessness most closely associated with delinquency—and parental divorce or separation the least. Tuckman and Regan (1966) discovered that children from divorced families were most often referred to outpatient psychiatric clinics for aggressive and antisocial behavior. Russell (1957) indicated that enuresis, extreme anger, and disobedience were found more frequently in homes broken by divorce or separation than in homes broken by death. Academic retardation, he said, was more often found in children whose homes had been broken by death. Children from broken homes generally manifested more behavior problems and more lying and stealing than children from unbroken homes. There is a welter of complexities to be considered here. What summary statement can be given? This, perhaps: The type of fatherlessness and the nature of the residual family's resources make every difference when one deals with individual clinical cases, but in the mass of cases the fine differences are less deeply etched.

Differential Reporting of Delinquent Acts According to Race, Class, and Family Type

Criticism of existing statistics on delinquency has been mentioned several times previously. Monahan (1957) stated that children from unbroken homes were much more likely than children from broken homes to be dismissed from adjudication by the intake interviewing staff of the juvenile law enforcement agency. Sterne (1964) pointed to differential reporting of delinquent acts among races and among social classes. Herzog and Sudia, in *Children In Fatherless Families* (1970), decried the unequal treatment of delinquent children from different backgrounds, including racial, socioeconomic, and familial. The more advantaged kids remain less restricted, less disadvantaged, even when they do delinquent things. Robins (1966) found that having a juvenile court hearing increased and confirmed children's sociopathy.

Sex of Delinquent

Little has been written to distinguish between delinquent acts committed by male and by female delinquents, although it is fairly well established that female delinquents frequently are committed for incorrigible sexual behavior, but males almost never are (Hetherington et al., 1971).

Grygier et al. (1969) found that the types of broken homes from which male and female delinquents derived revealed almost no differences. For both males and females, death and temporary absence were nonsignificant. Permanent separation was significant and usually involved the father rather than the mother. These findings were supported by Koller (1971). Elliott and Merrill, cited by Sterne (1964), had reported earlier that for delinquent girls from homes broken by death, it was usually death of the mother—not death of the father—that broke the home. Loss of a mother is more catastrophic than death of a child's father, we know, and perhaps especially for girls.

Ordinal Position

Nye (1958) wrote: "Family relationships, duties, responsibilities, and privileges and the amount of control exercised over children differ considerably with family size, birth position of the child, and by broken and unbroken homes" (p. 37). He found the least delinquency among oldest children and only children, describing both as "exclusive relationships which might facilitate both internalization of parental values and the development of indirect controls through affectional identification" (p. 37). Sterne (1964) disagreed with this, finding that only children from unbroken homes showed a significantly high number of delinquent acts. Koller and Castanos (1970) also disagreed with Nye when they reported that there is a tendency for the eldest child to be delinquent and for the penultimate one not to be delinquent. More recently Sherle Boone (1979) reported that firstborn and middle-born children in father-absent families are more likely to exhibit aggressive behavior than their father-present counterparts. Adams and Horovitz (1980a) found, in an impoverished group of firstborn males from fatherless homes, that aggression generally was low but higher only in the younger group of boys, both black and Cuban. Again there is conflict in the research findings. That impresses upon us even more strongly the necessity to control for these many variables, including ordinal position, when assessing the effects of fatherlessness on children.

Number of Siblings

Research generally suggests that the smaller the family, the less opportunity for it to spawn delinquent children (Nye, 1958). Koller and Castanos (1970) stated that the family size of their offender group was comparatively large. They also noted an excess of male children in these large families, relative to the control group. This finding gives another reminder that delinquency is never very far away from the lower-class male. Koller (1971) said of delinquent females that they were derived from large families with younger than average parents and the intermediate female children were most likely to become delinquent. Koller and Castanos had also noted the tendency for offenders who had experienced parental deprivation to have parents who were younger and themselves to be younger than their counterparts who had experienced no loss.

Recidivism

Monahan was cited by Sterne (1964) as one who, comparing delin- quents appearing once or more in court, found that there was a greater proportion of repeat appearances for children derived from every type of broken home in every group and in all instances *save one*. This exception was black boys of divorce. There were signifi- cantly fewer court appearances by those with both parents dead than by those with unmarried parents. Children who grieve "act in" and are less prone to "act out" during childhood.

Seriousness of Offense

Bacon, Child, and Barry (1963) attempted to determine the type of crime associated with the male youth's lack of a strong identification with a father figure. Forty-eight preliterate societies were examined. In these, a differential was established between theft and personal crime. Both types of crime were associated with failure of the male child to form a strong identification with a male role model. A high degree of socialization anxiety in childhood and a high degree of status differentiation in adulthood were significantly associated with theft only. Adult feelings of suspicion and distrust were more defi- nitely associated with personal crime.

We mentioned earlier that being a welfare recipient is associated with serious, not minor offenses. Children of foreign-born parents also commit more serious offenses. The older the delinquent youth, the more serious the offense. The more devoutly religious the Protes- tant family, the more serious the offense. Those are conclusions to be drawn from Sterne's 1964 study.

Sterne cited earlier studies as well as his own research findings on the hypothesis that boys from broken homes commit more offenses than boys from unbroken homes. Earlier studies included those of Breckinridge and Abbott, Weeks, and Slawson, all of whom found little difference in severity scores between delinquent boys from broken homes and delinquent boys from unbroken homes. Sterne found no support for this hypothesis, either, nor did he find that the type of home break was associated with the seriousness of the offense.

Conclusions and Clinical Implications

So what can we conclude about the relationship between father-absence and delinquency? Several theories of delinquency have been proposed and reviewed, including the Gluecks' (1956) theory of body type as related to delinquency; Miller's (1958) inclusion of Cohen's earlier speculations in a theory attributing the emergence of the lower-class street-corner group to the predominance of matriarchal households in this subculture; Aichorn's (1936) theory of impaired ego and superego development as being contributory to social mal-adjustment; Nye's (1958) social control theory that stressed the non-delinquent proclivity of small families that live in rural areas and attend church regularly; and Hetherington et al.'s (1971) theory of family types and specific delinquent behavior.

All the theories we have enumerated have their proponents and opponents, but what does solid research show? The effects of father-absence appear to relate to delinquent behavior mainly when we consider white middle-class males. But research conducted in this area seldom has been controlled, so it is difficult to determine whether this effect is one of fatherlessness per se or a sequel to the sociopsychiatric conditions under which father left. The one factor that does appear to have been well established is that there is a relationship between delinquent behavior and socioeconomic status—or at least between the reporting of delinquent behavior and socioeconomic status. Careful research in this area should clarify the myriad of conflicting theories that presently exist. If intervention is to be made for the purpose of curtailing delinquency, socioeconomic intervention probably would be the most fruitful course, with the most positive effects. Other clinical interventions might be useful with delinquents, but perhaps they become more effective to that very degree that they are "alloyed" with practical help for the delinquent and her or his family (Freud, 1919).

MENTAL DISORDER

Seligman et al. (1974) attributed mental illness among early adolescents to *parental deprivation,* a term that Howells (1970) dubbed a misnomer. *Mental illness* itself is a term that has been questioned by

Szasz (1974) and others. Howells and Layng (1955) suggested that children suffer emotionally just from being with their parents, and that separation can in fact be used therapeutically to allay the effects of harmful interactions. Proponents of "parentectomy" believe that removal of a child from noxious parents is indicated for asthmatic, antisocial, and numerous other disordered children. Hisop (1979) associated parental deprivation with irritable bowel syndrome. Munro and Griffiths (1968) suggested one must consider the "quality of deprivation" when assessing any deprivational effects. Other authors have asserted that "parental deprivation" is not associated with mental illness (Gregory, 1958, Langer, 1963; Pitts et. al., 1965; Munro, 1965; Koller & Williams, 1974; Kagel et al., 1978). The *Lancet* (1966) provided a review of the literature in this area, saying in essence that although some long-term effects have been identified, immediate effects of parental deprivation are still uncertain. Research to the present time may have cast a bit more light on this area, but at best the conclusions that may be drawn are only tentative. Michael Rutter's reviews in 1972 and 1979 concentrate on *maternal* deprivation but contain general caveats that should draw the close attention of the student of paternal deprivation. For example, intrafamilial conflict before the divorce may be more pathogenic than the switch to one parent only.

Another general term employed when describing paternal absence is *broken home*. It is as if a father can make or break a home. Hence, Newman and Schwam (1979) are two psychiatry professors who, in their discussion of "The Fatherless Child," concentrate on loss and mourning, keeping as their model the earlier most frequent form of father-absence, namely, the father's dying, even when they deal, outside the bereavement paradigm, with not "death, [but] separation of the parents (either prior to the birth or later), or severe psychological distancing from the family" (p. 357). Langner (1963) associated broken homes with mental disorder, as did many others before Langner. Douglas (1970) sensibly suggested that what happens after the break is a more important variable in the etiology of mental illness than is the break itself. This viewpoint coincides with that of Nye (1957), who argued that a good divorce is not as devastating to children in the home as is the family turmoil preceding or substituting for a divorce.

Petursson (1961) reckoned that psychiatric illness is due to a genetic predisposition coming under the influence of environmental factors, but omitted parental absence as a specified stressor. Losses may produce disorders other than neuroses, one suspects, and at times may produce no obvious disorder. Koller and Williams (1974) argued that if parental deprivation was high in the general population, it was still higher in abnormal populations. Cobliner (1963) wrote that among environmental factors exacerbating mental disorder, the principal one is a disruption in the family of orientation. This is related to social class, however. A physical separation from one's parent or parents becomes more harmful as the social-class ladder is descended. These results are questionable since we do not know whether it is physical separation or poverty that increases the risk of mental illness as socioeconomic status declines and economic deprivation worsens. Pitts et al. (1965) reported that both psychiatric illness and early parental death are found disproportionately often in the lower socioeconomic classes.

Kolvin et al. (1971a) noted that social class affects the type of psychiatric disorder manifested and that children with infantile psychoses tend to come from social classes I and II while children with late-onset psychoses come from social classes IV and V (Hollingshead & Redlich, 1954). Children with late-onset psychoses also tend more to have schizophrenic parents; that suggests an increased genetic influence as one descends the social ladder. To the extent that poverty diminishes one's survival chances, it may be seen as giving more force to hereditary influences.

Other authors have attributed psychiatric disturbance not to parental absence, nor to genetic factors, nor to socioeconomic status, but rather have blamed the quality of family relationships (Howells & Layng, 1955; Rutter, 1970; Kauffman, 1971; Parker, 1979). Howells and Layng (1955) wrote that children who are parentally deprived are children who are victims of inadequate parenting. Kauffman (1971) reported that emotionally disturbed, preadolescent boys perceive themselves more negatively within their family relationships and have stronger sibling rivalry than do nondisturbed controls. Rutter (1972) stated:

Whereas various patterns of child-rearing and parent-child separation are classed as low-risk factors, a child's family background is nevertheless a most important influence on his development. Of all the family variables that have been studied, discord, quarrelling, tension and disruption have been most consistently associated with disorder in the child. [p. 215]

Psychiatric disorder is a term referring to varied conditions and traits. Feelings of fear, dread, loneliness, depression, dissatisfaction, malaise, sexual unrest, and even alienation are rampant among modern children; those who have those feeling states are not necessarily mentally disordered. Yet there is suffering present in such children. As a convenience the epidemiologist takes a special interest only when such unhappy states afflict fewer than 10% of children, hallowing a statistical incidence as the way to divide sick from well, happy from unhappy. Beside incidence as a criterion, severity of signs or symptoms is another convenient yardstick to apply to children's sufferings: only those who suffer severely are considered to be truly disordered, "true cases."

Psychologists and psychiatrists have another convention among themselves when they deal with mental disorders in children, namely, dividing the children's problems into those that show a more or less stable underlying state, and those that change as the child's circumstances change—circumstances of growing and developing, circumstances of forming new friendships and new learning. The more durable markers are of *trait* and the less lasting markers are of *state*. To a degree, using *DSM-III,* the psychiatrist codes many of the more enduring features of children on the personality disorder axis, Axis II, but we are not permitted to have it easy so *DSM-III* also puts all the developmental disorders, some very serious and hardly treatable, on the same Axis II.

One of the general dimensions of the child's personality, predisposing but not truly indicative of disorder, is the self-concept. As we discussed in Chapter 1, the nuclear self-concept is laid down in its broad dimensions about the same time that the child learns core gender identity and, incidentally, at about the same time that the body image or body schema is constructed—between 16 and 30 months of age. The self-concept is one of the fundamental psychiatric facts. It is a composite of all of those feelings and attitudes that William James called the "sentiments of self-regard," a phenomenon that sparked renewed interest in psychiatrists thanks to Harry Stack Sullivan and his followers. Even the Freudian and Kleinian analysts are showing great fascination with the self since, under the rubric of a whole spectrum of narcissistic phenomena, they find the basic self-concept of deep importance and consequence in nearly all psycho-analytic therapy. Hence, the self-concept of fatherless children promises to be of general concern for all the mental health fields. We include only a small sampling of some of the work done on self-concept and fatherlessness here, prior to embarking on more specific diagnostic categories of mental disorder.

Fleck et al. (1980)—considering people much older than infants—administered part of a Parent Behavior form, plus a questionnaire about sexual experiences, an anxiety scale (The State-Trait Anxiety Inventory of Spielberger et al. 1970), and the Bem Sex-Role Inventory (Bem, 1974), to 160 females of college age, asking them about their recalled life situation when 16 years old. The finding that paternal warmth and acceptance at age 16 were correlated with *lessened* heterosexual activity when of college age agreed with earlier findings, but pulling together some findings relative to their "attractiveness to males"—hardly the acid test today of female self-acceptance—they discovered that their study group felt more attractive in association with their experience of holding hands, kissing, petting, coitus, frequent dating, frequent intercourse, and lower state anxiety in the dating situation. Falsification resulted for their hypothesis that those with high father acceptance would be more androgynous; insead those women were more *feminine* on the Bem inventory. Bannon and Southern (1980) did more, using 57 college women between ages 18 and 30 years, dividing them into four roughly equal, matched groups: 15 from father-present, intact homes; 15 whose fathers died early in their lives and who had no older brother; 15 whose parents divorced and who had no older brother; 12 whose parents had divorced and who had an older brother or brothers. Each woman was administered a self-concept scale and a questionnaire about her relations with men. They found surprisingly few differences among the four groups, save for the women who had difficulties in nurturant relations with male agemates, who showed significantly greater father-absence (without an older brother present). Self-concept differences existed at levels of significance only in respect to the social self subscale of the Tennessee Self-Concept Scale. Hence, any delayed or remote effects of fatherlessness on their opinions of themselves were not very potent among the women surveyed by Bannon and Southern.

With children themselves, and adolescents too, the picture of self-concept and fatherlessness needs, and has received, some qualification. Parish and Nunn (1981) and Parish and Taylor (1979) presented some updating reports on this topic. Parish and Nunn dealt with 132 late-elementary-school children who had lost father by death ($n = 20$) or divorce ($n = 112$), administering the Personal Attribute Inventory for Children, finding that children of divorce feel positively about themselves and in direct relation to their favorable opinions about mother, father, and stepfather while children from bereaved or intact families had their own opinions about themselves, in no consistent relation to their opinions about mother, father, or stepfather if present. Parish and Nunn commented that self-esteem, being fairly high on the Maslow hierarchy of motives, is eroded in children after divorce dependent on their having prior and more basic needs unmet. The autonomy of children was higher from bereaved families and from any family structure deemed "happy" by the children than from families after divorce. The authors judiciously observed, however:

> It would appear that both *family structure and process are important variables which may mediate autonomy. Further research is needed, however, to clarify other factors pertinent in this regard (e.g., parental warmth, socioeconomic variables, remarriage of parent).* [p. 107]

Parish and Taylor (1979) left rats and college students, the two most accessible populations for academic psychologists, and studied 406 midwestern elementary and junior-high-school students, ranging from third through eighth grades. After divorce, children's self-concepts lowered. Mother's remarriage improved them somewhat but highest self-concepts were found in children from nondivorced families. Does that show variation due to divorce or fatherlessness? Hedging in their interpretation that divorce = fatherlessness = lowered self-concept, these authors noted:

> *Divorce in actuality may not be the key variable which lowers self-concepts. . . . Individuals who have experienced the divorce of their parents could also frequently endure lowered socioeconomic conditions, the necessity of mothers working outside the home, the need for mothers to function as a solo parent without the support of a spouse in the home, etc. [p. 431]*

The reminder that fatherlessness or divorce may cover over more vital conditions than mere father-absence is useful, we feel. Also, tying more basic human values and motives to higher-order deficits seems opportune. That is in Maslow's tradition and part of his legacy: Physiologic needs must be met and feelings of security and belonging have to be implanted prior to heightening self-esteem or self-actualization. Was it not Brecht who had poor people chant, in *The Three Penny Opera*, "Give us bread before you offer us your morality"? Parish (1981) himself recently concluded, in a study done while he was a professor of psychology at Kansas State University, that "the longer one was raised without a father figure in the home, the more likely it was that he/she experienced depressed levels of moral judgment," and attributed the moral deficit not to father-absence alone but to the overall deprivation of resources and morale that may afflict the fatherless family. To us it would seem logical that deprived children would show impaired conscience and moral sense as well as ego injuries that show in impaired self-concepts.

Father-absence, specifically, has been associated with behavior problems in children (Biller, 1971, 1974), including encopresis (Schanegold, 1977; Bemporad et al., 1978) and night terrors (Herzog, 1980) and with complication of the decathexis process in adolescence (Oshman & Manosevitz, 1978). Kellam et al. (1977, 1979) reported on the basis of a longitudinal and community-wide study that mother-alone families were more at risk for social maladjustment and psychological malcontent of the child than were intact families. They qualified this finding, however, by indicating that it was not so much father's absence as mother's aloneness that seemed to germinate problems. In a later published study, using Cuban refugee and U.S. black subjects from an urban slum, Adams and Horovitz (1980) found (when race, social class, ordinal position, age, gender, and place of residence were controlled) that behavior problems were not associated with father-absence. "Moreover, the data seemingly indicate that poverty exerts a leveling influence that overrides the differentiating characteristics of ethnic and age grouping, family structure, father presence or absence, and linguistic and cultural heritages" (p. 135).

Again we see the imperative to control for multiple variables in assessing the effects of father-absence on, in this case, psychiatric disorder. The need to control for the following factors, in addition to those enumerated above, has been verified in the existent research: length of father-absence (Trunnel, 1968), age at time of father-absence (Rutter, 1970; Trunnel, 1968), number and sex of siblings (Kauffman, 1971), and type of father-absence (Gregory, 1958). Gregory, in a review of the literature on parental absence current to that time, criticized existing research for containing: "1. Comparisons between unlike samples, 2. Unrepresentative samples due to selection, 3. Chance errors in sampling, 4. Fallacies in deduction" (p. 440). That disapprobation of existing literature might still hold in some recent cases.

Specific Psychiatric Disorders

Psychoneuroses. Specific research regarding the correlation of disorders with father-absence concerns the psychoneuroses generally, including depression and suicidal behavior; and schizophrenia, including paranoia. Some authors implicate the broken home as a causative factor in the development of psychoneuroses (Madow & Hardy, 1947; Oltman, 1952; Petursson, 1961). Madow and Hardy (1947), who reviewed the literature current to that time, revealed that few, if any, statistical studies had inspected the actual percentages of broken families among groups suffering neuroses. On the basis of their study with neurotic soldiers, however, they concluded that the broken home *is* a contributing factor to the existence of neuroses in these young men prior to their entering the service.

Petursson (1961) noted that in a population of 439 psychiatric patients only 11.4% came from intact homes. Nonintact homes included those psychologically broken (with high parental discord and conflict) as well as those physically broken. Of the 190 psychoneurotic patients, only 32% came from physically broken homes—an insignificant number considering Munro's (1965) statistic that 46.7%

of the population at large come from broken homes. Howells and Layng (1955) and Howells (1970), who distinguished between psychologically broken homes and physically broken homes, found that physical separation of the child from the parent is not incriminated in the genesis of psychoneurosis.

Howells and Layng (1956a) suggested instead that a poor standard of mothering is causative of neurosis. They reported a tendency to allege harmful effects of separation when the child is under 2 years old and the separation is sustained longer than 2 weeks. The effects are temporary, however, as these children, separated when their age was under 2 years, tend to forget their parents and adjust to new adults. Oltman (1952) found that when comparing different psychiatric disorders, incidence of parental deprivation and broken homes is very similar among individuals suffering from dementia praecox, manic-depressive psychosis, alcoholic state, and "other psychosis" and in normal controls. However, the incidence is significantly higher among *psychoneurotics* and *psychopathic personalities*.

Other authors attribute psychoneuroses to genetic factors (Petursson, 1961) and constitutional components (Lourie, 1967). Petursson (1961) observed the frequency with which patients exhibited the same specific psychiatric disorders as had their parents, lending credibility to a theory of a genetic loading exacerbated by environmental conditions. Squaring psychoanalytic views with research by Chess and Thomas on temperament, Lourie (1967) proposed that there were certain instincts, organically and physiologically determined, which underlie every stage of personality development. These instincts (drives) are involved in homeostasis and metabolism; they are varied quantitatively and qualitatively within each individual, resulting in a unique configuration of constitutional components. The three categories of drives that Lourie invoked were: "instinct" for self preservation, "instinct" for race preservation, and instincts that he called aggressive drives. Constitutional components involved in the execution of these instincts are: activity level, intensity of response, level of sensory threshold, distractibility, persistence and attention span, and adaptability to change in routine. These components may be identified and evaluated in infants, the author suggested. Identification of early developmental cues may be utilized in the prevention of neuroses.

The studies reported here give some indication of the research done for this area. However, we must note, at the risk of overstating our case, that methodological errors run rampant in these studies. When parental absence is considered, frequently the sex of the absent parent is not even noted; much less are race, socioeconomic status, educational level, sibling composition, ordinal position, and other variables controlled. Madow and Hardy (1947) corroborated that there is a correlation between broken homes and low socioeconomic level and suggested that broken homes were associated with the emergence of neurosis. Howells and Layng (1956a) and Madow and Hardy (1947) noted the importance of the child's age at time of separation. Perhaps the most glaring error observed in studies using psychiatric patients is their failure to utilize a control group of normals. A survey of a neurotic or psychotic group is not very instructive unless we know how they compare to a normal or unselected or comparison group.

Depression. Some authors indicated that early parental loss is involved in the emergence of depression (Munro, 1966; Caplan & Douglas, 1969; Susz & Marberg, 1978). Munro (1966) compared a psychiatrically hospitalized population with a control group of general hospital outpatients, concluding that severe depressives are more likely and moderately severe depressives are *less* likely to have lost a parent by death before their sixteenth birthday as compared to general hospital outpatient controls. Caplan and Douglas (1969) found a relationship between early (before 8 years) object loss and later depression in children, although they did not differentiate the severity of the depression. They found that parental deprivation was more frequent among nondepressed neurotics than in the general population and still more frequent among depressed neurotics than among nondepressed neurotics. That is a move in the right direction.

Several studies implicate early maternal loss more than paternal loss in the causation of psychiatric illness generally (Earle & Earle, 1961) and depression specifically (Spitz, 1946; Haworth, 1964; Munro, 1966). Although interesting, these studies deal more with motherlessness than with fatherlessness so they will not be evaluated here. Hopkinson and Reed (1966), in replicating Brown's study with manic-depressives, found that parental deprivation in childhood was not a significant etiological factor in manic-depressive psychosis. The difference between their findings and Brown's was explained, they held, by the diagnostic criteria used. There are indications that manic-depressive psychosis is more strictly genetic in nature than is neurotic depression. There are fewer studies specifically devoted to father-absence in determining the onset of depression. Munro (1966) found that severe depressives, as compared with controls, reported a highly significant excess of disturbed relationships with both mother and father during childhood. He also found indications that depressives as a whole are more likely than normals to have lost a father by death from 11 to 15 years old, but this finding was not statistically significant. In this area of scholarly work, statistical significance is a must but, even so, it does not always accompany clinical significance.

Suicidal Behavior. Suicidal behavior has been associated with disorganized family structure (Bigras, Gauthier, et al, 1966; Bruhn, 1962), including broken homes (Dorpat et al., 1965; Winn & Halla, 1966), and with father separation (Winn & Halla, 1966). Bigras, Gauthier, et al. (1966) noted merely that in a sampling of adolescent girls who attempted suicide, 50% came from disorganized family structures. That was no more than should be expected. The precipitating event was in most cases a conflict with the parents. Bigras and Gauthier associated the suicidal behavior with paternal deprivation because father most often was passive and dominated by mother; she tended to be either overtly rejecting or cold and rigid. Bruhn (1962) distinguished the broken homes of psychiatric patients who had attempted suicide from the broken homes of psychiatric patients who had not attempted suicide by characterizing the former as containing a higher degree of marital disharmony. Feuding families lead adolescents to suicide, and we see that clinically, too. Dorpat et al. (1965) found that the majority of two populations, one having attempted suicide, and one having completed suicide, had come from broken homes. Death of a parent was the highest cause of broken homes among the completed suicides; divorce of parents was the highest cause of broken homes among the attempted suicides. In fact, though, it was only in 1965 that the major cause of broken homes changed from widowing to divorcing, so it would be difficult to assert that suicide attempters and completers differed significantly from the overall population in a decade of pivotal change.

Bunch and Barraclough (1971) commented on the frequency with which suicides occur within a month of their fathers' death anniversaries. Women were found to be more likely to kill themselves within 30 days of both their fathers' and mothers' death anniversaries.

Winn and Halla (1966) reported the following statistics for 70 children who had threatened or attempted suicide before reaching 15 years of age:

8% were from intact families

25% were illegitimate

50% had never known their real fathers

75% were not living with their real fathers at the time of admission to the psychiatric facility

15% had suffered permanent loss of a parent or parent surrogate by death

85% had experienced prolonged separation from a parent or parents

These 70 children were predominantly black or Puerto Rican and came largely from families in the lower socioeconomic strata. Over half came from the slum areas of New York City. We do not know what part the various factors contributed to their suicidal behavior.

Gertrude White-Coleman (1979) studied all suicides in Jefferson County, Kentucky, with findings that—whether fathered or fatherless—young males *completed* suicide more than females, and young females made more *attempts* than males; adolescents who attempted or completed suicide typically felt they could not talk with their parent or parents but were under the stress of trying to do so, even to meet the needs and demands of their parents. Her findings echoed many earlier ones that showed feelings of estrangement or isolation from parents to be a stress leading young people to suicide.

Schizophrenia. Schizophrenia has been attributed to heredity (Rosenthal, et al., 1971) in conjunction with environmental factors (Kety et al., 1971; Lidz, et al., 1958); to father-absence (Heacock, 1968; DaSilva, 1963; Huttunen & Niskanen, 1978); and to inadequate fathering (Lidz et al., 1956; DaSilva, 1963); to pathology in mother (Heilbrun & Norbert, 1971); and to disturbed family relationships between mother and child (DaSilva, 1963) and between mother and father (Lidz, et al., 1954), or to the pathologic communication patterns in the family group (Wynne & Singer, in Usdin, 1975). Lidz, et al. (1956) wrote that few fathers of schizophrenic patients have filled the paternal role usually expected in middle- and upper-class families, and that many of the fathers exerted seriously pathogenic influences on the family structure and the rearing of children. Lidz and his co-workers described three types of fathers of schizophrenic patients, one of these the passive father who is a nonentity in the home. DaSilva (1963) stated that the absence of the father, whether it be physical absence (through death, divorce, or long separation) or emotional absence (through lack of involvement), appears to contribute significantly to the schizophrenic illness of the son. Much like Meerloo (1968), DaSilva perceived the function of the father as being the cutting of the umbilical cord that was symbiotically uniting mother and son. If there is no father present, a surrogate father is needed to perform this figurative rite. He noted how in therapy the patient's father and the therapist are perceived by the schizophrenic child as depriving maternal figures, and a struggle ensues to obtain from father and the therapist excessive recompenses for the deprivation suffered.

It has been noted that both reactive and process schizophrenics demonstrate significantly less father and ideal-father identification than do normal control subjects. But no differences appear between the two schizophrenic groups on these measures. Heilbrun and Norbert (1971) noticed that the differences that *do* emerge between reactive and process male schizophrenics are in terms of their method of adapting to the behavior of the high control–low nurture (HC–LN) mother. Since it was mother, not father, who was highlighted, we leave that work.

Summary

Thus, we see that paternal absence has been associated with psychiatric illness generally. We do not know, however, whether the etiology of mental unhealth is more closely related to family discord preceding and/or following paternal absence, or to the poverty that often accompanies father's absence, or a combination of the above.

We do know that the incidence of psychiatric disorder increases as the social ladder descends. Whether this is an accurate measure of some of the consequences of poverty or the function of our definitions of *normal* and *abnormal* is uncertain. Thomas Szasz thought that the very concept of psychiatric disorder with its accompanying escalations of classifications of psychiatric disease was nothing more than a political weapon, used disproportionately often against poor people, women, blacks, and other oppressed groups.

Father-absence, specifically, has been associated with behavior problems in children. Although behavior disturbance has been commonly accepted as a repercussion of father-absence by some, it has been found that when other variables are controlled this cause–effect relationship does not hold true.

Parental deprivation, including inadequate parenting, has been associated with particular psychoneuroses, including depression and suicidal behavior, with diagnoses of psychopathic personality, and with schizophrenia. In studying schizophrenics there is a general proclivity to implicate mothers more than fathers, regardless of whether the latter are present or absent. In fact, no single form of psychopathology can be proven to be associated with father-absence at the present time.

CHAPTER SEVEN

Review of Research

This chapter, intended for researchers interested in fatherless children, offers both a summary of the directions taken by outstanding researches already published and a body of directions that seem most fruitful for future work.

The bulk of this chapter tabulates the main studies considered in Chapters 5 and 6, as a way to help the interested reader locate studies that focus on variables of particular interest as well as the methods and techniques then adopted. Relevant studies may be traced by a rapid scanning of the tables using the key affixed to them. Following this tabular material, the chapter summarizes some practical suggestions that we make about research on fatherless children. Concluding this chapter are brief considerations of the varied and complex research instruments—"tests and measurements"—used to study fatherless children that have not been described adequately in other parts of this book.

KEY TO TABLES

I. Characteristics of Children (Adolescent/Young Adult) Studied (Variables Specified or Controlled)

1. Age
2. Behavioral characteristics of child; temperament
3. Body type
4. IQ of child
5. Occupation of father/mother/other
6. Personality dimensions of child
7. Physical appearance
8. Preexisting pathology or juvenile offense
9. Race or ethnicity
10. Religion
11. SES (socioeconomic status)
12. Sex
13. Other

II. Family and Household Features (Variables Specified or Controlled)

14. Age of siblings
15. Family constellation: who are the adults in household?
16. Geographical location
17. Head of household: Stepfather/other male ever?
18. Main decisionmaker in household
19. Main wage earner in household
20. Maternal punishment history
21. Most influential adult
22. Number of siblings
23. Ordinal position of child studied
24. Paternal punishment history
25. Self-concept of child
26. Sex of siblings
27. Social isolation
28. Other

III. Characteristics Specific to Absent Father (Variables Specified or Controlled)

29. Age at which father left and/or duration of absence
30. Father present or absent
31. Number of contacts between child and absent father
32. Type of father absence: unspecified
33. Type of father-absence: death
34. Type of father-absence: desertion
35. Type of father-absence: divorce
36. Type of father-absence: separation
37. Type of father-absence: temporary separation from parent or child
38. Other

IV. Research Design (Specified/Interpreted by Author)

Characteristics of Sample:
39. Thirty or more in study sample
40. Control group of similar age, either matched or highly comparable

Time Dimension of Study:
41. Cross-sectional study
42. Longitudinal study
43. Decade studied: 1920s
44. Decade studied: 1930s
45. Decade studied: 1940s
46. Decade studied: 1950s
47. Decade studied: 1960s
48. Decade studied: 1970s
49. Decade studied: 1980+
50. Other or unspecified

Type of Study or Sample:
51. Book review
53. Case study
52. Case control
54. Cluster
55. Comparative
56. Correlation
57. Dependent
58. Descriptive
59. Essay
60. Factor analysis
61. Independent
62. Matched pairs
63. Large
64. Proportional

65. Quota
66. Random
67. Regression analysis
68. Repeated
69. Representative
70. Review of literature
71. Small
72. Stratified
73. Systematic
74. Other

Instrument Used:
75. Attitudinal
76. Behavioral
77. Questionnaire/survey
78. Standardized test/checklist/scale
79. Interview
80. Case studies/family histories
81. Records
82. Other

Individual Participating or Completing Information:
83. Child
84. Parent/primary caretaker
85. Other family member
86. Teacher/school counselor
87. Social service worker or other professional
88. Researcher
89. Other

Table 7.1. Academic Performance

Research Emphasis and Findings	I	II	III	IV
Albert, R. S. (1971)				
Paper reports an analysis of descriptions of children with IQs of 155 or better; distinguishes between gifted and exceptionally gifted groups; findings are discussed in terms of how certain parent–child relationships might contribute to the development of cognitive giftedness into high levels of creative behavior.	Secondary analysis (4, 43, 44, 58, 74)			
Becker, S. (1974)				
Asks the question whether children who have experienced father-absence will be more creative than children who have not experienced father absence; subjects divided into three groups according to family structure and to perception of parental influence and tested for fluency, flexibility and originality; most significant finding was that mother-influenced subjects, whether father was absent or present, were superior to father-influenced subjects in all three areas of creativity; contains review of literature.	13	21	30	39, 41, 55, 70, 74, 77, 78
Bernstein, B. E. (1976)				
Research shows that the effect of father-absence manifests itself as early as age 11 and is more pronounced among girls; analysis shows a sex difference—for boys, math skills were insignificantly affected by father absence; for girls, father-absence significantly depressed math scores relative to verbal scores.	13	16	30	39, 41, 55, 78, 83

Table 7.1. *(continued)*

Research Emphasis and Findings	I	II	III	IV

Bronfenbrenner, U. (1967)

Review of the literature indicates serious inadequacies experienced in school by disadvantaged children, especially black youth, which find their origins primarily in parental damage, father-absence, impoverished home environment, and dysfunctional patterns of child rearing; paper attempts to show that all these considerations apply with even greater force when the costs of equality and inequality are reckoned with in psychological rather than economic terms.

Review of Literature (70)

Burnes, K. (1970)

WISC test was administered to black and white boys from lower-class and upper-middle-class homes in order to determine group patterns of intellectual ability; results indicate significant differences among subtest scores—lower-class subjects of both races obtaining lower scores; a few differences in patterns are found between SES groups, not between races.

I: 1, 4, 5, 9, 11

IV: 39, 40, 41, 50, 55, 74, 78, 81, 88

Carlsmith, L. (1964)

Paper reports results of an investigation of effects of father-absence on young boys (with normal home life except for temporary absence of father during World War II) on patterns of math and verbal aptitude scores that subjects later attain on college entrance exams; findings related to sex identification theory.

I: 1, 5, 13

II: 15, 23, 28

III: 29, 30, 37, 38

IV: 39, 40, 41, 47, 55, 78, 81, 88

Table 7.1. (continued)

Research Emphasis and Findings	I	II	III	IV
Chapman, M. (1977)				
Assessed the effects of father-absence and stepfathers on cognitive performance; results concurred with earlier findings of greater field dependence and lower SAT scores in father-absent males but indicated that the presence of a stepfather was associated with attenuation of this effect; failed to find father-absence effects in females.	13	14, 15, 17, 26, 28	29, 30, 33, 35	39, 41, 56, 74, 77, 78, 83, 88
Collier, L., et al. (1973)				
Purpose of this study was to ascertain which of the following was most affected by the condition of father-absence or father-presence: IQ, achievement, self-concept, or personality; no significant differences indicated therefore the null hypothesis was not rejected; implications arising from this study suggest the need for further study of the effect of father-absence on black adolescents and that general assumptions cannot be made at the present time.	4, 13		30	39, 41, 55, 66, 79, 81, 83
Collins, M. A. (1969)				
Study compared standardized and teacher-rated reading and math achievement, intelligence, classroom behavior, absence mobility, personality and adult ideals of black children from father-present and father-absent homes in order to determine significant relationships among family composition, sex and these variables; no significant differences found between intact and broken homes; there were a number of sex differences indicated.	2, 4, 12	15		39, 40, 41, 55, 58, 77, 81, 83, 85

Table 7.1.   (*continued*)

Research Emphasis and Findings	I	II	III	IV
Duke, M. P., and Lancaster, W. (1976)				
Subjects from father-present and father-absent homes were administered the Nowicki-Strickland locus of control scale for preschool and primary-grade children (PPNSIE): results indicate that the father-absent group was significantly more external than the controls.		15	30	39, 41, 55, 75, 78, 88
Eisenstadt, J. M. (1978)				
A scientific theory is proposed to account for the historically eminent individual or genius by relating his or her development to loss of parents; a parental loss profile is described and a study of 699 eminent persons using this profile is reported.	Secondary analysis (74)			
Fowler, P. C., and Richards, H. C. (1978)				
Predictions of academic deficits due to early and continuing parental absence, as derived from Zajonc's and Markus's confluence model, were investigated; comparison of pairs (one father-present, one father-absent) suggests that father-presence facilitates the math performance of girls more than boys; results only partially support the confluence model predictions.	9, 11, 12	15, 22	29, 30	39, 40, 41, 56, 81, 86, 87
Henderson, E. H., and Long, B. H. (1973)				
Hypothesized that expectancies of teachers about academic performance have important effects upon pupils; study is second in a line of research directed toward such questions as: Do teachers expect less from black children?; discussion states that while racism exists among both black and white teachers, this study renders support for remedial programs.				39, 74, 75, 82, 86

225

Table 7.1. *(continued)*

Research Emphasis and Findings	I	II	III	IV
Herzog, J. D. (1974)				
Article focuses on relationships between father-absence and school performance among a sample of boys from Barbados; results fail to demonstrate the supposed "unmistakable influence" of father-absence; examples of findings—father-present boys do better in conforming to school's routine expectations, father-absent boys do better on novel tasks.	2, 4, 9, 11, 12, 13	15, 28	29	39, 41, 47, 55, 75, 76, 78, 81, 86
Jackson, R. M., and Meara, N. M. (1977)				
Study concerns the relationship between the adequacy of the father as an identification model and the achievement and occupational behavior of economically deprived rural male adolescents; statistically significant differences found with regard to the variables studied.	1, 12, 13	16, 28	30, 31, 35, 37, 38	39, 40, 42, 55, 76, 80, 89
Koch, M. B. (1961)				
Study compares two groups of normal nonproblem preschool children, one group from homes broken by divorce and the other from intact homes, on the basis of responses to a projective test of anxiety and the home situation as surveyed by interview methods; significantly higher anxiety scores existed for the broken home group; major differences between parents of group members were in attitudes toward the responsibility of child rearing.	1, 2, 4	14, 15, 26	30, 35	40, 62, 76, 78, 79, 83, 84, 89

Landy, F. et al. (1969)

Paper examines the effects of father night-shift work on the quantitative performance of 100 females; results indicate that children under age 9 were negatively affected.

Descriptive study (12, 29, 30, 38, 39, 41, 58, 78, 83)

Table 7.1. *(continued)*

Research Emphasis and Findings	I	II	III	IV
Lessing, E. et al. (1970)				
Purpose of this study was to determine the cognitive correlates of prolonged father absence as portrayed in WISC subtest and IQ scores; findings were discussed in terms of two explanatory hypotheses relating the effects of father-absence both to stress and to the loss of male identification model.	1, 4, 5, 11	15, 17	30	39, 47, 74, 78, 83
Lifshitz, M. A. (1976)				
Attempt made to assess what links family structure, cognitive processes, and social behavior; assessed relationships among family structure, social perception of self, parental figures, and social milieu and their behavioral integration in the classroom; all subjects described themselves as different from parents.	9, 11, 13	15, 22, 28	29, 30, 33	39, 41, 60, 62, 78, 79, 85
Mackie, J. B. et al. (1974)				
Study examines the influence that black fathers may or may not have on the intellectual development of their children in kindergarten and first grade; results indicate that fathers have less influence than many investigators would have us believe; also indicates that preschool education enhances the intellectual abilities of boys, but not of girls.	5, 9, 11, 12, 13	15, 17, 28	30	39, 41, 55, 79, 84
Martindale, C. (1972)				
Ratings of degree of psychopathology and of probability of cross-sexual identification were made on temporarily stratified samples of 42 eminent English and French poets; found that psychopathology and cross-sexual identification were highly related.	Content analysis (8, 30, 39, 50, 72, 74)			

227

Table 7.1. (*continued*)

Research Emphasis and Findings	I	II	III	IV

Maxwell, A. E. (1961)

	I	II	III	IV
Means, standard deviations, correlations, and factor loadings for a sample of children attending a psychiatric clinic are reported for the subtests of the WISC and the results are compared with the normative data given in the WISC manual and with normal British children; mean scores for psychiatric sample were found to be lower than those for normal children; a few associations between cognitive test scores and a number of "psychiatric" variables were demonstrated—the lack of a father in the home tended to have an adverse affect on children's performance on some WISC subtests.	2, 4, 8, 12, 13	28	29, 30, 33, 35	39, 41, 46, 56, 60, 76, 81, 88

Miller, R. (1977)

	I	II	III	IV
Report represents the first stage of an ongoing longitudinal study; investigates the development of competence in infants and preschool children with the goal of contributing toward the construction of a theory of educability based on "laws" of optimal development.	2			39, 42, 55, 56, 58, 76, 78, 88

Mischel, W. (1961)

	I	II	III	IV
Article explores the relationship between a person's choice preferences for immediate, smaller reinforcement as opposed to delayed, larger reinforcement and his or her motive systems; expected significant positive relationships between preference for delayed reinforcement and no achievement were found.	1, 9, 12, 13			39, 41, 55, 76, 77, 83, 88

Table 7.1. *(continued)*

Research Emphasis and Findings	I	II	III	IV
Moffitt, T. E. (1981)				
Results of scores from the vocabulary and arithmetic subtests of the WISC were analyzed for 60 Danish boys. Previous studies had indicated that boys with absent fathers demonstrated greater verbal skills than math skills, a reversal of the traditional male pattern. Although no such reversal was found in this sample as a whole, high-SES subjects did tend to display this reversal while lower-SES subjects did not.	1, 11, 12	15, 17	29, 30, 31, 33, 34, 35, 36, 37	39, 40, 42, 49, 56, 78, 79, 80, 83, 87, 88
Mumbauer, C. C., and Miller, J. O. (1970)				
A battery of tests was administered to two groups of 4-year-old children; results supported the hypothesis that culturally disadvantaged preschool children would be less efficient in intellectual performance than advantaged children of the same age.	1, 4, 5, 11, 12			39, 40, 41, 55, 78, 88
Nelsen, E. A., and Maccoby, E. E. (1966)				
This article investigates hypotheses centering around sex typing and the interfering effects of certain tension-producing experiences upon cognitive processes; answers to questionnaire analyzed in relation to differential verbal and math abilities; example of findings indicates that for boys, a high-verbal, low-math pattern was associated with reports of father-absence.		15, 20, 24	30, 38	39, 41, 46, 47, 55, 75, 77, 78, 81, 83

Table 7.1. *(continued)*

Research Emphasis and Findings	I	II	III	IV
Parish, T. S., and Copeland, T. F. (1979)				
Study consists of 206 male and female college students who filled out evaluative surveys for each of the following targets: "yourself," "mother," "father," or "stepfather"; students from intact families were found to have self-concepts that were significantly correlated with how they evaluated their mothers and fathers; students from father-absent families tended to demonstrate self-concepts that were significantly correlated with how they evaluated mothers and stepfathers (not natural fathers).		15, 17, 25, 28	30	39, 41, 56, 75, 83, 88
Richards, H. C., and McCandless, B. R. (1972)				
Data for this study were gathered over a 3-year period from more than 300 black and white prekindergarteners in poor, urban neighborhoods in Atlanta; a correlation matrix was generated from the data and factor-analyzed; results were interpreted to mean that coping by withdrawal indicates personality maladjustment and interferes with verbal facility.	1, 5, 9, 11	15, 22, 23, 28	30	39, 42, 47, 56, 60, 76, 78, 81, 83, 86
Roach, D. A. (1980)				
Four hundred and eighteen elementary-school children from Jamaica were examined in an attempt to establish their preference for conceptual style. The Conceptual Style Index and a questionnaire were administered. Analytic conceptual style was significantly and positively correlated with SES for girls but not for boys.	1, 11, 12	15, 17	29, 30, 31, 33, 34, 35, 36, 37	39, 40, 42, 49, 56, 78, 79, 80, 83, 87, 88

Table 7.1. *(continued)*

Research Emphasis and Findings	I	II	III	IV

Rouman, J. (1956)

Findings and conclusions based on case studies of schoolchildren in Los Angeles County; example of conclusions—working mothers contribute to only one-fourth of the number of cases in need of psychological help.

Case study (1, 2, 5, 6, 12, 13, 15, 17, 23, 39, 41, 53, 58, 80, 88)

Santrock, J. W., and Tracy, R. L. (1978)

The possibility that teacher ratings of children may indicate a stereotype on the part of teachers was investigated by showing 30 teachers a videotape that focused on the social interaction of an 8-year-old boy; the Bonferroni multiple-comparisons procedure indicates that teachers rated the divorced child more negatively on the following three variables reflecting affective state or relations: happiness, emotional adjustment, and coping with stress.

Descriptive study (6, 39, 58, 76, 82, 89)

Stodolsky, S. S., and Lesser, G. (1967)

Includes review of the literature on learning patterns in the disadvantaged; a specific case of research is included that examines the patterns among various mental abilities in 6- and 7-year-old children from different social class and ethnic backgrounds.

Descriptive study (9, 11, 13, 58)

Sutherland, H. (1930)

Purpose of paper is to study the connection between size of family and intelligence of children, specifically fatherless children, with the intention of separating hereditary from environmental factors; two groups of fatherless children were compared with control groups; in both cases the average intelligence of fatherless children was less and there was slightly less correlation between intelligence and family size.

I	II	III	IV
4	15, 22	29, 30	39, 41, 55, 56, 81, 88

Table 7.1. (continued)

Research Emphasis and Findings	I	II	III	IV
Sutton-Smith, B. et al. (1968)				
Effects of father-absence for varying lengths of time and varying growth periods are compared with the effects of father-presence, as reflected in college entrance scores on the ACE; generally father-absence has a depressive effect with the greatest effects during the early and middle years; boys without brothers more affected; also girls with a younger brother and only girls more affected than only boys.	12	15, 22, 23, 26	29, 30	39, 41, 55, 78, 81, 83, 88

Table 7.2. Sex-Role Identification

Research Emphasis and Findings	I	II	III	IV
Andrews, R. O., and Christensen, H. T. (1951)				
Present study uses the Winch measure of degree of courtship behavior and analyzes it in regard to its relationship to parental loss and courtship status; results appear to contradict the earlier findings of Winch who found the degree of courtship behavior to be retarded in males with absent father; present study points to the direction of an accelerated courtship for both sexes when the father is absent.	1, 10, 12, 13	15, 28	29, 30	39, 41, 46, 55, 62, 74, 80, 83, 88

232

Table 7.2. (*continued*)

Research Emphasis and Findings	I	II	III	IV
Biller, H. B. (1969)				
Matched father-absent and father-present kindergarten-age boys were studied in order to ascertain the effects of father-absence and degree of maternal encouragement of masculine behavior on boys' sex-role development; father-present boys were found to be much more masculine in projective sex-role orientation and slightly more masculine in game preference but were not significantly different in terms of a rating scale measure of covert masculinity.	1, 4, 9, 11	22, 26	30, 35, 36	39, 40, 41, 55, 62, 77, 78, 83, 84, 88
Boss, P. G. (1980)				
One hypothesis of this study is that wives of missing husbands (MIAs) whose personal qualities are androgynous will be more likely to reorganize and take over the missing father's roles than will those wives who are not androgynous. Results indicated that androgyny per se is not significantly related to psychological father-presence in MIA wives. However, both androgyny and psychological father-presence are significantly related to wife/family dysfunction, but in different ways.	13	15, 17	30, 37	39, 42, 48, 60, 75, 77, 78, 79, 84, 88
Brim, O. G. (1958)				
Article reports some relations among ordinal position, sex of sibling and sex-role learning by children in two-child families; findings based on further analysis of Koch's data relating personality traits of children to their sex, sex of sibling, ordinal position, and age difference from siblings; hypothesizes that cross-sex siblings will have more traits of the opposite sex than will same-sex siblings and that this effect will be greater for the younger, as contrasted with the older sibling.	2, 6, 9, 12, 13	14, 15, 23, 26		39, 40, 41, 58, 76, 78, 88

Table 7.2. (continued)

Research Emphasis and Findings	I	II	III	IV

Brown, D. G. (1956)

Present study represents an attempt to investigate and analyze the nature and extent of young children's preference for objects and activities characteristic of their own or opposite sex; findings include: (a) Large and significant differences occur between sexes, suggesting dichotomous sex-role patterns in young children; (b) a number of children showed a mixed preference pattern (tendency twice as frequent in girls); (c) some children showed a strong opposite-sex-role preference (also more common in girls).

Descriptive study (1, 5, 39, 41, 58, 78, 83, 88)

Burton, R. V., and Whiting, J. W. M. (1961)

This article presents evidence of the effect of the father's position in the family as it relates to the growing child's learning by identification and to the development of his or her sex identity; also hypothesizes that in societies with maximum conflict in sex identity, there will be initiation rites at puberty that will function to resolve this conflict in identity (hypothesis confirmed by the data); contains literature review.

Cross-cultural study (58, 70, 74)

Colletta, N. D. (1979)

Focused on differences in child-rearing practices of married and divorced mothers as a function of father-absence or as a condition of low income. Results indicated that income is a key factor in that child-rearing practices were more restrictive and demanding at the lower but not at the higher income levels.	5, 9, 10, 12, 13	15, 17, 22, 26, 28	30, 35	39, 48, 55, 78, 79, 88

Table 7.2. (*continued*)

Research Emphasis and Findings	I	II	III	IV
Colley, T. (1959)				
Attempt was made in this paper to construct a theoretical formulation that will be helpful in understanding and describing the nature and origins of sex identity; emphasis placed upon the part that both parental figures play in responding differentially to the child in terms of sexual identity; child then carries this differential of expectation into his or her interactions with others in later life.	Theoretical paper (74)			
Covell, K., and Turnbull, K. (1982)				
In a study of 173 male college students, it was found that male students with a history of father-absence are neither less masculine nor more feminine than those from two-parent families.	1, 9, 11, 12, 13	15, 17	29, 30, 33, 35, 37	39, 41, 49, 74, 75, 77, 78, 80, 82, 83, 88
Deaton, H. S. (1979)				
Analytic intervention in the life of a girl growing up in a chaotic environment (Freudian interpretation).	Case study (53)			
Epstein, A. S., and Radin, N. (1975)				
Interpersonal and task motivations were related to observed paternal behavior and cognitive functioning in 4-year-old white children; sex and social class differences were found; for all boys, motivation was an intervening variable between paternal behavior and the son's intellectual performance.	2, 4, 5, 11, 12, 13	24		39, 41, 56, 74, 79, 83, 84, 87

Table 7.2. (*continued*)

Research Emphasis and Findings	I	II	III	IV

Eysenck, H. J. (1971)

Purpose of study is to utilize the methodology of Terman and Associates to find out if differences exist on the Maudsley Sex Inventory between men and women similar in kind to those observed within a given sex between men (or women) scoring high or low on a psychoticism scale; support furnished for the view that the psychoticism scale appears to be closely related with the masculinity–feminity dimension.	6, 12, 13			39, 55, 69, 75, 78, 88

Fleck, J. R., et al. (1980)

Proposed that the psychological absence of the father is related to a higher frequency and extent of heterosexual behaviors, increased anxiety as personality trait, and increased anxiety in a dating situation. A positive psychological presence of the father was hypothesized to correlate with androgyny in adolescent females. Results indicated a significant relationship between father psychological absence and more frequent heterosexual behaviors as well as a personality trait.	1, 5, 9, 10, 11, 12, 13	14, 15, 17, 22, 23, 26, 28	29, 30, 31, 32	39, 40, 41, 74, 76, 77, 78, 79, 83

Gershansky, I. S., et al (1978)

The relationship between mother's and children's levels of psychological differentiation as measured by the Rod and Frame Test and the effects of onset and nature of father's absence on this relationship were explored for 209 children between the ages of 8 and 16 years and their mothers; significantly higher correlations between the scores of children whose fathers were absent from home and their mothers.	8, 9	15	29, 30, 33, 34, 35	39, 41, 74, 78, 83, 88

Table 7.2. (*continued*)

Research Emphasis and Findings	I	II	III	IV

Giele, J. Z. (1971)

Author states that change in the family demographic trends, and new consciousness about sex roles are linked; sex-role changes will require a much larger step from older generations and people unfamiliar and unsympathetic with these trends; if people can be shown that liberation of men and women is not a wild idea, then it is only a matter of time until we shall see further change of remarkable proportions; contains a literature review.

Theoretical paper (70, 74)

Goldstein, H. S., and Gershansky, I. (1976)

Study of the relationship between children's perceptual differentiation as measured by the Rod and Frame Test (RFT) and their self-concept differentiation as evidenced in their human figure drawings using a body sophistication scale; study utilizes a clinic population; relationship between perceptual differentiation and self-concept differentiation was significantly positive only for white females with a present father.

4, 9, 13   15, 25   29, 30   39, 41, 56, 78, 83, 88

Goldstein, H. S., and Peck, R. (1973)

Paper explored the effects of father-absence and mother's cognitive style on the cognitive differentiation of their children; aspect of cognitive differentiation examined was extent of field dependence, which was assessed by Rod and Frame Test; father-present black males and females and father-present white males were significantly positively correlated with their mother's level of differentiation, whereas none of the father-absent subgroups was.

8, 9, 12   15   29, 30   39, 41, 55, 66, 74, 78, 83, 84, 88

Table 7.2.   (continued)

Research Emphasis and Findings	I	II	III	IV
Herzog, J. D. (1974)				
Article focuses on relationships between father-absence and school performance among a sample of boys from Barbados; results fail to demonstrate the supposed "unmistakable influence" of father absence; example of findings—father-present boys do better in conforming to school's routine expectations; father-absent boys do better on novel tasks.	2, 4, 9, 11, 12, 13	15	29	39, 41, 47, 55, 75, 76, 78, 81, 86
Hetherington, E. M. (1973)				
Study finds that father-absence can manifest itself in a girl's behavior at adolescence; if the cause of the marriage breakup is a divorce, the girl may be clumsily neurotic with men; if it is death, she may be scared of men.	Descriptive study (58)			
Hunt, L. L., and Hunt, J. G. (1975)				
Article investigates how structural circumstances condition the meaning of the father–son relationship to the effects of father-absence; results indicate that father-absence has different consequences by race, with father-absence perceived as having more deleterious effects for white boys than for black boys; review of literature included.	5, 9, 11, 13	15, 25	30	39, 41, 54, 55, 72, 75, 79, 89
Johnson, M. M. (1963)				
Article attempts to make theoretical sense out of already available findings on sex-role learning in the nuclear family; major theoretical proposition suggests that it is identification with the father, in the sense of internalizing a reciprocal role relationship, which is crucial for producing appropriate sex-role orientations in both males and females.	Theoretical paper (70, 74)			

238

Table 7.2. *(continued)*

Research Emphasis and Findings	I	II	III	IV
Kaplan, H. B. (1970)				
Describes the relationships observed between selected childhood family characteristics and self-derogation scores of adult subjects; significant relationships were found among adult self-derogation and the number of siblings, birth order, and sex distribution of children; related literature is discussed.		22, 23, 25, 26		39, 41, 47, 56, 75, 79
Kestenbaum, C. J., and Stone, M. H. (1976)				
Case studies of patients who sought or went for treatment because of skewed development for which paternal loss appeared as one of several contributing conditions; implications of research suggest that the impact of paternal loss upon daughters appears varied and not easily predictable; failure to complete Oedipal resolutions and impairment of feminine identification were noted in all the cases.	Case study (53)			
Lynn, D. B. (1976)				
Review of the literature that found fathers generally more concerned than mothers with sex typing their children, particularly boys, although they may be more effective in enhancing their daughters' femininity; also includes a study of 90 boys that indicated that sons were more likely to imitate their fathers than their mothers or a man who was a stranger.	Review of literature (52, 70)			
McClelland, D. C., and Watt, N. F. (1968)				
Sex-typed reactions are contrasted in male and female normals and chronic schizophrenics; in general, the schizophrenics show sex-role alienation on tests that contain a self-image reference; contains a literature review; a theory is proposed relating schizophrenia to sex identity alienation in the early years of life.	1, 8, 10, 11, 12, 13			39, 40, 41, 55, 62, 78, 88

Table 7.2. (*continued*)

Research Emphasis and Findings	I	II	III	IV

Neubauer, P. B. (1960)

Case studies of four children who experienced parental loss; findings contradictory to much existing literature; found that Oedipal conflict was not resolved in one-parent families and an absence of Oedipal reality exists; contains review of literature.

Case study (51, 70)

Pollack, O. (1969)

Theoretical article on family structure and its implications for mental health; first analyzes family forms and their relationship to MH; also analyzes power relationships among various family members and their implications for MH; one conclusion states that when women will permit boys to become men and men will be able to help girls to become women, the power structure of the family of the future may become equitable on the spouse and parental level.

Theoretical article (74)

Santrock, J. W. (1970)

Article studies the effects of parental absence and its relationship to older siblings and a father substitute on the dependency, aggression and masculinity and femininity of preschool children; findings indicate that FA boys were more feminine, less aggressive, and more dependent than their FP counterparts but no significant differences occurred between FA and FP preschool girls.

	I	II	III	IV
	2, 9, 11, 12, 13	15, 17, 28, 28	29, 30	39, 40, 41, 55, 56, 76, 78, 79, 83, 84, 88

Table 7.2. (*continued*)

Research Emphasis and Findings	I	II	III	IV

Schrut, A., and Michels, T. (1974)

Article probes into the multiple causation of suicide attempts; case histories of nine suicidal women who share a history of an insufficiently frustrated ego structure based upon inadequately fulfilling parent–child relationship, influenced by mother's intolerance of feminine sexuality and men, and by father's indifference, hostility, or absence.

Case study (53)

Sears, P. S. (1951)

Paper investigates the effects of certain common variables on the doll-play aggression of young children; sex differences in aggression appear strikingly in the data; however, age differences within each sex do not appear strongly; sibling status has definite effects on aggressive behavior in dollplay.

I	II	III	IV
1, 2, 9, 12, 13	22, 23	30, 33, 37	39, 41, 74, 76, 78, 83, 88

Seegmiller, B. (1980)

Attempts to determine whether maternal employment affects sex-role differentiation in preschoolers, and whether this relationship varies as a function of the sex of the child, father's presence or absence, and/or the sex of the child's siblings. Significant relationships were found between the main effect for sex and the sex of the child × sex of sibling interaction.

I	II	III	IV
1, 5, 11, 12, 13	15, 22	30, 32	39, 41, 49, 74, 76, 78, 83

241

Table 7.2. *(continued)*

Research Emphasis and Findings	I	II	III	IV
Shill, M. (1981)				
Four groups of college-age males were administered TAT stories that were coded for castration anxiety. It was hypothesized that males from father-absent homes would have higher levels of castration anxiety. The findings substantiated the hypothesis and were statistically significant. It was also found that males who had lost their fathers through death rather than divorce experienced a higher degree of castration anxiety.	1, 6, 12, 13	15, 17, 22	29, 30, 33, 34, 35, 36, 37	39, 40, 49, 74, 77, 78, 83, 88
Sigusch, V., and Schmidt, G. (1971)				
Emotional and social aspects of lower-class sexuality in West Germany are examined on the basis of results of interviews with two comparable groups of males and females from six large cities; particular attention given to the relationship between sexuality and love; comparison between Scandinavian and American patterns of working-class sexuality shows that the West German pattern is laregly congruent with the Scandinavian pattern.	1, 2, 5, 10, 12, 13	16, 28		39, 40, 41, 45, 55, 65, 77, 79
Ucko, L. E., and Moore, T. (1963)				
This paper presents findings concerning a group of boys and girls tested in a previous study to assess parental roles as seen by young children in doll-play; children tested at 4 years and 6 years; tendency to call in the parent figures or to dispense with them, and the allocation to father and mother respectively of positive, negative, and authoritarian roles and of various combinations of these are considered; significant differences reported between sexes and ages.	12, 13	20, 24, 25, 28		39, 42, 55, 76, 82, 83, 88

Table 7.2. *(continued)*

Research Emphasis and Findings	I	II	III	IV
Wakefield, W. M. (1970)				
Sixty adolescents and their parents were chosen to test the hypotheses that (1) the adolescent has more positive feelings toward the parent who is more aware of the adolescent's feelings toward himself or herself; and (2) the adolescent perceives himself or herself to be more similar to the parent who is more aware of the adolescent's feelings about himself or herself; the data failed to support the hypotheses.	6, 12	28		39, 40, 41, 55, 74, 75, 78, 83, 84, 88
Weinraub, M., and Frankel, J. (1977)				
Article evaluates sex differences in parent–infant interaction during free play, departure, and separation; findings indicate that although there were no parent sex or infant sex differences in infants' free-play behavior, there were parent × infant sex differences in parental free-play behaviors; implications of these findings for understanding differential roles of mothers and fathers, the development of sex differences, and the determinants of separation distress are discussed.	1, 2, 12, 13	28		39, 40, 41, 55, 79, 81, 83, 84, 89
Wohlford, P., et al. (1971)				
Sixty-six black preschool girls and boys were studied in order to investigate the role of the older male sibling as a potential surrogate male role model for father-absent children; findings indicate that children with older male siblings were significantly more aggressive on the maternal interview aggression score and less dependent on both dependency measures than children with no older male sibling.	2, 9 11, 12	14, 22, 25, 26, 28	29, 30	39, 40, 41, 55, 74, 76, 78, 79, 83, 84, 88

Table 7.3.   Juvenile Delinquency

Research Emphasis and Findings	I	II	III	IV

Andry, R. G. (1962)

Examines concept of "maternal depriva-   Review of literature (70)
tion" and recognizes additional concepts
including pathogenic paternal factor in
delinquency.

Atkinson, B. R., and Ogston, D. G. (1974)

Comparative behavioral study of young and adolescent male children from fatherless and intact homes; no appreciable difference between groups was indicated.	1, 2, 9, 12	15, 16, 20, 24	30, 31, 32, 33, 34, 35, 36	39, 40, 41, 48, 55, 76, 77, 79, 83, 84, 86

Axelrad, S. (1952)

Comparative study of black and white delinquents within the same institution; verified hypothesis that courts commit on a differential basis.	1, 8, 9, 12	15, 16, 22		39, 40, 41, 44, 55, 80

Bacon, M. K., Child, I. L., and
Barry, H. (1963)

Forty-eight nonliterate societies sampled   Comparative study (41, 50, 55)
for frequency of theft and personal crime
and correlated with variables suspected of
being causal factors in crime development;
socialization anxiety in childhood and
status differentiation in adulthood were
significantly associated with theft.

Bartemeier, L. (1953–54)

Essay on Cornelian Corner and the contri-   Essay (45, 59)
butions of both mother and father to the
mental health of the family.

Table 7.3. *(continued)*

Research Emphasis and Findings	I	II	III	IV
Castellano, V., and Dembo, M. H. (1981)				
Focused on the relationship between father-presence or -absence and level of antisocial behavior with social egocentrism in adolescent Mexican-American females. Results indicated that females who scored high in antisocial behavior had significantly higher egocentrism scores than low-antisocial females. A significant correlation was also found between antisocial behavior and father-absence.	1, 2, 8, 9, 11, 12, 13	15	29, 30, 32	39, 40, 41, 49, 66, 74, 76, 77, 78, 79, 81, 82, 83, 84, 88
Eisner, V. (1966)				
Court delinquency records studied in a large city to determine effects of the number of parents in a child's home on delinquency rate; white juveniles living in intact homes had a lower delinquency rate than nonwhite males in the lowest SES quartile in the city.	1, 6, 9, 11, 12, 13	15, 16, 28		39, 40, 47, 63, 81, 85, 88
Fleisher, B. M. (1966)				
Attempts to discover whether low income is a cause of juvenile delinquency; found that while income alone does not explain delinquent behavior over time, the elasticity of the relationship between income and unemployment may "explain" about 15% of measured increase between 1952 and 1960.	1, 11, 13	16, 28		39, 46, 67
Gardiner, H. W., and Suttipan, C. S. (1977)				
Describes efforts to develop a scale for measurement of Thai children's perception of parental discipline on aggressive behavior; low positive correlation between maternal and paternal approaches to punishment of both public- and private-school children was found regardless of age and high positive correlation in the use of parental punishment in private school families.	1, 11, 12, 13	20, 24		39, 40, 41, 50, 62, 66, 76, 78, 83

245

Table 7.3. *(continued)*

Research Emphasis and Findings	I	II	III	IV
Glueck, E. T. (1962)				
Analysis of the role of 44 sociocultural factors in the dynamics of delinquency; an example of the findings indicates that an overcrowded home environment contributes to the development of traits that are significantly more characteristic of delinquents than nondelinquents.	2, 3, 6, 11, 13,	20, 24, 28		39, 40, 50, 60, 76
Goldstein, H. S. (1972)				
Analyzed differences that exist between intact and fatherless families with regard to childhood development of internal controls; found that children from intact families told stories in which punishment for aggressive behavior was much more frequent than children from father-absent families.	1, 2, 8, 9, 12	20, 24, 28	29, 30	39, 40, 41, 50, 62, 76, 78, 83
Grygier, T., Chesley, J., and Tuters, E. W. (1969)				
Part of a larger group study of delinquent children in training school; attempts to establish extent of paternal deprivation in a group of delinquent children to determine whether it may not be of equal significance with maternal deprivation in the etiology of delinquency; implications of study indicated that the importance of parents' roles has not been proved; also includes literature review.	8, 12	15, 28	29, 33, 34, 35, 36, 37	39, 41, 76, 77, 78, 80, 83, 88

Table 7.3. (*continued*)

Research Emphasis and Findings	I	II	III	IV
Hetherington, E. M., et al. (1971)				
Describes differences in family interaction patterns and parental attitudes in families with adolescent daughter/son classified as nondelinquent, or neurotic, psychopathic, or social delinquent; evidence opposes a unitary concept of delinquency and supports the usefulness of conceptualizing delinquency in terms of configurations of dimensions of delinquent behavior.	2, 8, 12, 13	15, 16, 28		39, 41, 50, 55, 66, 74, 75, 76, 77, 78, 83, 84
Hoffman, M. L. (1973)				
Comparative study of a father-present and father-absent group concerning seven moral attitudes and overt aggression; no differences were obtained for girls but evidence indicates that there are differences in the males.	1, 2, 4, 5, 9, 11, 12, 13	28	29, 30	39, 40, 41, 50, 55, 62, 75, 76, 78, 81, 83, 86
Horne, A. M. (1981)				
Findings indicated that families with an identified deviant child demonstrated more aggressive behavior by family members than did families for whom the target child was identified as normal. In deviant families, the mother-only family demonstrated the highest rate of aggression. In normal families, however, the mother-only normal family had lower aggression scores for siblings and total family members than did intact family siblings and total family members.	1, 8, 11	15, 17, 26	30, 35, 36	40, 49, 71, 74, 75, 78, 79, 83, 84, 85, 88

Table 7.3. (*continued*)

Research Emphasis and Findings	I	II	III	IV
Jenkins, R. L. (1968)				
Three groups of clinic children, separated by clustering of symptoms, were described; author indicated that overanxious children are likely to have an anxious, infantilizing mother; a critical mother or stepmother is typical for the unsocialized aggressive child; socialized delinquents are likely to come from large families; parental pathology is more typically paternal than maternal.	2, 8			39, 41, 54, 58, 63, 76, 88
Koller, K. M. (1971)				
Contributes to the literature of female delinquency; hypothesizes that early adverse experiences are related to female delinquency in particular and to behavior disturbances in general; conclusions of two groups studied indicate that the role of the absent father, the effect of the physical presence of the mother, and the influence of institutionalized life affected the development of subsequent delinquency.	1, 5, 8, 11	15, 20, 23, 26, 28	29, 30, 32, 33, 34, 35, 36, 37	39, 40, 41, 50, 55, 77, 88
Koller, K. M., and Castanos, J. N. (1970)				
Offenders from two prison populations (first offenders and long-term offenders) were examined and matched with a control group derived from the population at large; parental loss was common and statistically significant especially among long-term prisoners; found that offenders who experienced parental deprivation had younger parents and were themselves younger than their counterparts who had suffered no loss.	1, 6, 8, 11, 12, 13	15, 17, 22, 23, 26, 27, 28	29, 33, 34, 35, 36, 37, 38	39, 40, 41, 50, 62, 66, 76, 77, 78, 88

Table 7.3. *(continued)*

Research Emphasis and Findings	I	II	III	IV

MacDonald, M. W. (1938)

Social data and observations are described for a group of eight boys showing criminally aggressive and passive–effeminate behavior.

Case study (6, 8, 12, 15, 53, 76, 80, 88)

Malone, C. A. (1963)

Descriptive study of South End Family Project, which centers around relationships of pathologic family members with each other and the project staff; focus on perpetuation of impulse disorder.

Descriptive study (58, 76, 80)

Millen, L., and Roll, S. (1977)

Factor analysis of a questionnaire that measures son's feelings of being understood by his father; five factors were extracted from the data—three were positively correlated with son's self-concept; two were negatively correlated with number of somatic complaints.

	I	II	IV
	1, 12	25, 28	39, 50, 60, 75, 77, 78, 83, 84

Miller, W. B. (1958)

Descriptive study of one form of delinquency (law-violating acts committed by adolescent street-corner groups in lower-SES communities) and the motivation underlying these acts in which the gang participants adhere to certain forms of behavior; suggests that membership in street-corner groups involves a positive effort to achieve status, conditions, or qualities valued within the actor's cultural milieu; describes focal concerns.

Descriptive study (58, 76)

Table 7.3. *(continued)*

Research Emphasis and Findings	I	II	III	IV

Moerk, E. L. (1973)

Study attempts to demonstrate that profiles of children with imprisoned fathers were more similar to those of juvenile delinquents and less similar to a norm group than were profiles of children from divorced families; found that father-absence and father imprisonment per se were not the cause of negative psychological reactions.	1, 9, 11, 12, 13	15, 25, 28	29, 35, 37, 38	40, 41, 50, 62, 75, 76, 77, 78, 79, 83, 84

Monahan, T. P. (1957)

Proposes that in one large minority of the population there exists twice the average rate of socially broken homes and twice the average rate of delinquency while, in other groups, strong family cohesiveness shows below-average delinquency rates; feels apparent association cannot be dismissed.	9, 12, 13	15, 17, 28	29, 35, 37, 38,	39, 41, 46, 63, 76, 81, 88

Monahan, T. P. (1960)

Descriptive study that states that the age of the child at the time of family disruption and the nature of the break tend to define the way he or she is affected; the broken-home factor varies in importance and in type with advancing age of child.

Descriptive study (29, 33, 35, 58)

Montare, A., and Boone, S. L. (1980)

Hypothesized that paternal absence may differentially influence aggressive behavior. Aggression scores were obtained for 132 preadolescent inner-city males. Results indicated that when compared to their racial/ethnic counterparts living with both parents, father-absent Puerto Ricans were equally aggressive, father-absent blacks were less aggressive, and father-absent whites were more aggressive.	1, 2, 5, 9, 11, 12	15, 17	30, 35	39, 49, 60, 74, 76, 77, 78, 81, 83, 88

Table 7.3. (*continued*)

Research Emphasis and Findings	I	II	III	IV
Newman, G., and Denman, S. B. (1971)				
Hypothesized that males who had been deprived of their fathers during childhood would be more likely to express conflict by socially disapproved behavior and that loss of father is of greater significance than loss of mother in the genesis of antisocial behavior in the male; findings demonstrated that white males with absent fathers prior to 18 are more likely to be involved in criminal behavior categorized as "felonious."	8, 9, 12, 13	15, 17, 28	29, 30, 33, 34, 35	39, 40, 41, 47, 55, 62, 76, 80, 88
Nye, F. I., Short, J. F., and Olson, V. J. (1958)				
Questions whether delinquent behavior does occur differentially by SES; analysis shows that a disproportionate number of official delinquents come from lower SES categories.	1, 2, 4, 8, 11	16		39, 41, 50, 63, 74, 76, 78, 81, 82, 83
Rosen, L. (1969)				
Analyzed factors that were thought might be statistically significant in influencing the relationship between matriarchy and delinquency among lower-class black males; although there were significant differences for the total sample, no single variable proved to be a major factor.	1, 8, 9, 12, 13	15, 16, 18, 19, 20, 23, 28	30	39, 40, 41, 66, 74, 76, 77, 79, 83, 84

Table 7.3. *(continued)*

Research Emphasis and Findings	I	II	III	IV
Russell, I. L. (1957)				
Presents a comparative study of behavioral problems evidenced by children from broken and intact homes; tentative conclusions drawn from data are: (1) children from broken homes exhibit significantly more behavior problems, lying, and stealing than children from intact homes; (2) link to certain kinds of behavior associated with kind of home child enters after break occurs; (3) enuresis, anger and disobedience more frequent in homes broken by divorce or separation than in homes broken by death; (4) academic retardation more frequent in homes broken by death.	1, 2, 4, 9, 12	15, 17, 28	30, 33, 35, 36	39, 40, 41, 50, 62, 76, 80, 88
Shaw, C. R., and McKay, H. D. (1932)				
Authors question the link that exists between broken homes and delinquency rates; indicate that differences in delinquency rates between the delinquent and control group furnished an inadequate basis for the conclusion that broken homes are an important factor in delinquency.	1, 8, 9, 13	15, 16	30	39, 40, 48, 55, 81, 88
Song, R. H. (1969)				
Compares self-concept variables in two groups of delinquent boys—one from intact and one from broken homes; hypothesized that delinquents from intact homes would demonstrate higher self-concept, self-acceptance, and ideal self than delinquent boys from broken homes.	1, 4, 8, 9, 12	25, 28	30	39, 40, 75, 78, 88

Table 7.3. *(continued)*

Research Emphasis and Findings	I	II	III	IV
Sterne, R. S. (1964)				
Study of a group of delinquent boys that questions whether broken homes affect delinquent behavior; evidence shows that a break in the home is not generally a crucial factor in the severity of a boy's misbehavior.	4, 5, 8, 9, 13	15, 16, 22, 28	30, 33, 34, 35, 36	39, 41, 46, 55, 63, 76, 81, 88
Tuckman, J., and Regan, R. A. (1966)				
Referral problems for children in outpatient psychiatric clinics were compared for intact and for broken homes in which parents were widowed, divorced, separated, unmarried, or other; evidence suggests that the broken home should not be treated as a unitary concept.	2, 8, 9, 12, 13	15	33, 35, 36, 37	39, 41, 50, 55, 63, 76, 81, 88
Willie, C. V. (1967)				
Washington, D. C. study that hypothesizes that economic status and family status make both independent and joint contributions to deviant behavior; general conclusion suggests that juvenile delinquency will not be reduced in Washington or similar cities until there is a substantial increase in the nonwhite population's economic status.	8, 9, 11	15, 16, 28	30, 32	39, 41, 46, 47, 50, 56, 81, 82, 88

Table 7.4.   Psychiatric Effects

Research Emphasis and Findings	I	II	III	IV
Adams, P. L., and Horovitz, J. H. (1980)				
Study expands on earlier investigation of how psychopathology is related to father-lessness; no positive association between impoverished boys' psychopathology and their fatherlessness was found; data indicated that poverty exerts a leveling influence that overrides characteristics of ethnic and age grouping, family structure, father-presence or -absence, and linguistic and cultural heritage.	1, 2, 9, 11, 12, 13	16, 23, 28	29, 30, 38	39, 40, 41, 48, 62, 76, 78, 79, 84
Bannon, J. A., and Southern, M. L. (1980)				
Hypothesized that women with a father present during childhood would differ significantly from women with a father absent during childhood in terms of self-concept and ability to form relationships with men. Four groups of college-aged women were studied. Each group differed in the presence or absence of male family members (including father and older siblings). Results from the Tennessee Self-Concept Scale and a self-report questionnaire indicated that no significant difference existed among groups in most areas of self-concept and interpersonal relationships.	12	15, 17, 22, 23, 25, 26	29, 30, 33, 35	39, 40, 49, 55, 74, 77, 78, 83
Bemporad, J., et al. (1978)				
Article attempts to demonstrate that a thorough analysis of chronic neurotic encopresis (CNE) reveals a complex psychiatric disorder, one that is multifactorial in nature and etiology.	Descriptive study (2, 6, 28, 58, 80)			

Table 7.4. *(continued)*

Research Emphasis and Findings	I	II	III	IV

Bigras, J., et al. (1966)

Study confirms the hypothesis that paternal deprivation plays an essential part in the suicidal attempt of an adolescent girl; diagnostic problem of suicide in this population both central and complex.

Descriptive study (2, 6, 15, 17, 25, 28, 58, 76, 80, 84, 87)

Biller, H. B. (1971c)

Review of data suggests that mother–son relationship can have either a positive or negative effect on father-absent boys' sex-role and personality development; research suggests that mothers in homes where the father is absent or ineffectual often undermine the sons' feelings of masculine adequacy and ability to function interpersonally.

Review of literature (70)

Brown, F. (1961)

Hypothesizes that a depressive illness in later life is often a reaction to a present bereavement or loss that is associated with a more serious loss or bereavement in childhood; statistics support hypothesis.

1, 8	28	29, 30, 33	39, 41, 43, 63, 80, 82, 88

Brown, F. (1966)

Evidence concerning the relationship between childhood bereavement and subsequent psychiatric illness is reviewed and assessed; significantly increased incidence of childhood bereavement both of mother and father in the previous history of both female and male delinquents and criminals; also a significantly increased incidence of mental illnesses.

Review of literature (70)

Table 7.4. *(continued)*

Research Emphasis and Findings	I	II	III	IV

Bruhn, J. G. (1962)

Investigates factors of social disorganization that distinguish a group of attempted suicides with a history of broken homes from a group of psychiatric outpatients who have not attempted suicide but have a history of broken homes; four factors of social disorganization found to be more prevalent among attempted suicides from broken homes than among psychiatric outpatients from broken homes; broken homes causally significant only when other indications of social disorganization were also found.

	I	II	III	IV
	1, 5, 8, 12	15, 28	29, 30, 33, 35, 36	39, 40, 41, 47, 55, 62, 81, 88

Bunch, J., and Barraclough, B. (1971)

Hypothesized that more suicides than expected by chance would occur in a time period near the anniversary of a parent's death (0–30 days either side of the anniversary date); results proved significant for fathers' anniversaries, but not for mother's; more daughters than sons killed themselves near anniversary date.

	I	II	III	IV
	12	15, 16, 28	30, 33, 38	39, 41, 47, 58, 81, 85, 89

Caplan, M. G., and Douglas, V. I. (1969)

Focuses on the experience of early separation from a parent in children suffering from depressive symptoms; treatment waiting list of outpatient psychiatric clinic was examined and compared with a control group of nondepressive neurotics; results indicated a greater percentage of depression found in children who experienced parental separation or who had been placed in foster homes.

	I	II	III	IV
	8, 12	15	33, 34, 35, 36, 37, 38	39, 50, 55, 79

Table 7.4.   (*continued*)

Research Emphasis and Findings	I	II	III	IV
Cobliner, W. G. (1963)				
Results of data indicate that sheer physical separation from parents was a contributing factor in the etiology of mental disturbances; however it is the interplay between physical and psychological separation that is most conspicuous in the childhood experience of disturbed respondents.	1, 5, 6, 8, 11, 12, 13	15, 28	29, 30, 33, 35	39, 41, 46, 63, 66, 75, 77, 83
DaSilva, G. (1963)				
The role of the father as contributing to the maintenance of the illness of male chronic schizophrenics is studied through a clinical experience in which group psychotherapy is conducted with a group of 23 male chronic schizophrenics and another group with their fathers and mothers.	8, 12, 13			53, 74, 79, 80, 84, 87
Dorpat, T. L., et al. (1965)				
Part of a larger psychosocial study of an unselected and consecutive series of 114 persons who committed suicide and a series of 121 persons who attempted suicide; reports on the prevalence of broken homes in childhood within the two groups and discusses its significance in the etiology of suicidal behavior; incidence of death of a parent was highest for completed suicide group and most common cause of a broken home; most important cause of a broken home for the attempted suicide group was divorce.	8	15, 28	29, 30, 33, 34, 35, 36, 37, 38	39, 41, 50, 79, 80, 84, 85, 87, 89
Earle, A. M. and Earle, B. V. (1961)				
Investigates relationship between early maternal deprivation and the later development of personality disorder and patterns of psychiatric illness; found that early maternal deprivation is significantly related to the later development of sociopathic personality.	1, 8, 12, 13	15, 28		39, 40, 41, 50, 55, 62, 76, 79, 88

257

Table 7.4. *(continued)*

Research Emphasis and Findings	I	II	III	IV
Gershansky, I. S., Hainline, L., and Goldstein, H. S. (1980)				
Examined the relationship between onset and type of father-absence and children's levels of psychological differentiation defined along the perceptual dimension of field dependence/independence; 100 children between the ages of 8 and 16 were assessed using the rod-and-frame test. Results indicated that boys were significantly more field-dependent than girls. Significant relationships were also found between type of father-absence and between ages of children when the father left the home.	1, 8, 11, 12	15, 17	29, 30, 33, 34, 35, 36	39, 40, 49, 74, 78, 83
Gregory, I. (1958)				
Knowledge of the frequency of parental deprivation during childhood has been handicapped by comparisons between unlike samples, unrepresentative samples due to selection, errors in sampling, and fallacies in deduction; these factors are discussed and tables are presented with data from previous studies; concludes that further investigation will be necessary.	Review of literature (1, 70)			
Haworth, M. R. (1964)				
Study attempts to determine whether loss of a parent before the age of 6 would be reflected subsequently in children's responses to projective tests.	8, 9, 12	28	29, 30, 32	41, 48, 55, 62, 74, 78, 88

258

Table 7.4. *(continued)*

Research Emphasis and Findings	I	II	III	IV
Heacock, D. R., and Seale, C. (1968)				
Hypothesized that father-absence would have an adverse effect on specific areas of boys' personality development that would be reflected in the psychiatric diagnosis, symptoms and behavior on admission, adjustment in the hospital, adjustment to community life; findings report that the father-absent group showed a higher incidence of schizophrenia, poor peer relationships, higher school underachievement, better hospital adjustment, but poorer posthospital adjustment to community life.	2, 4, 8, 9, 12, 13	28	29, 30, 31	40, 47, 55, 76, 81, 88
Heibrun, A. B., and Norbert, N. (1971)				
Experiment tested the prediction that paranoid schizophrenics would be more sensitive to maternal censure cues than nonparanoid schizophrenics; results supported the prediction.	8, 12			39, 40, 41, 76, 88
Herzog, J. M. (1980)				
Case studies of boys from 18 to 28 months old are described. These boys all suffer from sleep disturbances (in some cases, night terrors) and each child perceived his father's presence or absence as a vital element in coping with that fear.	1, 12, 13	15	30, 35, 36	49, 53, 58, 80, 84
Hopkinson, G. and Reed, G. F. (1966)				
Study presents relevant findings with regard to a group of patients suffering from manic-depressive psychosis and compares them with Brown's figures for undifferentiated depressives and normal controls; implications of findings discussed.	1, 8, 12	28	29, 33	39, 41, 46, 47 53, 55, 80, 81, 82, 88

259

Table 7.4. (continued)

Research Emphasis and Findings	I	II	III	IV
Howells, J. G. (1963)				
Object of paper is to show that the point of view that states that "a bad natural home is better than any other home" is not well founded; states that the circumstances attending the separation are the most important factor in determining whether or not the child is deprived of the right care.	Descriptive study (58, 70)			
Howells, J. G. (1970)				
A direct study of separation experiences in young children reported; shows that separation per se does not lead to mental ill health later on.	Descriptive study (58, 70)			
Howells, J. G., and Layng, J. (1955)				
Seeks to find out the incidence of separation in a random sample of disturbed children attending a child psychiatric clinic and also in a control group of healthy schoolchildren; suggested that most disturbed children suffer emotionally from being with their parents.	8, 12	15, 28	31, 37, 38	39, 40, 41, 55, 77, 84
Howells, J. G., and Layng, J. (1956a)				
Article considers the effects on children of separation from their homes; mothers of a group of neurotic children and a control group of healthy children commented on effects that leaving home had on their children when they were under 5 years of age; findings suggest that conditions applying before, during, and after spearation are more important than the fact of separation in determining whether or not there will be harmful effects; includes review of 1955 research.	Descriptive study (70)			

260

Table 7.4. *(continued)*

Research Emphasis and Findings	I	II	III	IV
Howells, J. G., and Layng, J. (1956b)				
Investigation concerns separation from parents brought about by the normal happenings of everyday life in children living at home; findings indicate that illness is more frequent and lasts longer in mothers of neurotic children; work is the most common cause of father-absence; most common cause of child's absence from the home is his or her own illness.	8	28	30, 33, 37, 38	39, 40, 41, 79, 84
Huttunen, M. O., and Niskanen, P. (1978)				
Retrospective epidemiological study was conducted to test the role of maternal stress during pregnancy in psychiatric and behavior disorders; results suggest that especially during months 3 to 5 and 9 to 10 of pregnancy, maternal stress may increase the risk of the child for psychiatric disorders, perhaps mediated through the inborn temperament of the child.	1, 2, 8, 12	16	29, 30, 33	39, 40, 42, 43, 44, 45, 46, 74, 76, 81
Jackson, R. M., and Meara, N. M. (1977)				
Study concerns the relationship between the adequacy of the father as an identification model and the achievement and occupational behavior of economically deprived rural male adolescents; statistically significant differences found with regard to the variables studied.	1, 12, 13	16, 28	30, 31, 35, 37, 38	39, 40, 42, 55, 76, 80, 89
Kagel, M. A., et al. (1978)				
Study of intact and father-absent families; male adolescent disturbance in both groups found to be related to less warm, supportive, and expressive intrafamilial relations, less of a family orientation toward personal growth, and less successful participation in extrafamilial involvement.	1, 8, 9, 11, 12	22, 28	29, 30, 35, 36	39, 40, 41, 50, 55, 62, 74, 75, 77, 83, 84

261

Table 7.4. (*continued*)

Research Emphasis and Findings	I	II	III	IV
Kauffman, J. M. (1971)				
Results of test administered to 20 normal, 27 school-disordered, and 10 institutionalized emotionally disturbed preadolescent boys; data were interpreted as reflecting sibling rivalry and the operation of psychodynamic defenses.	8, 12	15, 22		39, 41, 74, 78, 88
Kety, S. S., et al. (1971)				
Study supports a genetic transmission vulnerability to schizophrenic-related illness among the biological relatives of adopted schizophrenics but not among their adoptive relatives; environmental factors also considered for development of clinical schizophrenic illness.	8	28		39, 41, 43, 44, 45, 66, 76, 80, 81, 88
Kogelschaatz, J., et al. (1972)				
A comparative study of 158 children, both clinic in- and outpatients, who were divided into four groups ("transitional" fatherless; "hard-core" fatherless, intact, and intact with a history of fatherlessness); demographic data were obtained for all groups of children and parents; an attempt was made to portray the differing life styles of entire households; authors suggested that a particularly crucial interaction occurs among: (1) the style of the household; (2) different economic positions; (3) households broken by divorce and desertion instead of death; and (4) households whose sociocultural values differ from the white middle-class norms.	1, 5, 8, 9, 10, 11, 12, 13	15, 16, 17, 18, 19, 21, 28	30, 32, 33, 34, 35, 36, 37, 38	39, 40, 55, 80, 84, 87

Table 7.4. (*continued*)

Research Emphasis and Findings	I	II	III	IV
Koller, K. M., and Williams, W. T. (1974)				
Suicidal, delinquent, criminal, alcoholic, neurotic, socially deviant, and normal groups were studied on variables related to early parental deprivation and other family characteristics; concluded that the vulnerability of selected individuals in certain families is compounded when these individuals are exposed to the unique specific effects of the various types of parental deprivation.		15, 22, 23, 26, 28	29, 30, 33, 34, 35, 36, 37	50, 54, 76, 79
Kolvin, I., et al. (1971a)				
Study that points to a conglomeration of personality oddities and absence of clarity of thought in parents of young schizophrenics or children with psychosis of late onset.	6, 8			39, 41, 50, 74, 76, 78, 80, 84
Kolvin, I., et al. (1971b)				
Findings of this study suggest that more parents of children with infantile psychosis belonged to social classes I and II (upper) and more parents of children with late-onset psychosis to social classes IV and V (lower), trend demonstrated by mothers of late-onset psychoses children toward a degree of social isolation; parents of infantile psychoses group had low rate of schizophrenia—LOP group had higher rate—suggesting a genetic link; boys more often psychotic than girls.	Descriptive study (13, 27, 28, 39, 58, 70)			
Langner, T. S. (1963)				
Study found that broken homes are not strongly associated with mental disorder in a randomly selected study group of 1,660; certain factors such as SES, sex of child, and sex of remaining parent can make experience more stressful; study refutes some often-accepted ideas.	1, 8, 11, 12, 13	15, 17, 28	29, 33, 34, 35, 36, 37, 38	39, 41, 50, 66, 77, 87

Table 7.4. (*continued*)

Research Emphasis and Findings	I	II	III	IV

Levy-Shiff, R. (1982)

Two-year-old boys and girls who had experienced father absence through death were compared with young children from intact families. Results indicated that reported and observed behavior of young children who lived in mother-headed families differed substantially depending on the sex of the child.	1, 2, 5, 9, 12, 13	15, 17	30, 33	39, 40, 49, 53, 74, 75, 76, 77, 78, 79, 80, 83, 84, 86

Lidz, T., et al. (1954)

Long-term study of the intrafamilial environment in which the schizophrenic patient grows up; found that in the 14 families studied that contained schizophrenic offspring the marital relationships of all parents were seriously disturbed.   Case study (9, 11, 53, 79, 84, 85)

Lidz, T., et al. (1956)

Long-term study of the interaction of all members of families of schizophrenic patients—seeks to recreate and analyze the family environment in which the patients grew up; pathogenic influences of paternal role discussed and fathers grouped into three or four categories.   Case study (9, 11, 53, 79, 84)

Lidz, T., et al. (1958)

Also part of an intensive study of the intrafamilial environments of 16 schizophrenic patients obtained largely through repeated interviews with family members, observations, and projective testing; approach includes psychodynamic aspects as well as sociologic and biologic considerations in preliminary form; major focus on personalities of parents.   1 Case study (53)

Table 7.4. *(continued)*

Research Emphasis and Findings	I	II	III	IV

Lourie, R. S. (1967)

Theoretical article that begins with the basic assumption that children are not born neurotic and discusses the components that go into a neurosis that have their origins in the first years of life.

Theoretical article (74)

Madow, L., and Hardy, S. E. (1947)

	I	II	III	IV
Group of 211 neurotic soldiers were studied to learn if the broken family was a factor in the background of neurosis; in the group from broken families before age 16, a higher percentage of neurosis was found prior to entrance in the army, a higher percentage from rural communities, migratory families, and from low SES; also a comparison of groups on standardized scale of neurotic traits shows a higher average number of symptoms in the unhappy sections as compared with the happy.	2, 8, 9, 11	16, 28	29, 30, 33, 35, 36	39, 41, 55, 76, 78, 80, 84

Munro, A. (1965)

	I	II	III	IV
Main emphasis of this article is on physical separation of parent and child, both temporary and permanent; findings suggest that children experience parental bereavement more commonly than generally realized; therefore, it is difficult to accept that parental bereavement *per se* can be an important predisposing factor in mental illness.	1, 10 11, 13	22, 28	29, 33, 34, 35, 36, 37	39, 41, 55, 79

Munro, A. (1966)

	I	II	III	IV
Study investigates whether individuals suffering from depressive illness were more likely than normals to have suffered from parental deprivation in childhood; example of findings—neither the death of the father nor the mother appears to have particular importance in the etiology of depression.	1, 8, 10, 11, 12	28	29, 30, 32, 33	39, 41, 50, 55, 62, 79, 88

Table 7.4. (continued)

Research Emphasis and Findings	I	II	III	IV

Oltman, J. E., et al. (1952)

| Data in this study do not confirm previous hypothesis that deprivation of parents occurs more frequently in schizophrenic patients than in normal subjects or individuals suffering from other types of psychoses; incidence of parental deprivation and "broken homes" was found to be very similar among individuals suffering from dementia praecox, manic-depressive psychosis, alcoholic, and "other psychoses," and in normal control subjects—higher in psychoneurotic psychopathic personality. | Descriptive study (8, 39, 58, 77, 80) | | | |

Oshman, H. P., and Manosevitz, M. (1976)

| Article studies the effects of stepfathers upon the more affectively based aspects of personality where father-absence has been shown to have explicitly negative effects; findings indicate that stepfathering is an important factor in mitigating the typically negative effects of father-absence; factors suggested that may account for positive effects of gaining a stepfather for the male child. | 6, 12 | | 29, 30 | 39, 55, 62, 75, 78, 83 |

Oshman, H. P., and Manosevitz, M. (1978)

| Study of parental perception of father-present and father-absent late adolescents; used stories created by respondents; findings suggest that father-present females produce more death and loss themes because they are actively coping with their fantasies of parental loss; no significant differences between father-present and father-absent males. | 1, 12, 13 | | 29, 30, 33, 35 | 39, 40, 41, 55, 62, 75, 78, 83 |

Table 7.4.   (*continued*)

Research Emphasis and Findings	I	II	III	IV
Parish, T. S. (1980)				
Hypothesized that the longer that individuals have been without their fathers or a surrogate, the more likely it would be that their needs may not be met and that their moral development would be impeded. Analysis of D and P scores on the Defining Issues Test (DIT) indicated that when the D score was used a significant inverse relationship existed between length of time father was absent and the subject's level of moral development.	1, 12, 13	15	29, 30, 33, 34, 35, 36, 38	49, 56, 77, 78, 83
Parish, T. S., and Nunn, G. D. (1981)				
Examined relationships between children's self-concepts and their evaluations of parents in families where father-absence had occurred, through either divorce or death. Children's perceptions of their families' current level of functioning were also examined. The results showed significant relationships between self-concept and evaluations of parents in "unhappy" and "divorced" family units.	1, 12, 13	15, 25, 28	30, 33, 35	93, 40, 41, 49, 56, 74, 75, 78, 83
Parish, T. S., and Kappes, B. M. (1980)				
Four hundred and twenty-one college students evaluated their natural mothers, fathers, or stepfathers on the Personal Attribute Inventory. Results indicated that parents of families broken by divorce were consistently more negatively evaluated than were parents from either intact homes or those in which the father had died.	1, 12 13	15, 16, 17, 28	30, 33, 35	39, 49, 67, 74, 77, 78, 83

Table 7.4. (continued)

Research Emphasis and Findings	I	II	III	IV
Parish, T. S., and Taylor, J. C. (1979)				
Self-concepts of 406 grade-school and middle-school students were assessed. Results indicated that children and adolescents who lost their fathers through divorce and whose mothers had not remarried demonstrated significantly lower self-concepts than those children from intact families as measured by the Personal Attribute Inventory for Children. Results also indicated that children and adolescents from broken homes where the mother had remarried had lower self-concepts than subjects from intact families. The latter findings, however, were not statistically significant.	12, 13	15, 16	30, 35	39, 40, 48, 67, 75, 78, 79, 83, 86
Parker, G. (1979)				
A nonclinical group was used to study any influence of early permanent parental loss and early parental separation on subsequent depressive experience in adulthood; findings consistent with the view that it is the quality of any parental contribution rather than continuity that is associated with subsequent depressive experience in adulthood.	12	28	29	39, 41, 74, 77, 89
Pedersen, F. A. (1966)				
Compares the extent of father-absence in the histories of 27 emotionally disturbed 11- to 15-year-old male military dependents and 30 comparable normal military children; no significant differences shown; a maternal pathology by father-absence interaction with the child's degree of disturbance is suggested to explain the nonunitary meaning of father-absence.	2, 8, 11, 12	23, 28	29, 30 37, 38	39, 40, 55, 76, 79, 83, 84

Table 7.4. *(continued)*

Research Emphasis and Findings	I	II	III	IV
Pitts, F. N., et al. (1965)				
Seven hundred and forty-eight consecutive psychiatric patients were examined at admission to the hospital for various evidences of parental deprivation and family history of psychiatric illness; no differences in parental deprivation in childhood found among various psychiatric and control groups but there were marked differences in the occurrence of psychiatric illness in family history.	1, 8, 9, 11, 12, 13	22, 28	29, 30, 33, 35, 36	39, 41, 72, 79, 89
Rosenthal, D., et al. (1971)				
Adopted-away children of schizophrenics were compared with 67 controls; evidence supports the theory that heredity plays a significant role in the etiology of schizophrenic spectrum disorders.	8	15, 28	29	39, 41, 55, 79, 81, 87
Rutter, M. L. (1970)				
Review of the literature on psychosocial disorders in childhood and their outcome in adult life.	Review of literature (70)			
Seligman, R., et al. (1974)				
Study of patients referred for psychiatric evaluation from an inpatient and outpatient medical adolescent population; a high frequency of early parental loss was found; frequency differed significantly at the .001 level when compared with control group sample; includes case studies.	1, 9, 11	28	33, 36, 37	39, 40, 41, 48, 53, 74, 80, 88
Schaengold, M. (1977)				
Review of the literature; investigators in five studies of encopresis have been described and explored; authors agreed that encopresis as a disorder has a multifactorial etiology.	Review of literature (70)			

269

Table 7.4. (*continued*)

Research Emphasis and Findings	I	II	III	IV
Sugar, M. (1967)				
Case studies of 20 pubescent boys with absent fathers and with the initial complaint of academic failure and behavioral problems, or both, were treated in an open group for periods varying from 2 to 15 months.	Case study (8, 12, 30, 53)			
Trunnell, T. L. (1968)				
Hypothesizes that (1) effects of parental absence on normal child development are reflected by correlations in form and severity of emotional disturbances manifested; (2) psychological efforts at restoring the missing father result in identifiable behavior patterns in the child; (3) parental absence is never a long psychotoxic agent; study indicates much more information needed about the types and significances of paternal deprivation syndromes.	1, 2, 8, 11	22, 23, 28	29, 30, 32	39, 41, 56, 76, 80, 82, 88
Winn, D., and Halla, R. (1966)				
Case studies that observe children who threaten to kill themselves; looks at a subgrouping of children who have in common the threat to kill themselves by running in front of a car or train.	Case study (8, 12, 39, 53)			

We probably need not reiterate our convictions that several of the tabulated studies do not see the forest for the trees, that some do judge a forest by a single windblown leaf or needle, and that a few studies make assumptions about the forest shade when there is no forest, only a cloudy sky on the prairie. The studies are not excellent ones, in the mass, and we include some that we have been involved in. But we feel that we have the beginning for a scientific corpus of theory and empirical facts that could stimulate additional research that could be good.

We turn now to considering some methodologic suggestions for any future researchers who try to learn about fatherless children and the world they inhabit. It seems that the best way to present these is in the form of a list of "requirements," or recommendations, to state it more mildly, for research on the topic of fatherless children.

1. *Behavior, not attitudes, needs to be studied.* Attitudes of fatherless children have been studied by use of pencil-and-paper tests as if they constitute a full equivalent of objectively witnessed behavior. We know that people seldom think, feel, or do what they say they think, feel, or do, in a standardized inventory or questionnaire. For instance, sometimes people have more race tolerance than they say they do; sometimes they have much more bias than they own up to on a test. So it is with fatherless children, their mothers, and other informants about their behavior: The questionnaire stance is not always reflected in real life. Rating scales of observed behavior are always a notch better than scales filled up *in vacuo* or *in abstracto*.

Naturalistic study of fatherless children's behavior in relation to mother, father (whenever any contact goes on), sibs, and peers is much richer than responses on the Blacky, IT scale, or the Draw a Person test. The father has been neglected in the lives of children, we acknowledge. It seems that when there is a father he is ignored; when there is no father and he cannot be taken for granted, his absence is made much of. Too, the mother's actual behavior in relation to the father, to her child(ren), to adult males of her acquaintance, and to other adult females makes for fruitful study. Hence, we lean strongly toward the methodologic injunction that researchers go to the fatherless child, to his or her real behavior, in the ecosphere of each child: home, school, and play group.

2.   No adequate study can be done without *control for the basic sociobiologic characteristics of fatherless children—economic class, IQ, sex* or gender, *age, physique, temperament.* When those variables, any of them, are left unattended, the research suffers immeasurable limitations on its ability to make strong conclusions about fatherless children. Economic class does pertain to the chances each child has to survive, to endure, to live in health instead of disease, to own property, to inherit wealth, to feel economically sound or secure. The psychology of individual differences as an academic discipline traditionally has stressed noneconomic variables, but includes some of the highly important ones. Differences in age, IQ, gender, physique, breadth of emotional expression, and emotional depth are basic psychobiologic differentiations that simply cannot be ignored or omitted in studying fatherless children.

3.   Secondary variables residing in children that add to the strength of any research with fatherless children include ordinal position and personality dimensions such as creativity, cognitive styles, academic skills, child's relations to grown-ups of both genders, and so on, including the child's self-picture. They have been tabulated in the foregoing tables of this chapter.

4.   More attention than has been typical needs to be devoted to features of the family or household. The size of the sibling group, the nature of the adults living with the child(ren), the history of maternal and paternal punishment, the kinds of discipline employed, the number of useful chores performed by each member of the household, the way decisions are arrived at in the household, and the degree to which the family is imbedded (or not imbedded) in a supportive network of community contacts and interactions—all those are important if we are to understand fully the intimate worlds inhabited by fatherless children and their families.

5.   Studies must include variables pertaining especially to fatherlessness, as we have done under the heading "Characteristics Specific to the Absent Father" in the key to the tables. The child's age when the fatherlessness commenced, the times of father's presence and whether he has been absent totally or intermittently, the reason for the father-absence (divorce, never married, desertion, death, work obligations, etc.), and as much information as possible pertaining to the father as a person need to be gathered.

6. Longitudinal studies should be given preference over any one-time cross-sectional studies of fatherless children. We need to gather data on fatherless families, and on their subset, woman-headed households, as well as on the boys and girls who live in such households. We need to gather that information over a time trajectory that will permit reviewing of their fate throughout childhood and on into adulthood and old age. That would be the type of research that would be supported fully in a child-caring society. This would be a more naturalistic approach, and could be economically designed and conducted. Our best example, probably, of such longitudinal research comes from Kellam and his associates who worked with the ghetto people in Chicago's Woodlawn region. Many more studies of families at risk, inclusive of fatherless ones, are required for both our theory and research.

7. Sample selection is especially risky business when work is done with fatherless children. We need to know a great deal about the children we are studying in the fatherless group, and we need furthermore to select matched groups of fathered children who share most of the former group's life circumstances. Ideally, the matching groups would differ only in respect of father-presence or father-absence. It also seems imperative that both fathered and unfathered children need to be followed over a span of time and then compared to a "surrogated group" whose mothers have sought father replacements for their children. Efforts should be made to set up comparable groups of fatherless children, dividing them only according to economic class, in order to learn how class operates within the fatherless group. Or, as another example, we ought to be able to know how some children cope successfully despite fatherlessness. Both fatherlessness and unhealthy coping exist in varying degrees, we have reason to believe, but that ought to be investigated systematically.

8. Studies of fatherless children must recall a simple rule: Correlations or covariances are not proof of causation and are not even approximations of causes. Statistical tests of significance help us to firm up our conclusions, as does analysis of variance, but those statistical tests never push covariance up to that realm of logic and proof where causes exert their influences on the lives of human persons.

9. On strictly logical grounds, a system approach, considering multiple variables that are mutually dependent, is superior to linear

cause–effect reasoning. There is no simple cause-to-effect lineup operating with fatherless children, it is almost certain. A conceptualization and a design of research that uses a multifactorial, complex of variables, conceptual scheme will be more fruitful in the long run.

10. More emphasis, as we have often stated, should be given to "invulnerable" children who are fatherless. Why do so many geniuses have childhoods that are fatherless? Who are the fatherless children who make it very well, although not being exceptionally creative in science or humanities? Is there anything other than economic class differences that distinguishes the successful copers from the fatherless children who do have serious problems?

INSTRUMENTS OF STUDY

Tests commonly used in studies of the effects of fatherlessness on school achievement, intelligence, sex role, and personality allow many possible injustices, and are, in fact, an important reason that we cannot clearly identify the effects of fatherlessness. We do know that fatherless children are likely to be poor and black, that many tests subtly or blatantly favor middle-class white people, that even those tests claiming impartiality may not be impartial enough for so wide a range of people as fatherless children, that testers' personal attitudes may distort the results.

We cannot assume that tests standardized on predominantly white middle-class samples or on mixed samples that represent only selected minorities will give valid results for members of any group not originally included. Culturally biased questions and questions presented in a child's second language obviously put the child at a disadvantage. Tests emphasizing verbal ability discriminate against people from relatively nonverbal subcultures. Difficult or ambiguous questions discriminate against members of subcultures more sensitive than the white middle class to feelings of frustration and defeat. Timed tests discriminate against those from cultures that do not prize hurrying. Most of the available information on fatherless children comes from tests with at least questionable validity. We present the tests for studying fatherless children in four large groups: *achievement, intelligence, sex role,* and *personality.*

Achievement

Infant and Preschool. Tests of infants (birth to 18 months) and preschoolers (18 to 60 months), individually administered, should cover motor and social as well as cognitive traits. Gesell and his associates at Yale presented in *Gesell Developmental Schedules* (1947) a systematic method to assess behavior development of young children, now the standard method. Most items require direct observation of a child's responses to toys and other stimuli augmented by information from parents.

The Bayley Scales of Infant Development (1955) include items from Gesell's test and from others, providing three tools for assessing children 2 months to 2½ years old: the Mental Scale, the Motor Scale, and the Infant Behavior Record. These scales asssess current development.

Scales based on Piaget's work, though applicable to older children, are more commonly used with young children; these experimental scales are rarely commercially available. The *Piagetan scales* have contributed a theoretical framework of developmental sequences and a flexible procedure with qualitative interpretation. Ordinal scales presuppose a uniform sequence of development through successive stages from infancy to adolescence and beyond: the sensorimotor, the preoperational, the concrete operational, and the formal operational stages. The scales describe what the child actually can do at each stage. The tasks focus on long-term development of specific concepts or cognitive schemata rather than on broad traits, aiming to elicit a child's explanation for an observed event. Scoring depends on quality rather than number of responses. An incorrect answer is as valuable as a correct one because it demonstrates the child's reasoning.

All tests using ordinal scales suffer from decalage, inconsistencies in anticipated sequences. Increasingly, data cast doubt on Piaget's continuities and regularities of intellectual development. The stage of a person's development too often varies with the task, not only when the tasks require different processes but also when they require the same process (Dasen, 1977; Goodnow, 1976; Horn, 1976; J. McV. Hunt, 1976; Tuddenham, 1971; Ward, 1972). Piagetan scales correlate substantially with standardized intelligence tests (Gottfried &

Brody, 1975; Kaufman & Kaufman, 1972); though they may yield a richer picture of a child, they do not yield a different picture than tests much easier to administer.

Richman and Graham's (1971) promising questionnaire, the *Behavioral Screening Questionnaire* (BSQ), for 3-year-olds, administered to parents, consists of 12 items concerning the child's eating, sleeping, soiling, activity level, concentration and dependence, relations to agemates and sibs, control, temper, moods, fears, and worries. Earls et al. (1982), working with 3-year-olds in Martha's Vineyard to validate the BSQ with clinicians' ratings of play sessions, reported that BSQ ratings agreed with clinicians' ratings of degree of psychopathology.

The *Wechsler Preschool and Primary Scale of Intelligence* (WPPSI), for children 4 to 6½ years old, includes 11 subtests grouped into a Verbal and Performance scale to give Verbal, Performance, and Full Scale IQ. The WPPSI was standardized on a national sample of 1,200 children, 100 boys and 100 girls in each of six ½-year age groups from 4 to 6½. The sample was stratified against 1970 census data on geographical region, urban/rural residence, proportion of races, and father's occupational level. Kaufman's (1973) careful reanalysis of the standardization sample showed that children with fathers in professional and technical categories averaged significantly higher than all other groups (mean IQ = 110), and children with fathers in the unskilled category averaged lower than all other groups (mean IQ = 92.1). Socioeconomic status was measured by father's occupation, leaving fatherless children unclassifiable.

Readiness and Achievement

Anastasi (1982) defines school *readiness* as the attainment of skills, knowledge, attitudes, motivations, and other appropriate behavior traits that enable a child to profit maximally from school instruction, what Hunt and Kirk (1974) called the "entry skills" that a child needs to cope with the first grade. In the past, readiness was physical maturation, a precondition for certain kinds of learning. We now know that other developmental qualifications are necessary: Unless children can make the necessary auditory discriminations, they cannot learn to speak by the usual procedures; without fine motor coordination, they are unable to manipulate a pencil.

Recent research increasingly recognizes the importance of prior learning, emphasizing the hierarchical development of knowledge and skills whereby acquiring simple concepts equips the child to learn more complex concepts at any age. As a counterpoint, educators and parents have been criticized for disvaluing the child's social development (Louisville, Kentucky *Courier-Journal and Times*, February 16, 1982, B1), a phenomenon which European and other humanists have considered to be distinctly American. Readiness tests, while much like intelligence tests for the primary grades, place their greatest emphasis on reading ability, specifically visual and auditory discrimination, aural comprehension, vocabulary, quantitative concepts, and general information.

In Kentucky, the public schools administer only one nationally standardized comprehensive test to serve both as a diagnostic measure and as a test of scholastic achievement of the normal population of school-age children (grades 1 through 12); it is the *Comprehensive Test of Basic Skills* (CTBS), designed to "measure the extent to which students have acquired skills that are required for effective use of language and number in everyday living and for further academic achievement" (McGraw-Hill, 1968–70). The CTBS was designed for and standardized on a wide variety of students. According to Buros (1978) several reviews found no glaring flaws in its validity. Kentucky's public schools also administer selected aptitude tests prepared for local use within school districts, including the *Specific Expectations in Reading* (SER), a criterion-referenced test to diagnose reading aptitude in grades 1 through 5; the *Prescriptive Reading Inventory/Reading System* (PRI/RS), a test to determine the need for remedial instruction in grades 6, 7, and 8; and the *Diagnostic Math Inventory* (DMI), another criterion-referenced test.

Under the Federal Education Act (Title I), Kentucky children who qualify as disadvantaged also take the series of *Metropolitan Achievement Tests* (MAT), a widely used attainment and readiness battery that orally tests such readiness skills as beginning consonants, sound–letter correspondence, visual matching, listening, and quantitative concepts. Several studies using the earlier edition of the MAT yielded correlations in the .70s with group intelligence tests. However, when checked against end-of-year achievement test scores, readiness tests yielded consistently higher validities than intelligence tests (Anastasi, 1982).

Some tests like the *Tests of Basic Experience* (TOBE) and the Boehm *Test of Basic Concepts* combine criterion- and norm-referenced approaches. Although both are reminiscent of Piagetan scales, TOBE has a broader scope and covers a rather heterogeneous collection of items in language, mathematics, science, and social studies while the Boehm more narrowly assesses knowledge of frequently-used basic concepts—widely but sometimes mistakenly assumed to be familiar to children entering kindergarten or first grade.

Several recent developments in psychometrics, psychological theory, and early childhood education converged in *CIRCUS*, a series of tests for preschool and kindergarten children (CIRCUS, 1973). The circus theme, which pervades the CIRCUS tests, was chosen because of its presumed intrinsic appeal to all children, regardless of sex, race, geographic location, or socioeconomic status. (See Table 7.5.) Testers need even more than usual controls for economic-class bias and examiner bias when working with fatherless children, for many fatherless children are members of groups frequently put at disadvantage by assumptions that spare middle-class children.

Table 7.5. *Representative Achievement Batteries*

Battery	School Grade Range
California Achievement Tests	K – – – – – – – – – – – – – 12
Comprehensive Test of Basic Skills (CTBS)	1 – – – – – – – – – 9
Iowa Test of Basic Skills	K – – – – – – – – – 9
Iowa Test of Educational Development	9 – – – 12
Metropolitan Achievement Tests	K – – – – – – – – – – – – 12
SRA Achievement Series	K – – – – – – – – – – – – 12
Sequential Tests of Educational Progress-Series III (STEP-III)[a]	4 – – – – – – – – – – 12
Stanford Achievement	1 – – – – – – – – 9
Stanford Test of Academic Skills (TASK)	8 – – – – – – 13
Tests of Achievement and Proficiency (TAP)	9 – – – 12

[a] CIRCUS extends STEP III down to the preschool level; the Stanford Early School Achievement Test (SESAT) extends the Stanford series back to the beginning of kindergarten (Anastasi, 1982).

Competency

Anastasi (1982) and others have noted growing concern about the low competency of many high-school graduates in reading, writing, and arithmetic, a concern that has led to popular demand for competency tests as a basis for awarding high-school diplomas. Objections to such tests center on possible misuses and misinterpretations and possible educational rigidities and bureaucratic controls. Most states have established policies about minimum competency testing, but policies vary widely in the time and grade level of testing, the use of results, and the degree of local autonomy in the development or choice of tests.

The concept of "functional literacy" underlies these tests (Sticht, 1975), a concept that may also encompass functional competence in speaking, writing, and arithmetic. Functional competence is practical, specifically the level and amount of reading required for a particular job or, more generally, the basic educational skills required to manage one's life (Anastasi, 1982).

The Basic Skills Assessment Program (Educational Testing Service, 1976), designed for grades 7 through 12, is a nationally available testing program developed by the Educational Testing Service in collaboration with a national consortium of school districts. Administered in the seventh and eighth grades, these instruments provide an early-warning system that allows time for remedial instruction. The four parts are a writing sample such as completing a form or writing a job application letter and three multiple-choice tests in reading, writing skills, and mathematics.

Rapid screening instruments include the *Peabody Individual Achievement Test* (Dunn, 1959) and the *Wide Range Achievement Test* (WRAT), both of which apply from the preschool to the adult level, individual tests giving each person only items suitable to his or her performance level.

Intelligence

Although many writers since the late 1960s have suggested deemphasizing individual testing (Barclay, 1971; Hughes, 1979; Meacham & Peckham, 1978), others predict a resurgence in individual psychological testing rather than a "near demise" (Fein, 1979).

Patterned after the original test developed in France by Binet and Simon, the first American version of the Stanford-Binet scale was developed by Terman at Stanford University, published in 1916, revised by Terman and Merrill in 1937 (Forms L and M), and revised again in 1960 (Form L-M); new norms for Form L-M were provided in 1972. The virtues of the Stanford-Binet went unchallenged for several decades; it was the criterion measure for validating multitudes of other intelligence tests. Its use for preschoolers went uncontested even after its popularity for older people began to give way. In spite of criticisms, many seasoned Stanford-Binet users are highly successful in obtaining what appear to be valid results with this scale. They like its capability to assess a subject's global intelligence (Terman & Merrill, 1960) and a variety of abilities and to integrate the results into a single IQ score that reflects the subject's "mental adaptability."

Binet originally defined intelligence functionally, as the capacity to judge, reason, and comprehend effectively, with emphasis on the ability to take and maintain a definite direction, to adapt in attaining a desired goal, and to criticize oneself (Terman, 1916). Binet believed that environmental factors influence intelligence and that intelligence tests assess a person's present status. In contrast, Terman viewed intelligence as genetically determined, a fixed trait. Terman's theory provided a basis for recent controversy attributing differences found in average IQs of blacks and whites to genetic differences. Terman also placed a heavier emphasis than Binet on the abstract, intellective nature of intelligence.

In some important ways Wechsler's views of intelligence and its measurement were more consistent with Binet's than with Terman's. The Wechsler scales have gained in popularity since the first in 1939, and each scale has been more carefully constructed and normed than its predecessor. While the WAIS may be used to test older adolescents and the WPPSI to test preschool children, the WISC and WISC-R are more commonly used to assess school-age children. The WISC was constructed for use with subjects from 5 to 17 and the WISC-R from 6 to 17 years. The WPPSI is preferred for children from 4 up to 6 or 6½. Wechsler's ideas about intelligence may be viewed as a challenge to Terman's concepts, especially with reference to Terman's emphasis on the abstract, cognitive nature of intelligence (Matarazzo, 1972). Wechsler (1958) stated that "intelligence, operationally defined, is the aggregate or global capacity of the individual to act purposefully, to think rationally, and to deal effectively, with his environment" (p. 7). Wechsler emphasized that general intelligence and intellectual ability cannot be equated—that general intelligence "must be regarded as a manifestation of the personality as a whole" (1950, p. 78). From this perspective, general intelligence can be social and practical as well as abstract. The structure, composition, and scoring of the Wechsler tests take into account these nonintellective aspects of intelligence.

Formats of the Stanford-Binet and Wechsler scales reflect the theoretical biases of their originators. A look at the Stanford-Binet shows that it is presented as a series of tasks classified by age levels (six tests at most age levels). The tasks aim to discern diverse verbal and performance abilities; all require some degree of general intelligence for their completion. The tests were allocated to a given age level on the basis of an assessment of the difficulty of the task for children of various ages. Generally, a task was assigned to the level at which an average child of that age could accomplish it. A child is tested down to a level where he or she can succeed at all tasks and up to a level at which he or she fails all tasks. By contrast, each Wechsler scale is composed of groups of verbal and performance subtests. The verbal tests (five or six) assess a different aspect of intelligence, usually getting at the more cognitive or school-related components. The performance tests (five or six) assess relatively independent abilities more often reflecting the nonintellective aspects of intelligence. This division grossly parallels the functions of the left and right hemispheres as revealed by recent brain research. Each test also measures some *g* or general intelligence. The score on each subtest places the subject's performance in relation with the average performance on the same tasks by persons in similar age groups.

The Slosson Intelligence Test (Slosson, 1963) is a brief individual test of intelligence adapted from items contained in the Stanford-Binet and the Gesell Institute of Child Development Behavior Inventory. The Slosson can assess mental age from 5 months to 26 years with a ratio IQ. The standardization sample, taken from children and adults in New York State, and the details of the test's construction are poorly described in the test manual. Validity coefficients with the Stanford-Binet reportedly range from .90 to .98. Examining studies not reported in the manual, Sattler (1974) found a median correlation with the Stanford-Binet of .90 but cautioned that these correlations were spuriously high because of the Slosson item adoption from the Stanford-Binet. He further noted that correlations with the Wechsler were uniformly higher with the Verbal and Full Scale IQ than with the Performance IQ. The Slosson is a valuable quick-screening device, but according to Steward and Jones (1976), interpretation should not go beyond broad categorization such as below average to average level of intelligence (p. 377). The Slosson cannot be used as a direct substitute for the Stanford-Binet or Wechsler scales, and its use without modification at the extreme intellectual ranges is inappropriate.

The Columbia Mental Maturity Scale, Third Edition (Burgemeister, Blum, & Lorge, 1972) measures the reasoning ability and perceptual discriminations of young children with 92 pictorial and figural classification items that require the child to select the pictures that do not belong. This format makes the test particularly useful for children with sensorimotor, speaking, or reading disorders. Results are expressed in the form of an age deviation score, maturity score, stanines, and percentile scores. The notable improvement in the third edition is in the standardization sample of norms—2,600 children residing in 25 states. We need predictive validity studies with impaired subjects; the Columbia appears appropriate for these special populations.

The Leiter International Performance Scale (Leiter, 1959) is a nonverbal/performance measure of intelligence that requires perceptual organization and discrimination abilities. The test covers the age range from 2 to 18 and provides results in terms of mental age and ratio IQ; the scale contains 54 tests that require the child to insert a response picture block into the appropriate frame. The norms (based on 289 middle-class children) are limited. The Leiter has other problems, too. Werner (1965) noted that the pictures are outdated, cultural fairness is questionable, the abilities measured are unclear, and there are a limited number of tests for each year level. Sattler (1974) questioned the reliability of the scale, the norm sample, and the failure to present standard deviations for the various age levels. Ratcliffe and Ratcliffe (1979) noted the great variability of the scores in comparison to the Stanford-Binet and Wechsler results. Yet, with all its faults, better standardization may improve the Leiter so it can fill a gap in nonverbal psychological assessment. The format of the Leiter appears particularly promising for hearing-impaired, bilingual, and Indian children.

The need to standardize testing of people with highly dissimilar cultural backgrounds has occupied researchers since mid-century. In the United States, each subculture fosters behavior consonant with its values and demands; cross-cultural tests have tried to rule out one or more cultural variations. Language is a good example: To test people who speak different languages, one needs tests using either translations or no language on the part of either examiner or examinees. To test people with different levels of education one must eliminate reading. Cross-cultural tests have often—though not always—tried to eliminate the influence of speed by giving no premium for faster performance or responsiveness. The test content too must be adjusted for cross-cultural testing; several nonlanguage and nonreading tests still require information specific to certain cultures, asking the child to understand the function of such objects as a violin, postage stamp, gun, pocketknife, telephone, piano, or mirror. Persons reared in certain cultures may lack the experience to respond correctly. Several tests that attempt to control such variables have been developed.

The Peabody Picture Vocabulary Test (PPVT and PPVT-R) is a useful quick-screening device (not timed but takes 10 to 20 minutes) for nonverbal or nonfluent children ranging from $2\frac{1}{2}$ to 18 years of age. Standardization has been done on some 4,200 children and adolescents from a national sample. PPVT-R's reliability when compared to the original PPVT is .70; the scores of the original Peabody compared well with Stanford-Binet scores but children showed a higher improvement following compensatory education on PPVT than they did on the Binet.

The Culture Fair Intelligence Test, developed by R. B. Cattell and published by the Institute for Personality and Ability Testing (IPAT) is a paper-and-pencil test available in three levels: Scale 1, for ages 4 to 8 and mentally retarded adults; Scale 2 for ages 8 to 13 and average adults, and Scale 3, for Grades 10 to 16 and superior adults. Cattell's tests have been administered in several European countries, in America, and in certain African and Asian cultures. Norms tended to remain unchanged in cultures moderately similar to that in which the tests were developed; in other cultures, however, performance fell considerably below the original norms. Black children in the low socioeconomic stratum tested in the United States did no better on this test than on the Stanford-Binet (Willard, 1968).

The Progressive Matrices, developed in Great Britain by J. C. Raven, were designed as a measure of Spearman's general ability, or *g* factor. Requiring the child to find abstract relationships and point to the correct answer, this test is regarded by most British psychologists as the best available measure of *g* and an excellent instrument to tap cognitive ability. Percentile norms for 1/2-year intervals between 8 and 14 years and for 5-year intervals between 20 and 65 years are based on British samples, including 1,407 children, 3,665 men in military service tested during World War II, and 2,192 civilian adults. Rimoldi (1948) obtained closely similar norms with 1,680 children in Argentina, and testing in several European countries likewise indicated the applicability of available norms. Studies in a number of non-European cultures, however, have raised doubts about the suitability of the test for groups with very similar backgrounds. In such groups, the test reflects educational background and gives altered results with frequent practice.

The Goodenough Draw-a-Man Test approaches cross-cultural testing differently, simply instructing the examinee to "make a picture of a man; make the very best picture that you can." The 1963 revision, the *Goodenough-Harris Drawing Test* (D. B. Harris, 1963), like the original test, emphasizes accuracy of observation and development of conceptual thinking rather than of artistic skill. Cultural differences appeared in a well-designed comparative investigation of Mexican and American children (Laosa, Swartz, & Diaz-Guerrero, 1974); mean scores increased consistently and significantly with socioeconomic level. These results unfortunately are typical of all tests initially designed to be "culture-free" or "culture-fair" (Samuda, 1975).

Out of contempt for tests' racial biases against blacks, the psychologist R. L. Williams (1972) originated the BITCH-100, a test of ghetto street vocabulary that yielded much higher scores for black than for white adolescents, an intriguing approach to a genuine methodological problem. Matarazzo and Wiens (1977) found that the *Blacks Intelligence Test of Cultural Homogeneity* did not correlate with the Full Scale WAIS nor with any of the 11 WAIS subtests.

Creativity

Tests for creativity may be particularly appropriate for fatherless children since fatherlessness appears so frequently in biographies of eminent artists and writers. From Thurstone onward, psychometrists have differentiated IQ and creativity, holding the latter to show divergent inductive reasoning, ideational fluency, and perceptual style. Thurstone (1951) and others, impressed by nonintellectual parameters of temperament, have reported that openness and receptivity to new ideas are signs of creativity.

The University of Southern California's Aptitudes Research Project (ARP) uses factor analysis to arrive at *Tests of Divergent Thinking*, for ninth graders and older people, and *Creativity Tests for Children* (published by Sheridan Psychological Services) for children in grades 4 through 6. *Torrance Tests of Creative Thinking* (published by Scholastic Testing Service) derives from the ARP tests (Torrance, 1965) and includes verbal, pictorial, and auditory batteries. These tests try to evaluate fluency, flexibility, originality, and elaboration, all dimensions of a creative mind.

Creativity requires not only divergent thinking but also sharpness of critique, so some tests of critical reasoning and old-fashioned comprehension and memory improve a creativity battery. Watson-Glaser's *Critical Thinking Appraisal* (published by Psychological Corporation) and some of the ARP scales (published by Sheridan Psychological Series) that include *Logical Reasoning* and *Pertinent Questions* can be used for high-school and older poeple. The Educational Testing Service (1976) has devised a promising *Kit of Factor-Referenced Cognitive Tests* to include several tests of reasoning power in young people.

In addition, haptic, phonic, and visual modes of perceiving and learning may be the basis for testing devices of great interest. Some children are highly verbal, others are not; some live and learn mainly visually, some auditorily, and some kinesthetically; some use all three modalities. Children show differences in cognitive and perceptual styles and the USC group have devised ways to tap such differences. But the major work to be done lies in the future.

Sex Role

In extensive psychological research on sex differences, several investigators have used self-report inventories to assess the respondents' sex-role concepts, preferences, and identification. The pioneer instrument for measuring masculinity–feminity (M–F), developed by Terman and Miles (1936), includes some self-report subtests along with other paper-and-pencil procedures. Items were selected empirically by the relative frequency of each response given by American males and females. Ruth Hartley (1960) found that children in their early school years perceive boys as aggressive, dominant, and independent and girls as passive, affectionate, and nurturant. Since stereotypes are more tenacious in young children than in adults, they make a burlesque of any instruments based on children's prevalent attitudes as sex-role orientation norms. The resulting inventory, labeled *Attitude–Interest Analysis,* included seven subtests: Word Association, Inkblot Association, Information, Emotional and Ethical Attitudes, Interests, Personalities and Opinions, and Introvertive Response.

The second-generation M–F scales of the next 2 decades include the M–F scales in the *Strong Vocational Interest Blank,* the *MMPI,* the *California Psychological Inventory,* and the *Guilford-Zimmerman Temperament Survey.* Although all follow Terman-Miles' model of empirical item selection and criterion keying, they differ in emphasis and content. These scales correlate poorly with each other, in the $+.40$ to $+.50$ range.

Another limitation of both first- and second-generation M–F scales is bipolarity; they assume that masculinity and femininity represent opposite poles of a single scale. Yet even the original results reported by Terman and Miles suggest that masculinity and femininity might be two variables whose intercorrelation falls far short of the implied -1.00. For instance, at higher educational levels, sex differentiation in M–F scores becomes less sharp, both men and women giving more responses characteristic of the other sex.

Henry Biller and Lloyd Borstelmann (1967) suggested a broader view of masculinity than children's attitudes provide, dividing the pertinent topics into *sex-role orientation* (now generally called core gender identity), which they contended develops in the second year of the boy's life; *sex-role preference,* which could be diametrically opposed to a masculine sex-role orientation; and *sex-role adoption,* which they defined as "the masculinity and/or femininity of the individual's publicly observable behavior." Only the third component, sex-role adoption, corresponded closely to Terman and Miles' masculinity in males. Biller followed these conceptualizations in quantifying different aspects of sex role. In *Father, Child and Sex Role,* Biller (1971) reviewed some of the tests which he felt would tap the numerous facets or dimensions of sex-roles, suggesting this tabulation:

Dimension	Instruments to Measure
Sex-role orientation or Core gender identity	Adjective checklists such as Heilbrun (1965) or Biller and Bahm (1971) Drawings, fantasy play, and TAT-like responses Human figure drawings and drawing completion tests like Franck and Rosen (1949) Brown's IT Scale for Children (1956)
Sex-role preference	Rabban Toy Choice procedure with eight feminine and eight masculine toys for children Terman and Miles inventory and their descendants: MMPI, Strong Vocational Interest Blank, Gough Femininity Scale— for adolescents Rosenberg and Sutton-Smith (1959) preference-for-games, technique that does not assume that masculinity and femininity are polar opposites
Sex-role adoption	Simple point scale ratings (as in Koch, 1956) Peer ratings of most and least masculine boys (Freedheim, 1960; Biller, 1968a; Vroegh et. al., 1967) Rating procedures that rate separately masculine and feminine (as in Biller & Liebman, 1971)—foreshadowing some concepts of androgyny

Among the best-known of the third-generation M–F tests are the *Bem Sex-Role Inventory* (Bem, 1974, 1977, 1981), used with adolescents and adults, and the *Personal Attributes Questionnaire* developed by Spence and Helmreich (1978), also available for children (Hall & Halberstadt, 1980). These tests eliminate certain shortcoming of earlier ones. First, the items are selected from judges' ratings of their relative desirability for males or females and the degree to which they characterize each gender in our society. This procedure helps sharpen the scale definition, clarify content coverage, and reduce chance variance in scores. Second, masculinity and femininity are treated as independent (and probably orthogonal) variables; persons high on both are classified as androgynous. Third, some efforts are being made to recognize multidimensionality both by identifying item clusters empirically and by considering situational influences at work on one person over time.

As currently used in personality research, the term *androgyny* characterizes the individual who manifests favorable traits ascribed to both sexes, for example, one combining assertiveness and competence with compassion, warmth, and emotional expressiveness. The androgynous person should be more flexible and more capable of adapting to varying situational demands than the traditionally sex-stereotyped person; it has been hypothesized that androgyny should be associated with effective interpersonal behavior and with psychological well-being. Research findings on this relationship, however, are mixed (Hall & Halberstadt, 1980; Jackson & Paunonen, 1980; Kelly & Worell, 1977; Worell, 1978). The relationship is probably complex, influenced by the sociocultural context and the criteria for effectiveness or well-being. The available instruments for measuring masculinity–femininity are still in a formative stage. Both the underlying personality theory and the test construction procedures are in the process of development. Some serious unsolved methodological problems remain (Jackson & Paunonen, 1980; Kelly & Worell, 1977; Worell, 1978). More information is needed, for example, on the factorial composition of the construct measured by different instruments and the adequacy with which the social desirability response tendency has been controlled.

Orlofsky (1980) concluded a review of the "androgynous sex-role orientation" instruments thus:

> *To date, the new sex-role measures have been used primarily for research, mainly with college populations. While they can be expected to have great potential in future clinical assessment, largely supplanting existing objective and projective measures of sex-role characteristics, such applications have not yet occurred with much frequency. They have yet to be adapted for work with children . . . and research is only now proceeding to develop norms for different socioeconomic and ethnic groups. [p. 669]*

Tests of sex-role orientation cannot be administered within most school systems today because parents react so negatively to any test that has the word "sex" in the title. All such measuring devices are politically suspect under the Buckley Amendment; the privacy requirements of many recent laws and court decisions consider these matters too intimate to be included in school records.

Personality

Psychological tests utilized to assess delinquent tendencies and predilection to psychiatric disorder are most often those tools that measure personality traits, projective tests, parent report and self-report inventories, and objective ("nonprojective") tests.

Projective tests can be used with children too young to complete self-report inventories, but their usefulness in many cases is directly proportional to the skill of the tester. Rachel Gittelman (1980), Eysenck, and others doubt the value of projectives as screening or diagnostic instruments because testers may overinterpret the pathology of children's responses and the tester's bias may distort results. For example, testing children from one-parent families, especially poor and black children, a white middle-class tester who views only the two-parent family as normal and healthy may err.

The Rorschach (Inkblot) Test for Children is probably the most frequently employed projective technique used with youngsters. It is recommended for children 3 and over. Invented by Hermann Rorschach (1921), the test consists of a series of 10 inkblots that the child examines one at a time in a precise sequence and interprets. The Rorschach test furnishes an unusual amount of information in a short time. The child's responses often indicate a diagnosis and a therapeutic approach. The Rorschach diagnoses borderline schizophrenia, often missed clinically, and it yields patterns of responses in some varieties of sociopathy or psychopathy and juvenile delinquency. The child's intelligence is associated with clarity in perception of form, accounting for the entire blot, number of original responses, and variety of perceived content. The child's cognitive, emotive, and perceptual responses to each blot indicate the method by which the child solves other kinds of problems.

The Thematic Apperception Test (TAT), developed by Morgan and Murray (1935), is second only to the Rorschach in clinical use. Recommended for children 4 and over, the test consists of a series of 20 drawings of people in various situations. The subject makes up a story about the pictures, necessarily expressing her or his motives, interests, and anxieties. The child inadvertently reveals level of intelligence; range of interests; unconscious tensions; attitudes toward death, violence, sex, and parents; and latent or repressed material. The TAT, like many projective techniques, lacks strict reliability, validity, and normative data base. It is easily distorted, so a high level of sophistication is required to administer and to interpret it. A useful adjunct, it does not provide a comprehensive profile of personality traits and must be supplemented and validated by other procedures.

The Children's Apperception Test (CAT), developed by Leopold Bellak (1949), a projective method for children 3 to 10, consists of a series of 10 drawings of animals in various social situations. The children tell stories about what they see in the drawings. The underlying rationale is that children can identify more readily with animal figures than with human figures, but this assumption has been disputed, and the CAT-H using human figures has been developed. Both tests elicit emotional responses from children. This test, too, lacks conclusive data on reliability, validity, and norms. The value of the test seems to lie with the tester and his or her clinical hunches.

The Blacky Picture Test, another projective technique using interpretation of pictures, explores personality dynamics and is recommended for children 5 and over. The Blacky pictures, designed as stimuli for a modified projective technique to study the psychoanalytic theory of psychosexual development, were published in 1950 by Gerald S. Blum as stimuli for exploring personality dynamics. Reliability investigations have, for the most part, demonstrated that the statistical significance of the Blacky dimension scores is not usually high enough to diagnose individual personalities. However, especially with boys, the Blacky pictures often provide adequate material for interpretations concerning attitudes toward siblings and parents, characteristic defensive reactions, and self-perceptions.

The Draw a Person Test (DAP), derived from the work of Karen Machover (1949), is recommended for children 5 and over. The underlying rationale for the DAP is that figure drawing is a projection of the child's self-concept, but unfortunately research does not support Machover's basic body image hypothesis. Drawings may also reveal the child's projection of his or her ideal self and attitudes toward significant others, life in general, and the tester. The sign–trait scoring, finding correspondences between signs in the drawing and traits in the person, for example between clawed hands and hostility, has not been supported by research.

The Kinetic Family Drawing Test (Buros & Kaufman, 1970) instructs the child to draw everyone in the family doing something as a group. These kinetic (action) drawings are more informative than drawings following traditional akinetic instructions. Young children usually express themselves more naturally and spontaneously through actions than through words, so action drawings provide an excellent method of exploring their world. Though difficult to score, drawing tests are nonthreatening, simple to administer, and useful when other techniques are limited by language barriers, cultural differences, and inability to communicate.

The IPAT High School Personality Questionnaire (HSPQ), prepared by Raymond B. Cattell and Mary D. L. Cattell (1953), is recommended for use with Children 12 to 18 by the Institute for Personality and Ability Testing (IPAT). A general test, it gives an overview of total personality, including these traits: reserved versus outgoing, less intelligent versus more intelligent, affected by feelings versus emotionally stable, phlegmatic versus excitable, obedient versus assertive, and disregardful of rules versus conscientious. This test lends itself to overinterpretation, but can be used with other tests and may indicate such qualities as leadership potential, neurotic inclination, and delinquent tendencies. It should by no means be used as a sole predictor of a young person's life course.

Another broadly focused test—this one for a younger age group—
is the IPAT *Children's Personality Questionnaire* (CPQ), developed
by Raymond B. Cattell and Rutherford B. Porter (1959), recommended for children 8 to 12. The test measures 14 personality traits
including reserved versus warmhearted, shy versus venturesome, and
relaxed versus tense. It can help predict such things as leadership potential and tendency toward psychopathology. The problems with
the CPQ are similar to the problems with the HSPQ; we lack validity
data. However, the test may focus on aspects of a child's personality
that need further exploration with other devices.

Another test for general personality prediction is the *Myers-Briggs
Type Indicator* (MBTI), devised by Katharine A. Briggs and Isabel
Briggs Myers (1943). The MBTI, recommended for use with children in grades 9 through 16 and with adults, measures four personality dimensions according to Jung's concepts: judgment–perception,
thinking–feeling, sensation–intuition, and extroversion–introversion.
It is commonly used for vocational counseling, personality research,
industrial placement, and academic counseling. For teenagers it gives
nonpathologic Jungian parameters. Although validity and reliability
data are better for the MBTI than for the HSPQ or the CPQ, it is designed for the normal population and may give inadequate results
with a disturbed person.

The Minnesota Multiphasic Personality Inventory (MMPI) developed by Hathaway and McKinley (1943), is the usual tool to assess
psychiatric disturbances in persons 16 and older, but the MMPI can
be administered to adolescents 12 to 15 years old with only slightly
diminished utility. There are 10 diagnostic scales—depression, hysteria, psychopathic deviate, hypochondriasis, masculinity–femininity,
paranoia, psychasthenia, schizophrenia, hypomania, and social introversion–extroversion—as well as scales that cross-check its internal
reliability. Extensive validity and reliability data have been collected
on each of the 10 diagnostic scales. The MMPI was normed on a normal adult, cross-section group that came from all over Minnesota,
from that state's every socioeconomic and educational level. It may
represent Minnesota well; however, the Minnesota population comes
largely from Northern European stock, is largely Christian in background, and has a relatively small number in several of the minority
groups. Thus, we question the use of the MMPI with people from
different ethnic and religious backgrounds.

Other tests that indicate child psychopathology are the *Child Behavior Profile* and the *School Behavior Checklist,* using parent reports and teacher reports, respectively. The Child Behavior Profile (Achenbach, 1978) is recommended for use with boys 12 to 16, and girls 6 to 16. It consists of social competence and behavior problem scales from the *Child Behavior Checklist* (CBCL), completed by parents or parent surrogates. Reliability and validity ratings are high. The checklist of 130 items has been extensively normed. Unweighted means analyses of variance (ANOVAS) have been performed on the scores of matched populations to assess differences in scores as they are related to age, SES, and clinical status. The Child Behavior Profile has been used predominantly to assess stability and change in children's psychopathology during and after mental health contacts and has contributed to understanding of children who act in (internalizers) and act out (externalizers).

The *School Behavior Checklist* (Miller, 1972), recommended for elementary-school children 6 to 12 years old, is designed specifically to assess deviant behavior with the following scales: low need achievement, aggression, anxiety, academic disability, hostile isolation, extraversion, and total disability. Identical scales are used for both sexes. Variations in scores resulting from race, IQ, age, religion, grade, socioeconomic status, and teaching experience of teacher have been computed. The test has been extensively normed and reliability ratings reach acceptable limits. The School Behavior Checklist has proved to be an effective tool in determining the general distribution of deviant behaviors in the urban elementary-school population of Louisville, Kentucky. A modified version of the School Behavior Checklist—the *Louisville Behavior Checklist* (Miller, 1979)—is available for parental endorsement of 164 observable child behaviors as witnessed or perceived by parents. The E-1 form is for children 3 to 6 years, E-2 for 7 to 12 years, and E-3 for 13 to 18. The aggression survey scale of this instrument was employed in the study of impoverished children, fathered and fatherless, reported by Adams and Horovitz (1980). They discovered no significant differences between fathered and fatherless in the degree of aggression and delinquent and nondelinquent pathology displayed. All the children they studied were male, firstborn, and impoverished; only the younger firstborn (below age 9) exhibited an increased psychopathology score. Many other uses have been made of the Louisville Behavior Checklist to detect various forms of psychopathology, including academic problems, fears, suicidal tendencies, antisocial behavior, hyperactivity, and so on; to check a parent's reports against teachers' and clinicians'; and to compare results of LBCL with Achenbach's Child Behavior Checklist and other instruments. Reliability and validity data are forthcoming for this screening instrument that now shows considerable promise.

Fatherless children's psychopathology can also be screened by standardized psychiatric interviews or by having trained observers rate children's behavior for psychopathology; the study can be done by working directly with the children and by interviewing their mothers. Several worthwhile instruments are available for this purpose.

Herjanic and Welner (Weissman et al., 1980) have devised the *Diagnostic Interview for Children and Adolescents* (DICA), which currently ranges from 6 to 17+ years and is administered directly to the subject. It is an excellent screening and diagnostic instrument that takes 1½ hours for each child.

The *K-SADS* is a "kiddie" version (by Puig-Antich & Chambers) of an adult rating Schedule for Affective Dsiorders and Schizophrenia (see Weissman et al., 1980). The Kiddie-SADS also requires 1½ hours of testing time and uses the child and parent as informants. It covers a wide spectrum of diagnostic categories, all consonant with *DSM-III*.

Kovacs et al. have designed the *Interview Schedule for Children* (ICS) to study childhood depression. The ICS gets information from 8- to 13-year-old children in almost as many pathologic domains as the DICA or K-SADS and takes only 35 minutes to complete. The same general point applies to the *Isle of Wight Survey Interview* (IWS) of Rutter and Graham (1968). Originated to study the total population of children between 7 and 12 years old on the Isle of Wight, it requires only half an hour to administer but its interrater reliability has not been good. The IWSI was a basis for epidemiologic study of psychiatric disorder in children; it had been surpassed by 1982.

Langer et al. (1976) developed a *Screening Inventory* (SI) that relies on parental report exclusively until the youth has reached 14 years of age. It is a better screening inventory than a diagnostic one but has shown some interesting cross-validation with the results of psychiatric interviews. Only about 22 minutes are required to administer its 83 items.

Kestenbaum and Bird (1978) developed the *Mental Health Assessment Form* (MHAF). Originally, it was a way to screen the offspring of schizophrenic parents and required 45 minutes to complete. For general screening it may prove to be a useful instrument but further validation and reliability studies are needed.

Moral Development

While Freudians (especially those who follow Melanie Klein) postulate that conscience or superego development begins in infancy, little evidence documents this stand except for occasional signs of infants' and preschoolers' guilt or shame concerning rules they have broken. According to this view, young children can suffer depression, even if they do not go into intrapsychic depressive and paranoid positions. Non-Kleinian Freudians, on the other hand, hold that real conscience must await the height of Oedipal development and that guilt and self-hatred (depression) cannot flower until the superego emerges during and after the Oedipal stage. Growing evidence suggests that both depression and mania can occur pre-Oedipally, and since fatherlessness alters the Oedipal experience, according to this view, fatherless children must develop abnormal consciences.

Most non-Freudians agree with legal theorists, sociologists, and others that a genuine "conscience of one's own" does not appear until around age 14. It would be interesting to know to what extent externalizers and internalizers are delinquents or neurotics, respectively, but data are scarce. Instruments to check matters of internalized moral standards are available, but standardization and studies of validity and reliability generally are missing. The WISC has several items to test moral judgment, for example, and there are some preschool and childhood adaptations of Rotter's (1966) scale of internal versus external locus of control; the moral judgment scale of Kohlberg (1974) seems to be the most comprehensive. Following Piaget, Kohlberg postulated six stages in moral development—from egocentric and premoral, to rule-following conformity, to self-accepted moral judgments. The scale is full of psychometric deficits and at present is not very useful for research about the moral judgments of fatherless children.

Standardized tests probably reveal that fatherless children differ from fathered children because they are less frequently white and middle class. We know that most tests apply inadequately to minority children; information about fatherless children from such tests, being distorted, must be eyed skeptically.

CHAPTER EIGHT

Policy Suggestions

RESEARCH

In one sense, when we made a plea in Chapter 7 for better designed research, we were making a bid for a change in public policy as it impinges on the scientific research community. Some excellent studies of fatherless children, such as that by Herzog and Sudia (1970) or the more recent one by Robert S. Weiss (1979) as well as most others, have been made possible by grants from the federal government. The principal benefactors for this scientific enterprise have been the National Institute of Mental Health (NIMH), the National Institute for Child Health and Human Development, the Office of Child Development, the Public Health Service, and the Bureau for the Education of the Handicapped. Sometimes the government agency's RFA (request or applications) is very specific, seeming tailor-made for only one or two applicants. Sometimes contractual arrangements with the former Department of Health, Education and Welfare, lately divided into the Department of Health and Human Services and the Department of Education, have empowered studies such as that by the sociologist Weiss. Public policy dictates what we know, what we study, what questions we ask, and the methods and techniques we employ. Governmental peer review committees prefer what is safe and not too upsetting to established theory and practice; consequently, innovative researchers and minorities find it hard to obtain funds. Methodologic toughness in peer review frequently masks a determination by the reviewer to be safe politically.

Research that gets funded often shows more methodologic narrowness than clarity of concept. Hundreds of studies have been amassed that appear to try to make up, by rigor and rigidity of technique, for their theoretical and methodologic shortcomings. Anything approximating experimental method or called "an experiment"—even if it is not—gets priority over practical projects. Funding goes more readily to a psychologist who wants to try an operant conditioning technique on six phobic adults than to a psychiatric social worker who wishes to study delayed stress in 100 girls who have been abused sexually by their fathers. So government grants occasionally seem to go to short-run dazzlers with gimmicks that do not challenge the prevalent ideology. It is poetic justice that some of these projects have received Senator Proxmire's Golden Fleece award. The kind of epidemiologic approach taken by persons like Kellam and associates at the University of Chicago's social psychiatry laboratory will be more useful in the long run than a few thousand funded small studies, but NIMH, for one, has only falteringly begun to support such longitudinal, community-wide researches, and few concern children.

When governmental agencies do support studies of children, fatherless or not, they do so as part of a categorical grant, that is, specifically for a targeted population—Medicare recipients, Head Start children, and so on. Some "requests for proposals" (RFPs) read like a laundry list of what will succeed. The issue that fatherlessness is prevalent although *not* accompanied by noticeable pathology in one of the census tracts of Jefferson County, Kentucky, for example, would probably not attract a governmental grant. (The area in question is made up of upper-class divorced women and their children, in the main.) General support grants are always an endangered species. Occasionally a granting agency will advertise acceptable priorities like these of NIMH (July, 1979):

1) *manpower for underserved people in a)* geographic areas—*rural,** *inner city,** *others with unmet needs*; b)* populations—*chronically ill and disabled, minorities,** *children,** *youth,** *the aged, juvenile and adult offenders,** *victims of violence*; c)* public mental health facilities*—*state and county hospitals, clinics, centers, correctional institutions.*

2) *increasing the numbers of minority psychiatrists and others in mental health delivery systems.**

3) *developing strategies for primary prevention.**

4) *increasing mental health skills and knowledge of primary care physicians.**

5) *linking training and delivery agencies together.**

The asterisks show areas that pertain to fatherless children as underserved, poor, often ethnic minority members.

The need for informed consent makes it difficult to undertake many studies that would be valuable, and often one is hard put to see any conceivable harm to the children involved. But if we propose to ask children about their sexual activities and fantasies, we have incriminated ourselves and raised hackles right at the outset;

the result is that we decide not to try research but to perpetuate our ignorance on that score. If we want to survey large groups of children, to ascertain what major stressful life events afflict children, we are hampered by the rule that informed consent must be obtained from parents and children in order to solicit the approval of the public school's *human experimentation* committee! We know the adults' stressors but we do not know about children. What life events increase the child's vulnerability to stress? (See Coddington et al., 1982). If we want to discover children's responses to sexual molestation, we find our work hampered by public servants who value not rocking the boat more than they value helping children. They hide their poor practice behind "confidentiality of the records." If we wish to find out about children who are incarcerated in various institutions, we find that we must butt our heads against a stony wall of concealment. Children are walled off from our need assessments and from needed services. We are told, "We don't keep our statistics that way." Children truly are nonpersons, "the parapeople—the recipients of paraservices, assigned to paraprofessionals, and always reached indirectly, through parents, through teachers, through pediatricians, through courts, through anyone except children themselves" (Adams, 1975, p. 18).

One of the authors (Adams, 1976) has described the numerous difficulties in studying black children's disproportionate uprooting as a result of court-ordered desegregation and has suggested that at the community level, at the grassroots, child-focused research and information bureaus may be required to get figures out of the closet wherever children are concerned. Adams (1975), already cited, has looked at the weak record and strong hope of the community mental health centers in conducting research concerning mentally disordered children. By law, research and evaluation are basic parts of a community mental health/mental retardation center (CMH/MRC), but although community mental health centers often claim that their major efforts on behalf of children go to "prevention, education, and research," the results are not impressive. Adams (1975) cited these shortcomings at that time:

> the weak position of the CMH/MRCs (about 400 of the 2,000 planned originally have actually been funded), the paucity of research done, the lack of evaluation of efficacy in many prevention and consultation

efforts, and so on. Some worthwhile values might have been mis-directed in practice, such as the mistrust of credentialism, impatience with the arrogance of many professionals, eagerness for institutional changes in our national life, a desire to help parents as well as their disturbed children, a wish to enrich the tribal and social aspects of atomized urban life, and others. The record of genuine accomplishments for any of the paraservices of the CMH/MRCs is not brightly encouraging. Certainly, no great social changes have been ushered in by the CMH movement, and the notion that CMH is Psychiatry's Third Revolution seems a bit ovedrawn in 1974. [pp. 29–30]

Anything we can say about community mental health and research concerning children applies equally to research concerning fatherless children: more ballyhoo than concrete results.

NEW YARDSTICKS IN HUMAN SERVICES

A new set of attitudes, it is suggested, must pervade the field of human services: *a change of focus from adults to children.* Human services budgets go mainly for adults with problems, not children; budgets give priority to the child within the adult, not the child. The adult alcoholic, even in an economy of scarcity, has preferential treatment over children. The adult drug addict, sexual psychopath, mental patient, and physically handicapped person receive the lion's share of human services today. A new viewpoint, looking to the welfare of children, is called for.

This reorientation would entail more and less than a change of heart in the taxpayers and voters of the United States: more, because the policy would assign public spending (institutional as well as mental) priority to the needs of children; less, because it would bring about practical institutional changes that need not wait for a rebirth of compassion in the body politic. Image building is part of this policy change, but the structured change that we envision is more than a change of image.

FAMILY IN THE FOREFRONT

The family itself, tied to the life cycles of children and adult caretakers, is an odd kind of institution and one that has not always served children well. Families are the points of convergence for material and spiritual things. In families, children are assigned statuses and roles along with the other family members. "Role" may be too dry a term since these roles pertain to gut-level events such as parental copulation, for fun as well as for procreation, childbirth, the emergence of independence, the experience of life-threatening events, adolescence, the simultaneous occurrence of aging and flowering and growth, and the acceptance of the death of cherished figures. There is nothing very antiseptic or dry about family life as children live it: It is very properly a mammalian arrangement with sensual and libidinal significances for all involved.

The family is both a setting for personal fantasies and projections, and a place for overt instruction of the young. Without realizing it, every individual family stratifies the child socially and orients the child to her or his position in the American economic class system.

Roles assigned and ascribed for intrafamilial life are informal and associational in nature, traditionally the area of a woman's expertise and interests. Family roles are not as formal as those in the marketplace or the government or the military, which are traditionally the realm of the male, the father in the family. Roles are about to change profoundly and already show marked alterations. The future is here, shocks and all. The woman is invading the man's zone of interest; the man is invading the woman's. Ancient patriarchal traditions remain operative, nonetheless, and children generally acquire traditional attitudes along with the modifications already realized. From the adults' standpoint, men and women are realizing more equality.

From the child's perspective, one of the most noteworthy changes in the American family is the greater, more active involvement of fathers in the domestic lives of their wives and children. The father's return to the family outstrips the woman's entry into the work force as a psychosocial fact in the lives of American children. That fact promises to make fatherlessness still more "nonstandard" and a more pathogenic influence on children than it has been in the past, another piece of evidence that childhood needs to become a national priority. The conditions of childhood in families are changing so that father-absence because of its concomitants and meanings will be felt more acutely, not less.

FAMILY FUNCTIONS

All characterizations of the functions of the family include maintenance of life (*subsistence*), because the animals large and small have
to be fed, bathed, sheltered, and given sleep and rest, and provision
must be made for disposing of their animal wastes. These matters of
subsistence and survival must be dealt with, for without provision
for them the adult members (and the dependent ones, the children,
in particular) will lack basic economic security. Then comes a related function of affiliation, love, *companionship*. In the past, men
were in and out, transient and intermittently salient, regarding companionship with family members but mother and children have always been thrown together. Now, if we discern correctly, the father
too will be a full-fledged family member, as much as his wife will be.
A third function of the family, perhaps the irreducible function, is
species continuity, begetting and *rearing children*. Parental sexual
behavior, including reproduction, is not of first-rank importance except as it sets the stage for the child-care function of most families.
For many current writers carnality reigns over family life and parental sexual feats assume a first-rate significance, ahead of child rearing.
With Rossi (1977) we disagree with the adult carnality proponents.
A fourth function has none of the large evolutionary sweep of the
third; it only has to do with tedious and practical everyday matters
that keep the motor going for the subsistence function. It is *housekeeping*, homemaking, some effort at orderly and expectable behavior in the daily living routines wherever adults are nurturing and
caring for children. Hence, child care, subsistence, housekeeping,
and companionship are the four basic functions of all kinds of families. They apply to fathered and fatherless households, to rich and
to poor, to black and to white. National policies will reinforce the
family's strengths only when these four functions receive the emphasis they deserve.

Obviously, a fatherless family requires some special efforts to
make it work in all four spheres. Weiss (1979) epitomized the fatherless (actually, in his terminology, the single-parent) family as presenting, regarding subsistence, *inadequate support;* regarding child care,
responsibility overload; regarding housekeeping, *task overload;* and

regarding companionship, *emotional overload*. Exorbitant demands are made on the single parent, Weiss reported, in all four functions.

In most fatherless households, the mother goes to work to offset inadequate economic resources; seeks auxiliary child-care arrangements while she is at work to lessen her feeling of total responsibility for the medical, physical, emotional, educational, and all other needs of her child(ren); shares the household chores with her children or relies on homemaker services of others to reduce her task overload. To cope with her emotional overload, from being on the hot seat alone with her child(ren), she seeks an occasional evening away or at home by herself, to unwind, to relax, to recreate, which is hard to do when her children's needs seem endless and total and she feels as if the pumping continues even when the well is bone dry. Sometimes home is her haven in a heartless world, but at other times it is no refuge, giving only increased demands from her consumer-children who, she knows, were never meant to repay or nurture a mother.

GOVERNMENT INTERVENTIONS, NOW AND THEN

Governments have always intervened in family life under the doctrines of *parens patriae* and *patria potestas,* the former originally a belief that the king owned all his subjects, and, as a kind of father figure overseeing all his children, he and his government could claim a right to interfere with parents' rearing of their children. The latter is a belief that a particular father has undisputed power over his family. The argument has long been that the state can intrude to protect children whose parents are abusive or neglectful, and to take over when parents find a child uncontrollable. But the state has always been reluctant to intervene against a father in instances of child labor, parent–child incest, family poverty, parental emotional abuse of their children, corporal punishment, parental religious teachings inimical to children, and many other injustices. In law, both statutes and court decisions have used "sanctity of the family" as a euphemism for parental ownership and control of children and have left the autocratic rule of parents untouched. A man is king in his own house.

If as a matter of public policy, children are to be valued, the children in fatherless families will have to have special governmental aid and support with relatively few strings attached. After all, they are *children at risk*. They are children (11 million strong) and they occupy a huge number (15%) of the total families of America. Their households, provided with added economic support, could do all the necessary things that intact, complete families do. Whether they are fatherless by choice or by an unsolicited fate, they are a potentially productive family group. With help, they may compensate for their deficiencies (but not their differences) and perform their functions better.

Economic support for fatherless families is so fundamental a matter that we must return to it after a few pages, but for now we turn to some other features of the new image of children as the linchpin of national policy making. Putting greatest value on children, whoever and wherever they may be, means that no selectively targeted population of children needs to be drawn out from the mass of children. We should no longer have to fight for programs for American Indian children as a special group (for example) but simply for programs for all children. In that way we reach those in any oppressed and impoverished conditions while "benignly neglecting" to target and stigmatize them.

Making children the basic reference criterion in public policy will not be done to extend the reach of the arm of the state into private lives, but to help the youngest and weakest, the generational group of children. State interventions have been most notably helpful to economic institutions up to now, by collusions through the military–industrial complex of war and defense profiteers, through governmental giveaways to oil companies, through subsidies to farm factories in the fields, Chrysler Corporation and others. The state, always keen on the marketplace and the battlefield, needs to change its basic emphases in order to enhance family life of all the children of America.

Impact studies, common nowadays, examine traffic patterns, housing geography, shopping areas, military bases, and, occasionally, environmental impact of new pollutants to be emitted from future industries. Impact studies under the new child-focused public policy would concentrate on families with young children and weigh the noxious and favorable impacts of any new policies on children and families. Fatherless children would benefit if there were such policy–image changes.

RENUNCIATION AND HIERARCHY VERSUS RESPECT

Looking into family life to upgrade the welfare of all children, the government may be well advised to consider parents vital guardians rather than owners of and sole arbiters over their children's lives. Are they doing what guardians must do? Guardianship by parents was proposed by James E. Block (1980); it warrants serious thought and perhaps ultimate acceptance. Accepting the guardianship model would certainly democratize the family by injecting a time-limited, developmental perspective into the relations between children and their adult caretakers. Today that relationship is authoritarian and drab; under the guardianship model it would change from an authority to an agency relation that would require the adult's optimal contribution to the child's optimal development, with gradual transfer of responsibility from the adult guardian to the growing child. Today parent–child relationships are pervaded and underpinned by law that makes appeals to property and authority, but with the guardianship model, the undergirding law would appeal instead to preexistent law governing guardianships—with emphasis on the needy one and the obligations of the guardian to provide for those needs only as long as necessary for the child, who by "status, or defect of age, understanding, or self-control, is considered incapable of administering his (or her) affairs" (Block, p. 42).

Many of the women known to us who head families of young children already have made very serious strides toward a family democratization, especially with children over 6 years old. Some of the clinical cases seen in practice have made guardianship both a reality and a talking point with their children. For example, one mother said,

I am not trying to lord it over my sons. As soon as they are able to do more for themselves and do not need me to ride herd on them, they know that I can back off. I have already backed off as soon as they were able to pick up on things I used to have to do for them. I know that what I want ultimately is for them to hatch, spring out of our family and lead happy lives of their own; that will allow them to be good to their children when that time comes.

That is the way one female head-of-household saw things. She had discovered the guardianship model on her own and delighted in the democracy it entailed.

Fatherlessness does not inevitably produce a more democratic family, since some women under pressure become like men, fearful and dictatorial, predicting evil when their children do not shape up fully enough or quickly enough. In our experience, the dirt-poor mothers without husbands are particularly prone to adopting authoritarian postures. Who knows what would happen if they were not so ground down in poverty?

From a sociopsychiatric vantage, subjugation and exploitation of children in any variety of family is detrimental (Cooper, 1970). Breaking of will by irrational authority messes up many youths, for their entire lives, and then through repetition corrupts succeeding generations. Erich Fromm (1944) hit the nail on the head about this usually pre-Oedipal neurotigenic insult that comes from irrational authority. Children who must encounter that arbitrary, irrational authority and bow down to it, especially in the extreme forms seen in both fathered patriarchal and lower-class fatherless families, orient their entire existence around the issue of pleasing their parents. This unnecessary burden would be released if parents and children related as guardian and ward, that is, knowing that the guardianship has reasons, circumscriptions, and limits.

Block (1980) wrote, "We must find alternatives to the last form of overt repression—the manipulation of infantile dread to engender renunciation and hierarchy—if we are to rekindle the faith of our young" (p. 440).

FATHERLESS CHILDREN AS CHILDREN ARE IMPORTANT

A humane national approach that gives societal support to all children, without singling some of them out for their condition of fatherlessness, would be the best thing for fatherless children. Yet under our present national administration, children probably will not be seriously advanced, so perhaps budget cutters could compromise and give certain special priorities to fatherless children as a specially targeted group. There are 11 million of them in the United States. They are often poor. To some extent that we cannot specify clearly, they are children at risk. Their risks are poverty, sickness, delinquency, alienation, and insurrection. The comprehensive approach to solve their problems, of course, would be to help *all* children, to make *all* children persons of deep societal concern.

Merely the health needs of children are striking (Harvard Child Health, 1977). Fom a base of 76.1 millions of people under 21 years of age, the estimate was that these numbers suffered from the following health problems:

Anemia	3	million
Mental retardation	2.8	million
Speech impairment	2.2	million
Physically crippling ills	1.7	million
Emotional disturbances	1.5	million
Learning disabilities	.75	million
Deafness	.5	million
Blindness	.2	million

That gives a total number of 12.65 million children with health problems in a country that claims to consider children "our most valuable natural resource." Just from the public health viewpoint, fatherless children are overrepresented in the ranks of the unhealthy.

Plenty of evidence based on existing research proves our point. As Benjamin Pasamanick (1971) wrote in his presidential address to the American Orthopsychiatric Association, entitled "A Child Is Being Beaten," we already know enough to move into vigorous social action. We need no more research to move us or to inform our hearts.

ECONOMIC SUPPORT FOR ALL CHILDREN

The family in a capitalistic nation is an economic unit. A thrifty instrumentality, it looks after the nurture and life maintenance of millions of young people. One of its major activities is its investment in that human capital (Sawhill, 1977). The family also decides how much work to do, who shall work and where, what goods to consume, and whether to have children who will, in turn, become economic producers. Families make, according to Sawhill, an accounting of costs and benefits as they reach their multiple economic decisions and weigh their choices.

Jerome Kagan (1977) reminded us that the family

keeps employment steady. Husbands and wives will retain their jobs with the same employers for long periods of time because they feel responsible for the family's economic welfare. If they do not have that responsibility, they might be more prone to occupational mobility and erratic patterns of employment. [p. 33]

Consequently, the family is an economic unit and an economically conservative one. Each family has to grapple with economic problems. The U.S. Department of Agriculture estimates it will cost $134,000 to rear to 18 years old a child who was born in 1979, comparing that to a cost of $34,000 for a child born in 1960. Supported by the general society, the family would have the opportunity to function better. Reasonable proposals for supporting the family group have included family subsidies or allowances, guaranteed family income determined by the number of children contained in the family, fatherless child insurance awarded in much the same way that Social Security benefits are dispensed to surviving children, paid maternity leaves subsidized for periods of time up to 2 years, Social Security credit given for homemaker work, and other schemes that we now review briefly.

Family Allowance

The most sensible way to allocate family allowances is in subsidies to children or to the mother as custodial parent. Family allowances, in the words of Maxwell S. Stewart (1970), were provided, at that time, by 62 countries:

every country in Europe, as well as by Canada, Australia, New Zealand, and many nations in Latin America and Africa. The United States stands alone among the advanced industrial nations in not adequately taking into account the number of children in a family in its

*social insurance program. Under most such programs, a case payment
is made to a family for each child above a specified number, regardless of the family's other income. Every child is protected, not merely
the poor or handicapped. [p. 32]*

Speaking precisely, the family allowance in most countries was pronatalist, extended to prop up a declining birth rate, and its opponents often say, as they say of welfare now, "It encourages fecundity
of the poor." In experience, in Canada and elsewhere, family allowances have not been accompanied by a climb in the birth rate, not
even in Catholic Quebec. In Sweden, where Liljestrom (1978) said
the threat of Sweden's declining population "serves Swedish family
policy as its official godmother," the increased birth rate was not as
remarkable a result as the family allowance's influence on redis-
tributing income and democratizing family life and the job world.
In Czechoslovakia and Hungary, family allowances are a less conspicuous part of generic family policy because the Czechs have
elected to saturate *young* families with supports and services in many
forms. The Czechs perceive the young family as needing more support than the older one, in which it is expected that the mother will
return to work, adding her income to that of the father. Because it
is ordinarily a two-income family, the older family is a more typical
target of social policy in many of the East European countries. Unfortunately for women, there too, working women are burdened
with two full-time jobs.

Kamerman and Kahn (1978) gathered one of the best compila-
tions of family policy as enacted in 14 different countries, including
Poland, Hungary, and Czechoslovakia from Eastern Europe. Those
last two countries, along with France, the country that (as early as
1913) began the whole experimentation with family allowances,
Sweden, and Norway, comprised the five countries with "explicit
and comprehensive" family policy. The United States came nowhere
near them.

A second group of five countries were classified by Kamerman and
Kahn as ones in which family policy was "a field"; a body of theories
and practices could be identified but they lacked the broad scope of
the policies of the first five. In the second five countries, family policy had carved out its identity as a field but had not become open,

direct, and explicit official practice applied to all other policy matters. The countries with "family policy as a field" were Austria, West Germany, Poland, Finland, and Denmark. Interestingly, all of them had family allowances usually granted according to fatherlessness and the number of children, acknowledging that, as in the United States, the larger families and one-parent ones are at greatest risk of being poor. Denmark is an interesting example of *family policy with a child focus,* yet Denmark lacks the comprehensive approach to family policy that is found in Norway and Sweden.

A third group of family policy nations, consisting of the United Kingdom, Canada, Israel, and the United States, are what Kamerman and Kahn dub the "implicit and reluctant family policy" nations. Each of them, however, except for the United States, has family allowances that are paid to the mothers (and/or fathers) of some dependent children. Britain, like Canada, has never given very sizable family allowances; but Israel has made child allowances the basis of its whole income-maintenance system since 1975. However, Britain (Land & Parker, 1978) has been forthright in formulating what its family allowance practices are designed to accomplish:

1. A pronatalist incentive—encouraging parents to have more children
2. A palliative or substitute for workers' demands for higher wages
3. Reduction of poverty among the nation's children
4. Improvement of the status of the mother in the national economy

Family allowances, or child allowances, stand little prospect of being adopted under the Reagan administration. If adopted, and funded so that each child received $50 or more each month, such a program would have a tremendously uplifting effect on children from many poor homes. Indeed, it would lift them out of the poverty class. It would probably cost at least $20 billion annually also; but it still would not suffice to take care of the children of the underclass who live in grinding poverty. For the latter, public assistance payments or other income maintenance would have to continue. These very practical and highly civilized arrangements for income transfer, to our general shame, seem visionary in the present anti-welfare, anti-human rights era. But presidents are elected for only 4 years per term and neither Rome nor revolutions are quickly built.

Guaranteed Income

However thorny may be the task of computing what a child costs, two facts are clear. One is that some children cost less than others to support and raise; the second is that it is difficult to devise a plan that will meet special needs, not giving exact equity to all children. Most nations provide extras for children with special handicaps or problems who make the family economic enterprise shakier than one average child would. In France, since 1978, the single-parent family gets a 50% supplement to its regular *complement familial* and receives still other concessions to help it survive. Income maintenance at a subsistence level is sought in many countries, sometimes through a family-based tax deduction or negative income tax. A plan of this sort could be put in place easily in the United States—through the Internal Revenue Service, it has been suggested.

Fatherless Child Insurance

We considered the plan of a fatherless child insurance scheme in Chapter 4. It has not had a good reception in the United States, but it would do for all children what it does at the present time, through Social Security, for all who are orphaned when the father dies. The orphan is rather well compensated, and without any stigma, as a survivor of a Social Security-covered parent; the child fatherless for any reason deserves as much.

Social Security Credits for Homemaking

A nation cannot have it both ways although the United States has put up a good try. It is difficult to encourage mother to remain at home in a traditional role, caring for children and doing the housework for her family, whether or not it includes a father, and simultaneously encourage her to seek gainful employment outside the home. Perhaps the point is simply that in a pluralistic society, women should have those options and others. If a woman wishes to devote 10 or 12 years of her life to child care and housekeeping, earning no wages outside the home, should she not have something to show for her valuable contribution to society? A fairer arrangement would give her Social Security credits for the full value of her time or even for a fraction, in case the policy were to prod her to get outside work.

Mother Seeking Gainful Employment

We have repeatedly indicated that women who head households cope most often by working outside the home, adding motherlessness to the fatherlessness that their children already experience. We have also stated that such women are often at the bottom of the occupational ladder when they enter the work force, and that they work 70 hours weekly since they have two jobs—neither of which can be dignified as moonlighting.

END SEX DISCRIMINATION IN WAGES AND JOB OPPORTUNITIES FOR WOMEN

Women who become heads of households and go out to work are oppressed by sex discrimination in the marketplace. From some jobs they are blatantly excluded; others are nearly impossible for women to obtain, and when the door is open women's wages are far below men's wages for the same work. Ending this familiar exploitation would help all families, fatherless families above all.

Controversy always lurks in the wings when women's inequality in the workplace is discussed. Many believe that women should not leave home and that, if need be, they should be subsidized to keep off the labor market. Some believe that a woman cannot feel fulfilled if she does not have children and spend the first 6 years of each child's life giving the young one attentive care. The maternity imperative, called by Nancy Felipe Russo (1979) the "motherhood mandate," is insupportable. We think that the 50% of married women who now work outside the home will not leave the marketplace even if asked sweetly to do so, and that we shall witness, as other nations have already done, an American family in the future that typically contains two adult wage earners. Olds (1979) found that working women who enjoy their positions are more affectionate with their children than mothers who are disenchanted with their daily work, bolstering the morale of a few who have encountered meaningful careers. Because capitalist economies require it and socialist economies require it, there is no going back.

Our argument is that women must have what the National Organization for Women has been demanding since its incipiency, and that is an option. Women who wish to be hearth keepers and child rearers should be supported financially while women who do opt to work elsewhere should be able to do so without being oppressed by sexist discrimination.

PROMOTE WANTED CHILDREN AS A POLICY

There are no better proofs of the importance of feeling wanted for a child than those demonstrated by fatherless children. When they are loved and wanted, at the microcosmic level by the mother in the family, they are fortunate, relatively speaking. If, in addition, they securely felt that the whole community, the entire country, the macrocosm, cared and would never neglect or exploit them, fatherless children would have far better lives. Children who are wanted have a prospect to live worthwhile lives. For that reason, we insist that wanted children should become a societal premium, and the wanting of children should be a national goal. A number of situations and circumstances flow from the premium being placed on the wanted child, and we shall consider a few of them.

Women are in the sensitive, critical position for bringing wanted children into the world. Hence, a number of prerogatives should be granted to women. The individual woman must take charge of her own reproduction as a ground rule for a decent society in which children are cared for properly (Kearney, 1979). Not husbands, not members of the moral majority, and certainly not clergymen who have chosen celibacy as a life style, but only the woman is equipped to make that decision. Like a priest, each woman should decide for herself whether to bear children. As corollaries to this basic rule:

1. We believe that the future augurs well for the child whose mother chose positively to bring the child into the world. The unwanted child is fated, by contrast, to be abused and neglected. We know that, even when "accidents" are accepted and women are brave about the consequences of carrying an unwanted, unplanned pregnancy to term, the child is under high risk throughout her or his childhood for abuse, neglect, mental disorder.

2. Family planning is a vital requirement for healthy childhood. Wider dissemination of birth control information and contraceptive devices is a must. Childbearing and child rearing are too important matters to be left to chance. Eligibility for contraception must continue to be granted to anyone who asks. Sexually active young people need only apply.

3. Abortions likewise should be available on demand. With teenagers who become pregnant and obtain abortions through a responsible family planning agency, a second pregnancy out of wedlock occurs at a much reduced rate; the young woman who has her baby (for whatever reason) is likely to be a repeater, and, alas, too often not for a second time only. So abortion services as a part of a human service agency have become excellent contraceptive information centers as well. Women who wish them should be able to have abortions. And, far from feeling bad for their "self-indulgence," they deserve the congratulations of all society and special praise from anyone who wants children to be welcome and to thrive. We know some women who want to have children, others who do not want to have them at the time they come, but who have religious scruples against abortion. We respect their different decisions, more when it is the woman's choice than when a man says he is speaking on behalf of women or children or a right-to-life group. Furthermore, when the right-to-life spokespersons begin to take up the cudgels for improving the quality of American childhood, we might take their opinions more seriously.

4. A greater array of social services and outright monetary supports should be made available to all women who have babies, espe-

cially to those who are unwed and bring up their children in father-less households. Many, many such women in the United States, black, lower-class women, have some of the largest families that can be found in the entire country. Here we do agree with the right-to-life party that says they should not be subjected to any special pun-ishments or disincentives for, after all is said and done, we do not care that their children are illegitimate. That they are children gives them the credential we revere. Never-married women need special encirclings of support. And for some of the services that have been proposed we refer the reader to the discussion given in Chapter 4.

5.   What about negative incentives for people who have large families advocated by some of the zero-population-growth spokesper-sons? We have little enthusiasm for this viewpoint, even while we understand the need somehow to turn down any tendencies toward overpopulation. With such unfair sharing of the economic goods of the United States, and with such maldistribution of wealth, with ownership and control of wealth in the hands of private profiteers, there is no space for decent provisions for children as a group. Only after structural changes in the economic life of the nation would we consider seriously any measures to reduce the prolificacy of welfare mothers. Perhaps when that occurs, some ways that will allow the in-volved women to make freer choices can be found, but we shall have to wait a while, it appears.

DAY CARE AND DIRECT SERVICES FOR CHILDREN OF WORKING MOTHERS

In most of the enlightened (and that is relative, we know) nations of the world, day care has been financed for the kids of working moms. Most countries have not waited, as Richard Nixon advised in his veto of the child development bill, for a great national debate to occur about removing child care from the home hearth and setting up "impersonal agencies outside the family." In the United States there has scarcely been a start in implementing day care. The evi-dence is that it can be beneficial physically and socially to children who are in good day care, and it is an unquestioned boon when it is not just a passive day-care operation but a comprehensive child growth center (Rossi, 1977) as day centers seem to be in Denmark.

To give the devil his due, Richard Nixon's public stand is one that some of the Eastern European nations (and Denmark) have been coming to more and more: a recognition that single parents prefer the smaller, more informal day care that they can get close to their homes and a more opportunistic recognition that income transfers and child-care leaves to families allow the families to perform child-care functions more wholeheartedly and at a lower cost to the public purse. Maternity leaves with pay for periods up to 3 years are allowed in some nations. That sends a believable message that child care is valued and that children are valued.

Housing, health, mental health services, education, and legal protection are all issues calling for direct and costly services to be given directly to children if child life is accounted a societal concern. An increasing number of the world's countries offers an entire array of family and child services at public expense. All are important, as more mothers enter the work force. But the reader may ask what these policy matters have to do with fatherless children and their social psychiatry. Our retort cannot be fully reasoned and argued here, but in short it says that advocacy for children—at home, at school, in the neighborhood, in the juvenile courts, in children's institutions, and in the political domain—is a necessary part of the functions of a child psychiatrist, or any other child mental health specialist. Policy affects clinical practice strongly. In the next chapter it will be seen how easily psychotherapy blends with advocacy.

CHAPTER NINE

Treatment Suggestions

Child advocacy leads a psychotherapist directly into political involvement as surely as anything we have been stating about public policy. Therapy involves educating, comforting, and advocacy, according to Paul Adams (in Sholevar, et al., 1980). Bratter (1973) also stressed advocacy by the therapist. That means that we advocate for the benefit of each and every child we see in therapy, for children individually and collectively. Justine Wise Polier (1977), a former jurist, took a more doctrinaire position that advocacy must always leave the individual and go for the mass only. She made a good point: For a lawyer the test case and the class action have greatest payoff. But there may be some possibility of a middle ground, having advocacy include what we do both for the individual child seen in a clinical setting and for the masses of children who need a voice and representation even if they remain unseen. William Blake (see Donne & Blake, 1941) offered a reminder for all advocates when he wrote, "He who would do good for others must do so in Minute Particulars. General Good is the plea of scoundrels, hypocrites and flatterers" (p. 961). Child mental health clinicians know minute particulars very well. Sometimes they need to think about the masses of children also.

Since fatherlessness is not a homogeneous state, not much is written about therapy with fatherless children and adolescents. What there is, is often devoted to a single case or two, not suitable for a variety of father-absent circumstances. For example, what helps the boy child whose father is imprisoned for having assaulted the child sexually is hardly designed to be apt therapy for the girl child whose father has died of cancer. Perhaps it is better not to lump fatherless children together, not to stigmatize the fatherless as needing special therapeutic approaches and confine ourselves to individual cases. Therapies endorsed for fatherless children range from individual psychoanalysis to mental health lectures, from intensive individual counseling lasting 2 or more years to TA or Gestalt workshops over a weekend, from family group therapy to guided group interaction (GGI) for delinquents under the supervision of courts. We consider some of these therapy approaches briefly before offering general guidelines and case vignettes to illustrate therapy recommended for a range of fatherless children.

GROUP PSYCHOTHERAPY, MAINLY WITH DELINQUENTS

Group therapy has been a method widely employed in the treatment of delinquent children. This mode of rehabilitation is employed by training schools, by group homes, and by neighborhood or community groups: Reality Therapy, guided group interaction, certain Gestalt and Synanon techniques frequently employed by "training school" staff, that is, people who staff correctional facilities for delinquent youths. Max Sugar (1967) described some of the dynamics that activate group therapy with a group of fatherless pubescent boys, referred to therapy for academic failure and/or behavioral problems. Sugar described the group early on as being "characterized by marked sensitivity to separation, intense transference, and an almost exclusive relation with maternal authority rather than peers" (p. 65).

> *Early in treatment, the therapist was viewed partly as a nonthreatening, supportive mother-figure, and this role was the positive aspect of the patients' attitudes and transference reactions. . . . As the group progressed therapeutically, their predominant attitudes and behavior changed so that the transference to the therapist as a father-figure became more positive and the mother transference became minimal.* [*p. 65*]

Thus, in the opinion of Sugar, therapy consists in large part of providing a male role model with whom the father-absent boy can identify, thereby attaining a suitable superego and a resolution of the Oedipus complex.

The Highfields experiment, described by McCorkel et al. (1968), smacked more of behavior modification than did the group psychoanalytic approach of Sugar. At Highfields, group therapy was used to promote a spirit of camaraderie among the delinquent boys, aimed at helping them provide peer counseling to each other and build a support system against further involvement in delinquency. When recidivism rates of boys from Highfields were compared with recidivism rates of boys from the Annandale training school, Highfields was shown to be more successful, with the most marked differences appearing among black boys and white boys from broken homes.

Arnold W. Rachman (1974) presented a case for the therapist's taking up a fatherly role in group therapy of lower-class delinquent adolescents, most of whom had negative interactions with and images of their fathers. "The therapist must take a stand in the relationship as an adult authority who is giving, caring, concerned, just and supportive. Moreover, he must convey both his authority and his caring directly and accurately to the adolescent males with whom he is working." Rachman divided the therapist's presentation of self as benign father during the three phases of the group's life: the early phase of corrective emotional experiencing, the middle of "encountering a caring adult," and the final one of terminating, "leaving the group with a positive image of an adult authority." His theoretical model was based on psychoanalytic principles. Rachman was unusual in disclosing his own feelings of fear, inadequacy, and helplessness in anticipation of forming the group he led, his impulses to act out especially when the group went on field trips, and his effective use of consultation or supervision. Since the work was so taxing, Rachman suggested that the younger therapist may have an edge of advantage for such work! Max Sugar (1975), described in Chapter 6, has also recommended group therapy with fatherless children.

For delinquents, GGI, guided group interaction, using some of the Synanon techniques, has been widely used in correctional facilities and by court workers with youths. The kind of father portrayed by the GGI leader is realistic, hard-boiled, preaching the young person's accountability for his or her own life. It would be good if children and adolescents *could* take charge in that manner.

GROUP THERAPY FOR FATHERLESS
SLUM CHILDREN

Describing group therapy with 28 delinquent boys in two groups (aged 11 to 14 and 15 to 17 years), Salvatore V. Didato (1970) wrote that 26 of the youths "had experienced some disruption in the family unity, such as the death of a parent, a desertion, a separation, a remarriage of a parent, or outright abandonment of the child to a relative or friend. Some of the boys were out-of-wedlock children." Apprehended and adjudicated delinquents show an impressively high rate of fatherlessness all around the world. Of their mothers, Didato stated that they "were unable to discipline their children. . . . In general, they were overtaxed by family responsibilities. They were intellectually and culturally impoverished, and seemed to offer no enthusiasm for living to their children." The burnout following task overload presents formidable hurdles to any purely mental therapy aiming to restore good morale to such mothers and their offspring.

Didato's aims were to keep affects high and powerful but ex-,pressed in other than antisocial ways, discussed in the group and made the basis for both reflection and empathy building. As have many, he observed that the lads initially showed affective blunting; a good antidote to blunted feelings is strong feelings that are verbalized in a group setting. Didato used Aichhorn's strategy of "surprise without causing fear" and heightened the "bummed-out" youths' involvement within themselves and within their group.

Delinquent both from group experience and from social disorganization, these young people can form groups through identification with a nonthreatening adult as therapist, learning how to initiate their own rules and discipline and to do organizational development in a fairly democratic way. Makarenko in the USSR, A. S. Neill and Homer Lane in Britain, Kurt Eissler in Europe and the United States, August Aichhorn in Austria, and José Gutierrez in Colombia have all arrived at the same general conclusion: Therapists (or teachers or counselors) who do not play authoritarian games but respect the delinquent's potential for self-governance are rewarded by a dropping off of delinquency and a picking up of the adult's real values. Apparently, the father transference contributes a small part to the trust built up; the heightened feeling and self-inspection make up the grander portion of the favorable changes, whether in a group or dyadic setting. Minuchin and associates (1967) have reported beneficial results, even in fatherless slum families, from "dislodging of affect" during family group therapy sessions. Stirring up affect is a goal and technique of many therapeutic modalities. Encouragement of strong feelings is particularly potent in older child and adolescent encounter groups, Gestalt therapy groups, transactional analysis groups in which behavioral contracting occurs or stars are introduced for modeling purposes, and in psychodrama. Many of these have been used and described by Irvin A. Kraft (1980) and others.

FAMILY GROUP THERAPY

Ira Glick (1979) and other family group therapists who attempt to intervene not at the individual level but at the level of the family system have made worthwhile contributions to working with father-less families, lower-class slum families, and what Joel Feiner (1979) has called "underorganized families." Glick pointed out that one must evaluate the actual family system, for "there is a bias that the single parent is going to do terribly and that the kids will too. We *don't* know that yet with any certainty . . . we don't know a lot about child development and outcome yet for either intact or single-parent families." Glick found that after a divorce one of the best things to get started early was "to help the children to take on some responsibility for family work, for example, washing dishes, and set-ting the table." Glick assented to the view that working with mother-headed families is not easy and about their greater burdens and fewer supports he commented, "If you have to *work* at making an intact marriage successful, you have to *work twice as hard* to make a single-parent household function successfully."

Most of this chapter reflects the interest and experience of the au-thors in working with fatherless children in individual psychother-apy, but we also involve the full family in the treatment efforts. At times we keep strictly to the family as a group, and at other times we intersperse family sessions with individual interviews. Nowadays most child mental health clinicians move flexibly and freely from individual child to family group.

INDIVIDUAL PSYCHOTHERAPY AND ADVOCACY

Timely and apt psychotherapy can help fatherless children on an in-dividual basis. By now it is certain that we do not view fatherlessness itself as an affliction calling for treatment, similar to a neurosis or psychosis. Instead, we see it as, at times, a grave inconvenience and cause for mourning, at times a source of serious economic instability, but at times a relatively salutary change for the mother and the chil-dren and occasionally only a normal and healthy variant that does not produce or attend much human suffering. Probably a minority of fatherless children will ever seek therapy.

Some guiding rules for individual psychotherapy with fatherless children pertain to the therapist's being on guard against countertransferences, not being prejudiced about the nature of the case, not seeking to replace the missing father, not overconcentrating on the child's relationships with others, and being open-minded about ways to involve others in the child's household and environs. Ten of these guiding rules are presented.

Guide 1: Don't Borrow Trouble. Since the image of father has such a pervasive power among psychiatrists and other mental health professionals, those therapists often look for father symbols, father figures, father modes where none may be. They borrow trouble, even invent it. Many fatherless children will never enunciate a patriarchal rhetoric, no matter how much a therapist wishes to implant a representation of a mother–father–child triangle in the heads of all who have encountered good psychotherapy. Some fatherless children, by the same token, will have to be simply counted out when a paternal deity is advertised and sold out of this or that sacristy.

The nonexistence of a father is a rather natural concept for a child born out of wedlock; it could be the same for a therapist. It is not a void or a deficiency for that child; assuredly it is not the child's responsibility. Instead, it is only a difference, giving a kindly therapist a new occasion to behold an expression of human diversity. The child can hardly comprehend fatherlessness as a lack since so many of our felt needs represent demands to reinstate former gratifications now missing from our lives. Of course, a perennially fatherless child *may* yearn for a father. Children read, listen, and make comparisons.

Since childhood is full of frustrating meetings with naked power, one should go ahead and learn from the child the amount of exposure to a father or other disciplining adult, what it has been like, and what it has meant. The child's interactions with disciplinarians should focus our inquiry and our reparative efforts. We could say that we dwell on the child's relations with *significant others,* whoever those others really are. Those others are *not* fathers for many fatherless children. Yet the child may have felt the sting of the lash repeatedly; not only fathers can coerce children.

Oedipal problems may be at the core of a fatherless child's neurotic patterns when there has been some exposure to a dreadful father; but if there has been no father to internalize and to stimulate the child's internal representations, the child's difficulties will have to be chalked up more sensibly to pre-Oedipal or non-Oedipal forces. Frantz Fanon (1967) made some extravagant claims for black children growing up in Martinique—they have no *Oedipal* complexes; they never turn onto a homosexual path.

> *But, putting aside the question whether the ethnologists are not so imbued with the complexes of their own civilization that they are compelled to find them duplicated in the people they study, it would be relatively easy for me to show that in the French Antilles 97 per cent of the families cannot produce one Oedipal neurosis. [p. 152]*

The truth may be more moderate, but the vital point is that Fanon's claim is nearer the truth than the doctrinaire viewpoint that everyone everywhere grapples with Oedipal issues in both reality and fantasy.

A 10-year-old boy whose father had died produced a slip of the tongue once during a therapy session, addressing the male therapist as *father*. The therapist—much like Fanon's ethnologist—was about to jump to some foregone conclusions but good sense prompted him to stop to ask the child what the slip meant: "You called me father. What is that about?" The child answered, "Our priest at school is the only man but you that I see much of. I called you father the way I do Father." Out, dad, and in, priest. That is the way real children are. Therapists need to ask, not to make grand dynamic assumptions.

A resident in child psychiatry at a well-established and well-recognized university program told one of us, "Sometimes I wonder if the big cloud of the Oedipal complex is as ubiquitous as we seem to make it in every case conference we hold. Or is it that we use the Oedipus complex as a template that may only let certain parts of the child come through?" Paul Chodoff (1966) attributed to Frieda Fromm-Reichmann his view that the Oedipus complex is characteristic of a minority of children and families, even raising the possibility that middle-class Viennese Jews at the turn of the century may have had a distinctive gift for spawning Oedipus complexes. Any psychotherapist who has partaken of that small culture or that emotional-hothouse family style should be careful not to impose expectations of Oedipal difficulties onto work with fatherless children. The children may, but may not, have Oedipal conflicts.

As we ask an adopted child about her or his fantasies of the biologic parent who is unknown and never seen, we may ask the fatherless child about fantasies and imagery of the nonexistent father. Asking, we should be ready to wait until the child formulates, aided by drawings or doll-play, what the bona fide fantasies are. We disserve the child and the psychotherapeutic process if we attempt to cram the child's mental representations into the mold of our familiars. Our family is not the child's family; our complexes are not the child's. Nor are our myths, attitudes, and values, nor even our aspirations and expectancies, the child's.

Guide 2: Search with an Open Mind for Actual Core Conflicts. Fatherless children are more like children than otherwise, to paraphrase Sullivan's dictum regarding the schizophrenic patient: "Schizophrenics are more human than otherwise." The fatherless child's conflicts have a human face: They usually concern anger, sexual lusts, fears and dreads, feelings of inferiority, sadness, shame, power struggles, and the stings of being subjugated by authority. Their lack of a father may not be an explicit complaint; it rarely is so, even with children who once had a father. Hence, with a child who knew a father once but no longer has a father in the household, the therapist must dig out the child's recollections and feelings about father, as well as about father-absence. Only when the child has talked about the absent or missing father can we evaluate the child in a true light. One easy way to start is to encourage the child to talk about how the present situation compares with the former, prior to father's absence.

One of the surprises for the knowledgeable worker with fatherless children is the children's special nostalgia for a father. Of course, one seldom misses or craves something one has not savored, so "father-hunger" is most felt by those who have had a father previously. However, children who have never known their fathers believe, almost as a kind of false consciousness, that everything is better for fathered children, an ideology that they appear to acquire early, certainly by the time they reach elementary school. Occasionally the ideology of the traditional nuclear family really does pervade the thinking of the fatherless families. (See Guide 10 about this.)

Once a child has revealed some of the father-longings she or he harbors, the therapist may proceed with the therapeutic work, including teaching, giving aid and comfort, and child advocacy (Adams, 1982). Although fatherlessness may appear to rule out psychodynamically oriented work, that is not so; children without Oedipus complexes or fathers can be helped as well as other children by a dynamic approach.

Guide 3: Gender of Therapist Is Not Always a Crucial Matter. Several young female therapists of our acquaintance say almost at once, if assigned a fatherless child (whether female or male) for clinical work, "I believe that child would be better with a male therapist." One of us (PLA) teasingly pursues their suggestion by asking how the genitals matter, what dimensions are called for, if circumcision is required or prohibited, and so on. When they retort that not genitals but masculinity is in question, the counter is, "What masculinity score is the lower limit?" Finally, they see that fatherless children need effective therapists, not father substitutes, when they come for psychotherapy. Kraft (1980) makes the same point insistently for dynamically oriented peer-group psychotherapy: Gender of therapist is of no real import.

A male therapist is not always better and not always appropriate. Whether male or female, the therapist knows he or she will be viewed by the child through transference distortion as somehow like other adult figures the child has known. Whatever the therapist's gender, the child should be given every opportunity to talk about these transferences. Especially valuable is ferreting out interactions with other adults of the therapist's gender because, at least in the early days of treatment, the child will make equations (distortions) that may be strongly influenced by a specific gender and say so, and why. So talk of grown-ups and gender could be a salient part of the therapeutic work without our feeling compelled to give a father substitute to the child.

If the child needs contact with adult males, the therapist does well to encourage the child and the mother to make more contacts with males who can be "real objects" in the child's life. The need for a man is not often that imperative, however, and most families of fatherless children provide abundant opportunities to associate with males. Neither fatherless girls nor boys, in most of the cases seen by child psychiatrists, suffer a lack of male figures. There are enough men to go around, men who will be the child's grown-up friends, the mother's friends too.

Not having a man in their lives does hurt some mothers. For them, the shrewd therapist can give some suggestions of places to meet men. Churches make good dating bureaus in the southern United States. In other areas it may be a bowling league, a grange meeting, a high-school ballgame, a community meeting in the housing project, a neighborhood improvement association in the ghetto. For some women, Parents Without Partners could be a congenial meeting place. The most militant feminists of our experience usually do not want to deprive themselves or their children of male companions, acknowledging that biologic dimorphism is not offensive even if sexism is.

Guide 4: Remember Survival Economics and Deal with Economic Matters in Therapy. Therapists often are not poor people themselves and may not have had any experience with poverty. Therefore, they must overcome the shock of the new and learn from their poor patients what poverty entails. As one young black unwed mother said, "If there is anything I am good at, it is how to be poor, and to survive." Their feats of economic endurance are amazing. Often a husbandless mother miraculously pastes together a series of sources of financial support for herself and her children. Kogelschatz et al. (1972) described the ways a husbandless mother can make do with part-time work, moonlighting work, taking in a boarder, cottage industry undertakings, welfare payments, loans, gifts from relatives and friends—and IOUs. All those are legal ways that become scarcer still in times of economic depression, harder to obtain and ever more taxing of the ingenuity and creativity of women who head families. While their inventiveness does not gainsay the need for solid societal support, as discussed in Chapter 8, we may be forgiven for praising the economic adeptness that some of these mothers display. Differences, often demeaned, sometimes deserve to be lauded.

Frequently, special practical arrangements have to be made for impoverished fatherless children who come for psychotherapy. Sources of money for bus fares are not the least of such practical considerations. Finding resources for one's patient is a humbling advocacy function. We can take small costs for granted when we work with mainly middle-class or third-party-endowed working-class patients; the underclass needs more practical accounting. Home and school visits are highly educational for therapists of poor children and may even move the working alliance forward. Section 8 housing, food stamps, AFDC, free agricultural commodities may be unobtainable without our suggestions and guidance. Also we need to get to know the welfare workers and others who influence and help fatherless families. Child advocacy makes strange bedfellows.

Finally, as with all differences that may be complicated by countertransference and pseudotransference, being fatherless needs to be considered in detail from the child's standpoint. Children without fathers may be imbued with a patriarchal ideology; that should not surprise us. Children without fathers liberally compare themselves to children with fathers; that affords us a volume of rich material from the child's own set of values. The child should be allowed (and even facilitated) to consider what, if anything, seems to make fathered kids better off. If the attitudes and valuations are there, they need to be unearthed. If brought into the open, they can be considered in perspective and made a part of an expanded ego-domain. This question of father ideology is the theme of Guide 10, in fact.

Guide 5: Strive to Get the Picture As It Is Factually and in Fantasy. This rule is an extension of part of the previous one but has special merit for the therapist whose background is of limited diversity and empathy.

A home visit to a fatherless child has been described interestingly and at length by Tobias (1979), a foreign medical graduate (FMG) in child psychiatry training, who concluded that a home visit was indispensable to her learning of cultural and subcultural nuances. What Carmelita Tobias said of the FMG applies equally to the more narrowly reared USMG.

The approximate time involved including travel is about one and one-half hours. . . . In order to understand a child, one has to learn the child's family and his milieu. Likewise, in order to understand the family, one must be a participant observer in the household and gain more intimate knowledge of and empathy for the child in his family. . . . I believe that foreign medical graduates, in particular, can derive many benefits from home visitation. The FMG gets a quicker view of his patient's intimate sub-culture and the numerous but distinctive values attendant on home life anywhere in the world. It enhances the FMG's enculturation into psychiatry as a field and into the United States as a national style of life. I felt I was a welcome and helpful psychiatric visitor in the home visits I made.

School visits also help to forge a better understanding or an empathy with fatherless children and their family members. School visits are set up by the therapist with the school personnel who actually know the child and family involved. The guidance counselor and the homeroom teacher, the therapist, the mother and the child are often the parties to the school visit. If mother or child cannot be present, then the meeting should be cancelled. The therapist conveys to all who are gathered that the child is in the forefront, and the child is not ignored or talked about as if he or she were not present.

Perhaps contemporary schoolteachers do not know as much of families' lives as they did in an earlier day; their abandoning the psychoanalytic model has brought a relative neglect of family life and a decline in teachers' know-how for work with parents. Today, most teachers use behavior modification, and they also enjoy educating parents; their resistance toward any other approach is notable. We let such teachers keep their religion but occasionally try to let a little of the child's inner world enter into the picture, allowing the parent some significance other than as shaper of the child's behavior at home and at school.

Teachers too are a disadvantaged group, relatively; they are underpaid, often unorganized and demoralized, usually females who soon can be induced to treat husbandless mothers in a positive way. Teachers are indispensable co-workers for child therapists.

Going with a poor person to the doctor is one way to convert the hard-to-reach poor into very workable patients or clients. To go with a husbandless mother to her doctor's appointment or to her clinic appointment is instructive for any clinician. The indignities to which poor people are subjected stand out in many public health and hospital clinics—they are called by their first names, subjected to long waits and the red tape of registration and eligibility interviews, going from one line to the next. As if by design, the services are hard to reach but the poor are called that.

Visiting the play area to which the child gravitates can give the therapist valuable insight into the ways of the neighborhood where the child lives. The therapist introduces himself as "_____'s friend" and lets it go at that; but the child may amplify that the visitor is his doctor. And friend.

Conferences with collaterals in the human services fields can be both informative and adjunctive to the therapy with the child and the family. Many fatherless families have said that the psychiatrist's expression of interest has "upped our stock with the welfare worker." It helps in tangible ways when someone from the mental health establishment takes a keen interest in a fatherless child and his or her fate in the welfare or social services establishment, but that is dealt with next.

Guide 6: Be Prepared to See the Family in Its Community Context. The mother-headed family is a microcosm of its neighborhood and larger community in many ways. A wealthy suburban neighborhood can contain well-to-do families after divorce who are barely distinguishable from intact families; an urban ghetto's fatherless households likewise do not stand out from their neighbors very much. Fatherless families, more often poor, are more often found in poor neighborhoods, especially in large cities, where they quickly appear to be "at home." Aggression, violence, suspicion, mistrust, sorcery, and obfuscation all move centripetally and centrifugally between the fatherless family and its community, as easily as do sociability and civic participation. Only a shortsighted therapist jumps to the intrapsychic while excluding the external forces impinging on the family; the same can be said of those who look exclusively to the macrocosm while ignoring the persons with all their values, complexes, and intimate worlds.

In a community where murders, sex abuse, muggings, burglaries, and forcible entries are rampant, one should not think paranoid a mother who seems to be highly concerned that her young children do not roam afar and insists that they keep the outside doors of the dwelling double-locked. In a community with 40% unemployment, a wise clinician will not be shocked that fatherless children seem detached, fatalistic, lacking in enthusiasm for school, diminished in verve and motivation to train for good jobs. Their success models are pimps, pushers, prostitutes, and workers in an underground economy, all too often, so whence come inner incentives to be industrious, thrifty, planful, or legal? In an inner-city community residual after white flight, poor blacks and Hispanics may be hard-pressed to build up a meaningful network of stores, churches, schools, clubs, lodges, neighborhood associations, parks, and playgrounds. Poor people often have underorganized families, seeming often to need an expert in organizational development more than a mental health specialist; moreover, they live in communities lacking any viable organization. Fatherless families, if poor, lack the adult who conventionally would be their intermediary to the outer world—but the outer world is not there for any vital contact or support. Underorganization and disorganization abound so the families are isolated, alienated, and disengaged, inside and out. As Minuchin et al. (1967) depicted them, they resort to extremes of "disengagement" in their own communication styles or, if the mother is a more valiant type, to "enmeshment" with its interactions fast acting, tough, loud, and often brutally overpowering because the mother feels too overburdened to try gentle reflection and explaining to her children. She is often devoid of extended family, friends, or true neighbors.

Clinicians need, we believe, to think more and do more about community-wide prevention—social policy—in order to help fatherless families more fully.

Guide 7: Attend Vigilantly to the Child's Interactions; Clarify and Identify Them. Dorothy Block's splendid book called *So the Witch Won't Eat Me* (1978) is filled with astute observations of the child's overt behavior and of subtle changes in the play sequences and spoken fantasies of the child in treatment. It is such painstaking and sensitive therapy that is best for fatherless children. Her message is that the child has sensed the parents' infanticidal longings and takes very elaborate steps to defend and restore lost securities, both dreading annihilation and fearing loss of love. Block correctly holds that childhood lived out with an agenda of "Child, be pleasing to your parents" is a tortured existence. Her thesis is relevant to fatherless children. Almost as if of necessity, the lower-class mother who is husbandless must take shortcuts and employ dispatch in extracting overt conformity and compliance from her offspring; as often as not, she overenculturates, and her children suffer from being hyper-coerced, from being made to feel unworthy and unwanted, and from holding the view that the only safety comes from obedience to the mother's will in order to earn her love. Of course, although mother or child can't foresee this, impoverished life is no milieu for ex-tracting obedience forever. Thus the impoverished mother requires overconformity but faces the eventuality that her offspring will get into street life and quickly be immunized against all her admoni-tions. A therapist can help her to moderate her fearful strictures now.

Transference is, as we have stated already, much more ubiquitous than father transference. Hence, the therapist needs to wait, listen-ing with the third ear, for the first signs of the child's bringing infan-tile or unconscious materials into the therapy sessions. In some ways, the transference of the fatherless child is easier to monitor than that of the fathered child, its analysis just as curative.

A premenarcheal girl named Marie gave us an example of des-perate transferences in work with a fatherless child. After severe physical abuse by her parents, Marie became a ward of the state hu-man services agency; they paid for plastic and orthopedic remedi-ation of her crippling induced by abuse. After two adoptions that the prospective parents called off, she wound up in the public social services agency. At 11, she was adopted by a single parent, a young woman who was divorced and wanted to do the parenting that she could see that Marie needed. Toward the male therapist, Marie seemed intent on engulfment, always seeking to sit on his lap and to have him put his arms around her, not average behavior for an 11-year-old. Toward her adoptive mother's boyfriend Marie alternated between attention seeking, demanding his show of love, and throw-ing out angry remarks such as, "Go away. Don't stay here tonight and sleep with my mommy." When the adoption was about to be final, after every conceivable adoption agency delay and mix-up, Marie announced to the therapist that she did not want to be adopted by her mother but wanted the therapist to adopt her in-stead. She unburdened herself of congeries of distortions and trans-ferences. Complicated strategies of confronting, identifying, explaining, and clarifying, along with some reassurance and interpretation, saw Marie over the period of her adoption. Something seemed to have been resolved within her, as well as in her outer world, during that time.

Shortly afterward, nevertheless, Marie began, on every occasion available to her, to seek out children 3 and 4 years of age, becoming bossy and physically cruel to them almost before she had given them a good looking over. They cried, alarmed and puzzled by her behavior, and she had to be torn apart from them. She found the concept of identification with aggressors acceptable, useful, and even helpful because she changed her overt behavior after exposure to the idea, the concept. She decided she could identify with children who are victims instead of with her, and their, adult aggressors. In Marie's case, her mother deprivation probably was more influential than her fatherlessness. Indeed she may grow up completely, perennially fatherless and live rather well if her more basic lacks can be redeemed. A psychotherapy that is as expert and deep as possible can aid her healthy development.

Guide 8: See the Members of the Family Who Actually Dwell Together. Neither a gravedigger nor a sectarian be. Do not try to exhume a father (who has deserted a mother who does not want him back) simply because contact with the child's father seems like a good idea for children in intact or recently divorced families.

We know that Kellam and associates found over seven dozen family types living in the Woodlawn area of Chicago. Yet for a given child in treatment, the only family type is the one experienced, so it is wise to see everyone who dwells in the household or who has enough exposure to the household to make an impact on it. Those children in therapy who have a maternal grandmother in the home or nearby need a therapy that includes her. The wisdom of seeing the grandmother has been expounded by Maurine LaBarre et al. (1960). Those children who reside with a mother and her maternal uncle need the great-uncle included; those who live with an aunt need the aunt and her children included. We do not give up and opt to see the child only, when a child is motherless, merely because we are geared to a mother-and-child approach. That would be too sectarian.

Another sectarian ideology, favoring family group therapy, would almost unbury the mentally defunct and absent father to include him in the therapy network. Family therapists of that stripe can very cunningly conceal, but hold, a pro-father perspective. They pursue the father so absurdly that they use a family group approach for everything, for example with fathers who have sexually abused their daughters, often making dad feel okay but bestowing a load of guilt on both mother and daughter. This sectarian view reminds us of Abe Maslow's comment that, to people whose hammer is their only carpenter's tool, every problem looks like a nail.

There *are* cases of fatherlessness due to divorce in which the father can be brought for a few sessions, simply to try to humanize the postdivorce air for the benefit of the child(ren). Still, when a father is nonexistent or noxious there is no reason to send a search party to involve him in the therapy process.

Guide 9: Be Prepared to Give More Than Usual Attention to Siblings.   The fatherless household may befuddle many a middle-class therapist simply because it is so large. The statistics do not escape the consciousness of the lower-class black child, for example, whose mother is under 40 and has 8 or 10 children by one or more boyfriends but has never lived with any man in a durable relationship. Black or not, the child is surrounded by siblings. And the mother, overloaded in multiple ways, vacillates between overcontrol and neglect. One child said: "I have seven brothers and sisters. A brother and two sisters older than me and three sisters and a brother younger. Both my brothers and one of my sisters has the same daddy I have; the other four come from two different people that used to like my mama." Hence, for this lad there were two sibling subsystems that had vital meaning to him—in one he had true sibs and knew it, in the second he felt less kinship since "they don't have the same daddy I have." Yet they were all interacting sibs feeling more in common than with their mother and fathers.

One way for mothers as single parents to cope is to unload some of their duties and onerous tasks onto the children. The chores have to be shared, the sheer labor divided among all the family members who are capable of doing any of it or learning how. Indeed, if the mothers have not done it already, before tumbling while trying to be heroic, it is a good thing for the therapist to help her and her children to divide up and reassign the homemaking chores.

The children in a fatherless household have a greater significance for one another. The sib group has an existence of its own and a therapist should not regard it as resistance when such a child spends greater time and effort talking about siblings. Child psychiatrists notably come from small middle-class families, not from large working-class or lower-class ones, and must realize that a partitioning of the generations within a family may be more pronounced when the mother is overwhelmed than where there are two kindly and empathetic parents to share—in a child-centered spirit—in the joys and travails of parenthood. We saw in Chapter 5 and Chapter 6 how older sibs can take on functions of nurturing and training a younger brother or sister and that, although the evidence is mixed, older sibs may compensate for some aspects of father-absence by serving as role models to their juniors within a fatherless household. Siblings must be reckoned with and made a part of the psychotherapy so their constructive influence can be reinforced.

Clinical experience has shown us, on the other hand, that other children in fatherless households also may brutalize and exploit younger sibs unconscionably. Whether the older siblings are benign or malignant, they appear to be intermediary screens or filters through which more than one version of the parental values are transmitted to younger sibs. If the mother clings to her infanticidal core and relates to one or more of her children through projective or narcissistic identification, or role reversal, an ambience of cruelty affects everyone. Even if she wants to serve her children thoroughly and to aid them through helping empathy, discouragements and frustrations abound to keep daily life less than blissful for all of them. Her salience is great and sibling salience mounts too. The siblings help to reconfirm the maternal attitudes; they sometimes give escape and redemption from them. The mother who heads a household carries heavy responsibilities and may not manage to evade a youth revolt within her own family. Seeing the entire family is the only way to detect and solve the problematic patterns of sibling and bigenerational interactions of the fatherless child patient.

Guide 10: Keep Open-Minded and Skeptical about Family Structure and Functions. The clinician who works with fatherless families needs to drop comparative analysis—always thinking, "If only a stable and well-paid man were in this family . . . ," always comparing this family to fathered ones. It is better to take each family afresh and evaluate it anew for strengths, weaknesses, and potentials for repair and growth. Otherwise, our own autobiographies assert themselves too forcibly, our zeal burns out too quickly, and we do not help the living and breathing families who seek our help. We resort to prejudices, stereotypes, and illusions—to attributing the family's therapeutic failure to "just the way things are." We need to guard against blaming the victim.

Fatherless families themselves are imbued with false consciousness, we recall. Mother and child(ren) do tend to glorify the dead or otherwise absent adult male. Idealization of a fathering that was very slim in reality comes easily to people who find themselves deprived and who seek an easy explanation for their suffering. Of this belief that all troubles hinge on the absent father, Stern (1980) stated:

> As every clinician knows, a single mother's concerns are hardly confined to or concentrated on the effects of father absence on the development of her boy(s); her many other problems by far override any worries she may have about the deprivation of male identity figures and play and recreation companions for her boy(s). . . . Nevertheless, . . . when a single mother indicates concern about these issues, she is expressing a feeling that is normative in our contemporary society, or at least in parts of it. Such concerns, therefore, need to be appreciated and probably accepted by the therapist, for a denial of a normative concern is hardly reassuring to a client. With respect to doing something about the situation, in some cases the most that can be done is to help the mother to live with it. [pp. 83–84]

On the contrary, not taking patients' words at face value, we should stress the greater value of a questioning attitude of the therapist. We are not espousing the amiable debates adopted for the cognitive therapy of depression, for example, nor harsh and hostile repudiation of the mother's (or child's) father-hunger point of view. Instead, a patient, quiet listening and "acceptance" is called for, combined with a problem-solving drive as shown in questions such as "How so? It must be tough at times. When lately did you notice this? What was happening? Have there been times when you or your son were able to overcome this lack, at least in part? Tell me about that. What do you see as one or two practical ways to lessen the hurt you feel?" To get a person going in demystifying her life and that of her children is the point of therapy with fatherless families.

THERAPY WITH SOME TYPES OF FATHERLESS CHILDREN

Fatherless by Divorce

Even if divorce did not produce psychiatric problems in their children, postdivorce parents have become keen applicants for child psychiatrists' services. Some practitioners find that specialized type of work (forensic child psychiatry) both fascinating and lucrative. Children of divorce, pawns of their split parents, are frequent clients of psychotherapists.

The custodial parent's permission must be secured before even an evaluation can be undertaken; otherwise, a lawsuit looms. But parents frequently call on the child psychiatrist fishing for a case against the former spouse, who at the time of the divorce was given custody gladly. The child psychiatrist, rather like the judge, tends to insist that whatever *is* should be, provided there is not a hint of danger in the child's present setting. Our child advocacy would advance, undoubtedly, if we wisely evaluated all sides and recommended fairly for the child's welfare. Solow and Adams (1977) boldly proposed that the disputing parents turn over custody decisions to the child psychiatrist, indeed the preferable option in some cases.

In the diagnostic phase, or early treatment period, while the child is being evaluated, a family history is taken—to include the divorce—as seen through the eyes of the child. The Kinetic Family Drawing may also be done, and a separate one that includes the now-absent father. The Sentence Completion and House-Tree-Person tests are also good tools for eliciting psychiatric data. The child gladly takes the opportunity to talk about the divorce, usually articulating a wish to have both parents and to love both parents. The child may resent the mother, usually the custodial parent, believing that she caused the divorce—hence, the fatherlessness—or prevented the father's having more time with the child. Or, even more likely, the child resents the father for his absence and for his difficulty in being a father while not married to the custodial mother. Such findings come out early in the work and liberate the child, who is pleased to meet a more neutral adult who listens to her or his feelings. The child likes the new game without the old rules and unrealistic values.

Psychotherapists help better when they recall that a conflict-laden, hateful marriage is really worse, for both parents and children, than a divorce. So the postdivorce period may be an emotional relief time for the fatherless child even when neither child nor parent may countenance that cessation of tension. But the therapist must accept the feeling of deserved respite as a viable reaction when a divorce remedies a marriage of brutal struggle.

Children of divorced parents have learned experientially that they cannot control the activities of grown-ups. But they don't stop trying. For if they could have their own way they would often opt for no divorce, claiming both of their parents. Hence, it is not startling when children of divorce develop grandiose views, determinedly setting out to reconcile their irreconcilable parents. Their grandiosity is a measure of their powerlessness in face of strong wishes. A clever therapist aids the child to acknowledge that parents, rather self-governing creatures, make up their own minds about marriage and divorce, and that in the final analysis much about the decision to marry or divorce is "none of your business." Only after the child has accepted some of the limitations on his or her power in these matters can fruitful therapy occur.

For the sake of the therapist, holding aside the child's welfare for the time being, the decisive designation of a custodial parent is a help, a fact taken into account by the Freud-Solnit-Goldstein thesis (Goldstein et al., 1973). A child is made more secure, however practical considerations may militate against its coming about, by knowing where home is, who has the say-so, and what parent is to be the regular parent for the child. Without custodial stability, therapy cannot proceed sensibly or smoothly. Naturally, there are other ways than the one urged by Goldstein et al. to dispose of the living arrangements for children of divorce. But the parents must adopt some plan and practice it before the child can use psychotherapy to any extent beyond a friendly holding operation.

Shared custody is a big new thing among certain middle-class people. "Even-steven" has an equalitarian ring; an even split sounds just. Parents sometimes choose to go for parity, 50%, cozily quid pro quo for the parents, but tremendously confusing for the child. The enshrinement of parental rights, even in their sharing custody, does not always work out well for the children, and shared custody is an experiment fraught with hazards, surely. However, sometimes joint custody does work for children. "If the parents can negotiate so amiably, why did they get divorced?" both child and child psychiatrist may ask, but their premises may be called simplistic by lawyers and judges—and determined parents.

A 4-year-old girl with an IQ of 180 was brought to a child psychiatrist in what could aptly be called a gross stress reaction, a "generalized anxiety disorder" according to *DSM-III*. The parents had divorced and agreed to joint custody. The father, an intellectual man, acquired a house right across the street from the mother. He knew that the mother was in truth the custodial parent and had organized a life for herself and the little girl that was mainly beneficial for his daughter. Yet he proclaimed his rights to visitation at his beck and call, threatening the mother with renewed court action if she opposed his visitation at any time he wished it. Under the guise of sharing custody and outmothering the mother, the father began performing vaginal examinations on his little daughter; he cloaked his sexual abuse under the guise of "cleaning her vagina" when the little girl reported his actions to her mother. He ranted against the mother's "neglect of the girl's vaginal cleanliness" and discounted the mother's objections as emanating from her "puritanism about everything sexual."

The therapist (a woman) tried to intervene, to reassure the child that she had every right to object to her father's abuse, but the father could not be brooked. He threatened the mother with "back to court" if she did not let him continue his practices with the daughter. Moreover, he threatened to seek full custody of the child for himself if the mother did not stop taking the child to the child psychiatrist. The therapist reported his case to protective services and made every effort to help the child but the protection agency found that what the father did—although admitted to be a bit bizarre—was not harmful to the girl. The court said there was no reason to change the child's life from its former status of shared custody by her parents. The therapist realized that child therapy and child advocacy may be hampered in the 1980s and had to yield, contenting herself with being available to the mother if needed. Joint custody did not cause the little girl's problem, but the case shows that, whatever adults may like, children may dislike the arrangements dictated by adults.

Postdivorce visitation between father and child should be accepted by therapists as the child's right (Benedek & Benedek, 1977) unless proven otherwise. In cases of father–child incest, or other abuse and exploitation, visitation is either uncalled-for or done only under such close monitoring that it quickly becomes only a formality, a bit of nonsense that benefits nobody. A father who left the family because of his abrogation of fathering is better absent than present, even for brief visits. That the child appears to have an attachment to her or his abusing parent does not gainsay enforcing no contact. Abused children share a general human fascination for sadistic violence and carnality; bonding to an abusing father comes easily to a child but professionals need not call it a healthy attachment, however strong.

In general, the therapist does best to concentrate on mother and child, not on father, after a family has undergone a divorce and the child is in the mother's custody. Whenever abuse has occurred, there is less reason than normal to encourage a family group approach to a fatherless child's problems with self and others. Otherwise we blame the victim—and, of course, the mother! Whether we like it or no, therapy deals in values, choices, tastes, and preferences. Child advocacy may lead us to some unpopular values at times but we can attempt to be eclectic and flexible about the values to which we are committed. Then perhaps, our unconventional values won't make us useless to the children we serve, apart from making us uneasy. Family therapy for father–daughter incest is only tomfoolery, in our experience, much ado about a unit that has died beyond reclamation or resurrection. Yet family group therapy is in and child advocacy is out for many workers in the mental health field.

Each child of divorce has her own unique patterns, or his own manner of coping with his particular world. We may err when we generalize about "children made fatherless by divorce," but we are not off base when we stress the necessity to study each child afresh, to explore his own household, his own private fantasies.

Fatherless by Death

The child whose father has died is in some ways more fortunate emotionally than other fatherless children. The father-orphaned child has a time-limited grief with which to cope. Clarifying the cause of the father's death will be needed: A child whose father was mugged by an unknown assailant is more stunned and outraged than the child whose father died after a prolonged bout with cancer. The child whose father died in prison, electrocuted for his crime, has less conventional esteem to go on than the child whose father died in a popular war. In the United States, only the Vietnam War is not perceived as a good and popular war; only the Vietnam War veteran took part in a war ultimately lost ignominiously by the U.S. troops—despite repeated promises by the generals that the war would be won next year. Children orphaned by the Vietnam War are the only children in memory who speak only with shame to mild pride about their deceased warrior fathers. In our therapy sessions we have to learn whether dad's death was, so to speak, a good death for the child.

The bereaved child does not grieve as an adult does; grief patterns depend heavily on the developmental age of the child. The therapist must recognize the patterns to determine, along with the child, precisely what the father's death means. The fact that the grief will end, that life goes on, until another death, is not cheerful news to the grief-stricken orphan. It is the truth, however. Like the developmental hope that we have for all children whom we work with in psychotherapy, our optimism for the orphaned child is best kept to ourselves until the child acknowledges that the work of mourning is drawing to a close. Our change work still consists in demystification and candor, not in spreading false cheer.

A 3-year-old whose father had died, explaining to a child psychiatrist what death means, described the way people who died did not breathe, as if they were somehow engaged in a permanent feat of breath holding. Then, she said, they got put into a coffin and buried. Then what? Nothing, the worms eat them up and that is all there is to it. She did not seem at all anxious about an interpretation of death that would inspire some apprehensiveness in most adults. The therapist wisely avoids ideological consolation of bereaved children and bypasses the training in false consciousness that usually spews from adults to children when such topics are considered.

A working-class lad of 13 years had been father-orphaned 2 years earlier. The father had been physically abusive and the boy, mixing grief with his fascination for being beaten, kept asking an older brother to "whip me to show love." That was a verbal and conceptual formulation told him by his father before dying; the boy said he believed that physical beating was indeed a way to demonstrate interest and loving concern. The mother had been left with a large family, and Jack, the patient, was her youngest. Jack had become a discipline problem at school, where he had fallen 3 years behind. The reason he was referred to child psychiatry was his school refusal backed up by threats to kill himself, and an angry bravado about what he would do to anyone who opposed him. The family life was grossly unstructured; the mother worried that Jack was being turned into a mama's boy, but she had asthma and feared she'd die suddenly as the father had done. She said it was not the right thing to do but she felt like keeping Jack close to her even on school days.

In working with Jack and his mother, the therapist had to deal with the themes of death, death fear, separation, and individuation (for mother); with separation anxiety, feelings of failure and inferiority, of shame and emerging heterosexual feelings, and antisocial leanings (for Jack). With both mother and son the work concerned actual privation, mother's chronic fatigue, and feeling entrapped in a home that was beginning to be an empty nest. This was a case where death of the father permeated the entirety of the therapeutic endeavor.

Fatherless by Illegitimacy

The child born and reared out of wedlock needs only to be able to give us an understanding of what the contact with the father has been: if it has been extensive or nil; whether there has been a good enough replacement for the natural father; what the child imagines and thinks about the absent father; whether the child feels any stigma about the unwed parentage; how the mother's perceptions of the absent father flavor the child's emotional coping. Even the child's birth order makes a difference. In some neighborhoods, people overlook one slip-up but scorn a second or third conception out of wedlock. Certainly, the economic problems compound for unwed women and their children as the children number more than one. In other neighborhoods, despite a moral majority, only the first illegitimate child seems shocking, and by number three or four it seems chronic and acceptable even if some doubt lingers in the mind of the preacher or schoolteacher—or child psychiatrist.

Psychotherapists need to recall that the stigma of illegitimacy now is milder than it was in the original families of the therapists themselves. Times have changed, but less for the working class than for either the underclass or upper-middle class. The working class still retains many familistic virtues and a very traditional family ideology. We must study these attitudes afresh with each new child brought to us for help, for each has his or her own perceptions and images regarding the father-absence and what makes for a good family.

The statistics on children born out of wedlock are not very soothing; for some ethnic and economic groups multitudes of such children grow up fatherless in households headed by women and suffering all the economic disadvantages that accompany that condition. The 1980 census shows, according to preliminary reports, that some 1.1 million single (never married) women are "maintaining families with no spouse present" and about 1.5 million children live in these families. In 1981, at least one in every six births involved an unmarried woman with a total of 600,000 such births (Dept. of Commerce, Bureau of the Census and Department of Health and Human Services, National Center for Health Statistics, cited in *Information Please Almanac*, 1982).

A case of a 13-year-old black girl shows some problems of welfare agencies striving to make do with inadequately trained, overworked, and underpaid staff (most of them young women too). The welfare department decided when Corita was newly born that they would manage, by intensified efforts, to help the little girl's aunt to be a fit parent for Corita after her mother, a prostitute, had abandoned her. The aunt persisted in physically abusing the child and the welfare department first removed her at 18 months for a brief period, the first of many, with the aunt resuming beating her each time she returned. At 6, when the welfare people stopped whistling in the dark,

Corita began her 10-year search for a stable foster home. She had not found one by age 13, so the welfare department finally terminated parental rights in order to allow the child to be adopted! Anyone can guess the difficulty in 1981 of placing for adoption a 13-year-old black female child.

Corita had an indomitable flair. Undoubtedly her IQ of 140 was useful to her. She used the therapy sessions to talk of her life, her hopes, and sometimes her feelings about the people she encountered every day. She had always insisted, "I don't have feelings," but when a white taxi driver refused to pick her up because she had a welfare coupon and was black and young, she got angry and began to own up to some of her feelings of humiliation and rage. In the next session she announced to her white therapist, a male, that she had been thinking about it, and she proclaimed, "I do want to be adopted. I want to have me a home, a father, to be adopted. I decided I don't care, even if they're white." She stopped there and a knowing smile lighted up her countenance. For Corita had had no father, but worse, no mother after her unwed mother abandoned her at birth. A series of partial parents was all she could refer to, yet her fantasies were structured by her longing for a father, even if he were white—as was her therapist.

Donald, a boy of 9 years who was born out of wedlock, had had no father living in the household until his mother—when Donald was 8—decided to cohabit with a boyfriend who quickly took up the appellation of "my daddy but not my real father, you know." Donald had been someone entirely special until his mother decided to have a man at home. His mother had been loving but not always a steady force, but when she lapsed and went off on toots his maternal grandmother took Donald very easily and gracefully into her husbandless home and showered the adoration of a doting grandmother on the boy. The grandmother had become increasingly conventional with passing years and she came to propound a very traditional intact-family ideology.

Donald attributed his school behavior problems not to fatherlessness but to being fathered, having a man in his mother's home. Donald's mother agreed, eventually got rid of her male companion—declaring him to be "no-account anyhow"—and restored the family balance to the familiar one for herself, her son, and her mother, who still maintained her separate dwelling. The therapist understood that one had to stretch the imagination immensely to see the boy as wanting a father; Donald obviously did not want one. He was a masculine boy, however, and had already established some heterosexual activities without his mother's knowing. He wanted, as do many ghetto children, to be a professional athlete when he grew up; he felt only negativity about a male living with his mother, whether married to her or not; Donald showed no Oedipal problems. His school misbehavior and unruliness subsided after he had been seen once weekly in play therapy for 6 months. His mother had become pregnant again and decided to go to term and to keep the baby, but had achieved the insight that a man would not alleviate her sorrows, economically or emotionally.

The lives of some children, on a day-in, day-out basis, have been devoid of adult male accompaniment. No father later becomes dethroned; the children have been fatherless all their lives. Donald was one. Instead of sanctifying our own projections about humanity or fatherlessness, we as therapists can help these children more fully if, by containing our countertransferences that go masked as science, we simply find out from the little children what it all means.

It is well for the therapist to recall that his or her own particular family constellation might have been idiosyncratic in its own way; one special person should be able to empathize with another who is special. To a child, every accustomed idiosyncrasy seems normal enough. Furthermore, it is well for a therapist to be radical and get to the roots of the matter, rather than rolling over and over in conventional wisdom or nonsense. In the radical view, the true view in this case, usually the mother, the basic caretaker, is the young child's guide and source of satisfactions. The core gender identity, of the child of either gender, is structured between 16 and 30 months of age. So, even for fathered boys and girls, we should recall that the mother does most to shape the "sentiments of self-regard," as William James called them. Mothers contribute not only to the formation of female identity but also to the structuring of the male ego and self-concept. That really should not be a novel notion for psychotherapists. After all, everything that goes to the roots is not brand new.

Fatherless by Desertion

Generally, the most derogated of absent fathers is the father who absconded, leaving the mother and children deserted. Although many women seem relieved to be rid of their rascal spouses, they seldom lose an opportunity to bad-mouth them. They convey an ideology against the father, against the adult male, into their children's daily lives. A therapist helps the child to find his or her real feelings without adopting mother's hard line. The child reflects what the mother feels, but from a therapist the child needs the freedom to understand, "You can have your own feelings." The therapist may have to question and analyze some of the child's statements about the father— derogatory or laudatory—so that they lose their compulsivity and fit in with the child's forward movement.

Rodney, aged 7 years, gives an example of the deserted child who used the psychotherapeutic relationship to form a revision of his mother's attitudes about his father. The lower-class family had survived, remaining intact despite poverty and insecurity, until Rodney was in first grade. At that time father took off and the mother folded up in feelings of abandonment and depression. She continued with her job that provided her with insufficient income to support Rodney and herself so she had to move into her mother's home where two of her sisters were already ensconced in an all-female setting.

Rodney was a hyperactive child who showed indications of suffering from MBD, or attention decifit disorder (ADD). For that, Ritalin had been started by a physician but the schoolteachers confiscated the medication, insisiting that it was against the rules for children to bring drugs to school. The mother did not know how to oppose their authoritative comments and arbitrary action. The medication had helped only slightly, in the first place, but sometimes every little thing helps, his mother knew. Rodney's EEG, obtained by the child psychiatrist who began treating the child and the mother, showed Rodney had a left temporal lobe seizure focus. Dilantin greatly modified his aggressive, cruel behavior but his attention deficit persisted until Ritalin was reinstated. The school finally permitted him to take his medication on schedule and he became a docile scholar for a change.

Rodney was her only child, and the mother expected him to console her, provide her with companionship and security in this world of woe. Rodney did not take up role reversal willingly. He was anything but comforting. Cruel to his peers and to animals, Rodney was inexpressive in the playroom except for brutal fantasies of disembowelment and torture. Yet he said he wanted to be a fireman when he grew up "so I can save people's lives." After his medication regimen was in place, Rodney was considerably transformed: He was able to concentrate, behaved better in school, began liking school better, commenced nurturant play with a baby doll in the playroom, originated a play sequence in which he hid the father doll and then engaged in a dramatic search for him. Once when he finally found the father doll he had him speak: "I walked off in my sleep. I didn't know what I was doing. I hate mama and my mean kids too." He seemed to be identifying with the absented father.

Some deserted families, by the time that we see them clinically, have elaborated a more eulogistic myth of the absent father. Sometimes the myth grows out of the woman's belief that desertion is a fact of life that she girds herself to face and surmount. Sometimes the mother shares the father's wish to abscond, to be childless and carefree. She may envy him and say candidly that she cannot blame him. Sometimes the mother is more affluent than her husband and is pleased not to contribute to his support any longer. Sometimes she adopts a stoical realism, concluding that her husband married too soon, cut short his adolescent moratorium on decision making, was not ready for responsibilities, meanwhile harboring the hope that at some future date he will return to pick up his responsibilities and demonstrate a basic worth that she had not doubted. Sometimes, too, a mother will make a career of vindictiveness. She proclaims, "I'll make him pay for this!" as she mounts nationwide searches for her deserting spouse, falling back for the first time in her life into a view of the family that is so reactionary it would make a Phyllis Schlafly blush, and so vituperatively demanding of male support and sharing the burden that it would seem excessive to a Gloria Steinem. The range of human thinking about problems like desertion is truly enormous. We should try to accommodate the broad span of viewpoints that we find in the families with whom we work, not try to make them be like us.

Only in his mature years could one prominent expert in the psychology of religion bring himself to feel detached from blaming his father who had deserted the family (Wayne Oates, 1980). The wounds from a father's desertion are slow to heal. Connie exemplified how long it takes, longer when deception enters the family's myth making.

Connie was a narcissistic, chronic runaway woman of 15 years who had been brought up by her mother and maternal grandmother after her father deserted the family when Connie was only a few weeks old. The mother buttered up the story of his elopement by telling Connie that her father died. That meant that this mother had no hopes or plans for the father's reinstatement into the life of the family. Connie's therapist had to work with all three generations who made up the household in order to establish some basic honesty about the father's departure, to help relieve the mother's chronic depression and neglect of her daughter, and to combat the grandmother's eloquent creed that all males are vile but that Connie, as the product of her father, and a runaway like her father, shared in his ignoble heritage. Connie = bad male = her father.

Connie's wounds and conflicts were thoroughly imbedded in her character structure; treatment could not be done in the trice called for by the welfare department that had taken over Connie's care. Connie wound up going from one agency and institution to another while the bureaucracy blew hot and cold. Only in the bureau's uncanny timing of each of its uprootings did it not err: it invariably interfered in her psychotherapy program, pulling her out of the children's hospital just when she seriously began any psychotherapeutic work.

Fatherless by Imprisonment

To complete this brief survey of treatment principles for fatherless children, we present a case of a 13-year-old male whose lower-working-class father was imprisoned for a sex crime. Reginald had lived in more than 30 foster homes and institutions such as shelters and group homes since his schizophrenic mother had murdered a younger sib when the boy was 5 years old. That may seem like a bad enough beginning.

Reginald had good reason to hate his father, but he also loved him and tried to protect him. Under pressure from the paternal grandmother and other relatives, he had perjured himself during the latest trial of his father. What Reginald lied about was (to be truthful): His father had forced Reginald to have sexual intercourse with a younger sister while the father performed sodomy on Reginald. Reginald had lied in the courtroom but his sister stuck to the truth; Reginald was rewarded with a motorcycle for his courtroom report and the sister consoled herself with the rewards of a clear conscience. Reginald's therapy centered on his identifying with his father's aggression, his loyalty to his father, his ultimately turning against his father and seeing him as a rather vile person, and his need for some self-esteem despite what both of his parents had done to him or had had done to them.

Reginald was like many another fatherless child in his reading of the golden rule to adults: *Don't do unto others what others did to you and what you did to yourselves.*

Fatherless children exemplify *the child's estate* more than conditions unique to fatherlessness. They have parents, one or more, who dominate their real worlds and their fantasies. Their parents, together with parent surrogates, inflict both the realities and fantasies of grown-ups on the children. The adults do not see children as they are, or as they are becoming, but often only as shadows of other relationships in which the parents have been immersed. Adults pass on their problems to children, even unto the third and fourth generations.

We close now, having considered the state of our art regarding fathering, father-absence of varied types and kinds, the effects on children of not having a father, suggestions for research methodology, and suggestions for a national policy concerning children. We ended with some treatment suggestions in this chapter: Don't borrow trouble; search for real core conflicts; don't worry about a male therapist for a fatherless child; remember to deal with survival economics; get fact and fantasy both; view the family in its community context; have special regard for overt behavior and its meaning; know everyone who lives in the household; be very cognizant of sibs; keep skeptical about family structure and functions. Although stated as commandments, our guidelines are meant to be practical hints to guide the psychotherapist who desires to help fatherless children. Many fatherless children do need help.

Comprehensive
Bibliography

Abelin, E. *The role of the father in core gender identity and in psychosocial differentiation.* Paper presented at the annual meeting of the American Psychoanalytic Association, April 1977.

――――. The role of the father in the separation-individuation process. In J. B. McDevitt & C. F. Settlage (Eds.), *Separation-Individuation.* New York: International Universities Press, 1971.

Achenbach, Thomas M. *Developmental Psychopathology,* (2nd ed.). New York: Ronald, 1981.

――――. DSM-III in light of empirical research on the classification of child psychopathology. *Journal of the American Academy of Child Psychiatry, 19,* 1980, 395–412.

Adams, P. L. Children and paraservices of the community mental health centers. *Journal of the American Academy of Child Psychiatry,* Winter 1975, *14*(1), 18–31.

――――. Dental symbols and dreamwork. *Psychiatry and Pedontics,* November 1963a, 24–28.

――――. *Dynamics of some adult attitudes toward children.* Submitted for publication, University of Louisville, 1981b.

――――. *Functional analysis of the lower-class partial family.* Unpublished paper, University of Florida, 1972b.

――――. Functions of the lower-class partial family. *American Journal of Psychiatry,* February 1973, *130*(2), 200–203.

――――. Individual psychotherapy with children. In P. Sholevar (Ed.), *Treatment of emotional disorders in children and adolescents* (Vol. 1). New York: Basic Books, Inc., 1980a.

――――. The influence of new information from social sciences on concepts, practice and research in child psychiatry. *Journal of the Amerian Academy of Child Psychiatry, 21,* 6:553–542, 1982.

――――. Local community change for service to children. *Child Psychiatry and Human Development,* Fall 1976, *7*(1), 22–30.

――――. *Outline for single parent families.* Unpublished paper, University of Florida, 1972a.

――――. Personal recollection, University of Louisville, 1980b.

――――. *Tele-analysis and kiddie lit.* Paper presented at the annual meeting of the American Academy of Child Psychiatry, New Orleans, 1972c.

――――. *The pitfalls of early parenting.* Paper presented at the regional meeting of the American College of Psychiatrists, Louisville, November 1978.

――――. What women's inequality means to children and adolescents. *American Journal of Social Psychiatry,* April 1981c, *1*(1), 6–8.

――――. Women in non-traditional families. In J. Spurlock & C. Robinowitz (Eds.), *Women in context: Social and cultural issues.* New York: Spectrum, 1983.

354

————. Women's and men's attitudes toward the female breast. *Medical Aspects of Human Sexuality,* October 1979, 54–58.

Adams, P. L., & Horovitz, J. H. Coping patterns of mothers of poor boys. *Child Psychiatry and Human Development,* Spring 1980a, *10*(3), 144–155.

————. Psychopathology and fatherlessness in poor boys. *Child Psychiatry and Human Development,* Spring 1980b, *10*(30), 135–143.

Adams-Tucker, C., & Adams, P. L. Role of the father (Chap. 12). In M. Kirkpatrick (Ed.), *Women's Sexual Development.* New York: Plenum Publishing Corp., 1980.

Aichhorn, A. *Wayward youth.* New York: Viking, 1935. [Original in German, 1923.]

Albert, R. S. Cognitive development and parental loss among the gifted, the exceptionally gifted and the creative. *Psychological Reports,* 1971, *29,* 19–26.

Altus, W. D. The broken home and factors of adjustment. *Psychological Reports,* 1958, *4,* 447.

American Psychiatric Association. *Diagnostic and statistical manual of mental disorders—DSM III* (3rd ed.). Washington, D.C.: Author, 1980.

Anastasi, A. *Psychological testing* (5th ed.). New York: Macmillan, 1982.

Andrews, R. P., & Christensen, H. T. Relationship of absence of a parent to courtship status: A repeat study. *American Sociological Review,* 1951, *16*(4), 541–544.

Andry, R. G. Paternal and maternal roles and delinquency. *W.H.O. Public Health Paper,* 1962, *14,* 31–44.

Associated Press. The "marriage penalty": Legislators seeking to amend tax law that makes "living together" profitable. Louisville *Courier-Journal & Times,* Sunday, July 8, 1979, A-13.

Atkinson, B. R., & Ogston, D. G. The effect of father absence on male children in the home and school. *Journal of School Psychology,* 1974, *12*(3), 213–221.

Aug, R. G., & Bright, T. P. A study of wed and unwed motherhood in adolescents and young adults. *Journal of the American Academy of Child Psychiatry,* October 1970, *9*(4), 577–594.

Axelrad, S. Negro and white male institutionalized delinquents. *American Journal of Sociology,* 1952, *57*(6), 569–574.

Bach, G. R. Father-fantasies and father-typing in father-separated children. *Child Development,* 1946, *17,* 63–79.

Bacon, M. K., Child, I. L., & Barry, H. A cross-cultural study of correlates of crime. *Journal of Abnormal and Social Psychology,* 1963, *66*(4), 291–300.

Badaines, J. Identification, imitation, and sex-role preference in father-present and father-absent black and Chicano boys. *The Journal of Psychology,* 1976, *92,* 15–24.

Baker, S. L., Cove, L. A., Fagen, S. A., Fisher, E. C., & Janda, E. J. *Impact of father absence: III. Problems of family reintegration following prolonged fa-*

ther absence. Paper presented at the meeting of the American Orthopsychiatric Association, Chicago, March 1968.

Baker, S. L., Fagen, S. A., Fisher, E. G., Janda, E. J., & Cove, L. A. *Impact of father absence on personality factors of boys: I. An evaluation of the military family's adjustment.* Paper presented at the meeting of the American Orthopsychiatric Association, Washington, D.C., March 1967.

Bandura, A., & Walters, R. H. *Social learning and personality development.* New York: Holt, Rinehart & Winston, 1963.

Bane, M. J. Marital disruption and the lives of children. *Journal of Social Issues,* 1976, *32*(1), 103–117.

Bane, M. J., & Masnick, G. *The nation's families: 1960–1990.* Boston: Auburn House Pub. Co., 1980.

Bannon, J. A., & Southern, M. L. Father-absent women: Self-concepts and modes of relating to men. *Sex Roles,* 1980, *6*(1), 75–84.

Barclay, A., & Cusumano, D. R. Father absence, cross-sex identity, and field-dependent behavior in male adolescents. *Child Development,* 1967, *38,* 243–250.

Barglow, P., Bornstein, M., Exum, D., Wright, K., & Visotsky, H. Some psychiatric aspects of illegitimate pregnancy in early adolescence. *American Journal of Orthopsychiatry,* 1968, *38,* 672–687.

Bartemeier, L. The contributions of the father to the mental health of the family. *The American Journal of Psychiatry,* 1953–1954, *110,* 277–280.

Bartlett, C. J., & Horrocks, J. E. A study of the needs status of adolescents from broken homes. *The Journal of Genetic Psychology,* 1958, *93,* 153–159.

Bartollas, C., Miller, S. J., & Dinitz, S. *Juvenile victimization: The institutional paradox.* New York: John Wiley & Sons, 1976.

Bayley, N. *Bayley Scales of Infant Development.* New York: Psychological Corp., 1969.

Bayley, N. On the growth of intelligence. *American Psychologist,* 1955, *10,* 805–818.

Bayley, N. Behavioral correlates of mental growth: Birth to thirty-six years. *American Psychologist,* 1968, *23,* 1–17.

Beck, A. T., Sethi, B. B., & Tuthill, R. W. Childhood bereavement and adult depression. *Archives of General Psychiatry,* 1963, *9,* 129–136.

Becker, S. Father absence and its relationship to creativity. *Graduate Research in Education,* Spring/Summer 1974, 7(2), 32–52.

Bell, R. R. *The one-parent mother in the Negro lower-class.* Paper presented at the meeting of the Eastern Sociological Society, New York, 1965.

Bellak, L. *The TAT, CAT, and SAT in clinical use* (3rd ed.). New York: Grune & Stratton, 1975.

Bem, S. L. The measurement of psychological androgyny. *Journal of Consulting and Clinical Psychology,* 1974, *42,* 155–162.

Bem, S. L.   On the utility of alternative procedures for assessing psychological androgyny. *Journal of Consulting and Clinical Psychology*, 1977, *45*, 196–205.

Bem, S. L.   *Manual for the Bem Sex-Role Inventory*. Palo Alto, Calif.: Consulting Psychologists Press, 1981.

Bemporad, J., Kresch, R. A., Asnes, R., & Wilson, A.   Chronic neurotic encopresis as a paradigm of a multifactorial psychiatric disorder. *Journal of Nervous and Mental Disease*, 1978, *166*(7), 472–479.

Benedek, R. S., & Benedek, E. P.   Postdivorce visitation: A child's right. *Journal of the American Academy of Child Psychiatry*, Spring 1977, *16*(2), 256–271.

Benedek, T.   The psychosomatic implications of the primary unit: Mother-child. *American Journal of Orthopsychiatry*, 1949, *19*, 642–654.

Bennett, E.   Your child: Fathers show youngsters how to manage their aggressive impulses. *The Houston Post*, Friday, November 19, 1982, F-1.

Berkov, B.   Illegitimate births in California. *Milbank Memorial Fund Quarterly*, 1968, *46*, 473–506.

Bernard, J. C.   *Remarriage: A study of marriage*. Tampa, Florida: Russel, 1971.

Bernstein, B. E.   How father absence in the home affects the mathematics skills of fifth-graders. *Family Therapy*, 1976, *3*(1), 47–59.

Besner, A.   Economic deprivation and family patterns. *Welfare in Review*, 1965, *3*(9), 20–28.

Bieber, I.   *Homosexuality*. New York: Basic Books, 1962.

Bigras, J., Gauthier, Y., Bouchard, C., & Tasse, Y.   Suicidal attempts in adolescent girls: A preliminary study. *Canadian Psychiatric Association Journal II* (suppl.), 1966, 275–282.

Biller, H. B.   A note on father-absence and masculine development in young lower-class Negro and white boys. *Child Development*, 1968, *39*, 1003–1006.

———.   Effect of absence of father on sexual identification. *Medical Aspects of Human Sexuality*, May 1975, 179.

———.   Father absence and the personality development of the male child. *Developmental Psychology*, 1970, *2*(2), 181–201.

———.   Father absence, maternal encouragement, and sex-role development in kindergarten-age boys. *Child Development*, 1969, *110*, 539–546.

———.   *Father, child and sex role: Parental determinants of personality development*. Lexington, Mass.: Heath, 1971a.

———.   Fathering and female sexual development. *Medical Aspects of Human Sexuality*, 1971b, *5*(11), 126; 129–138.

———.   *Paternal deprivation: Family, school, sexuality and society*. Lexington, Mass.: Lexington Books, 1974.

———.   The mother–child relationship and the fathre-absent boy's personality development. *Merrill-Palmer Quarterly*, July 1971c, *17*(3), 227–241.

Biller, H. B., & Bahm, R. M.   Father-absence, perceived maternal behavior, and masculinity of self-concept among junior high school boys. *Developmental Psychology,* 1971, *4,* 178–181.

Biller, H. B., & Borstelmann, L. J.   Masculine development: An integrative review. *Merrill-Palmer Quarterly,* 1967, *13,* 257–294.

Biller, H. B., & Liebman, D. A.   Body build, sex-role preference, and sex-role adoption in junior high school boys. *Journal of Genetic Psychology,* 1971, *118,* 81–86.

Biller, H. B., & Weiss, S. D.   The father-daughter relationship and the personality development of the female. *Journal of Genetic Psychology,* 1970, *116,* 79–93.

Birns, B.   The emergence and socialization of sex differences in the earliest years. In S. Chess & A. Thomas (Eds.), *Annual progress in child psychiatry and child development.* New York: Brunner/Mazel Pub., 1977.

Birtchnell, J.   Depression in relation to early and recent parent death. *British Journal of Psychiatry,* 1970c, *116,* 299–306.

Birtchnell, J.   Early parent death and mental illness. *British Journal of Psychiatry,* 1970a, *116,* 281–288.

Birtchnell, J.   Recent parent death and mental illness. *British Journal of Psychiatry,* 1970b, *116,* 289–297.

Blair, M., & Pasmore, J.   Family planning for the unmarried. *Journal of the Royal College of General Practitioners,* 1969, *18,* 214–218.

Blanchard, R. W., & Biller, H. B.   Father availability and academic performance among third-grade boys. *Developmental Psychology,* 1971, *4,* 301–305.

Bloch, D.   *So the witch won't eat me: Fantasy and the child's fear of infanticide.* Boston: Houghton Mifflin Co., 1978.

Block, J. E.   Beyond parenthood: Toward a guardianship model for parenting. *Social Policy,* March/April 1980, 41–46.

Blum, G. S.   A study of the psychoanalytic theory of psychosexual development. *Genetic Psychology Monograms,* 1949, *39,* 3–99.

Blum, G. S.   *Revised scoring system for research use of the Blacky pictures.* Ann Arbor: University of Michigan, Department of Psychology, 1951.

Bombeck, E.   Father's day was every day when you stop to think about it. Louisville *Courier-Journal & Times,* Sunday, June 15, 1980, G-5.

Boone, S. L.   Effects of fathers' absence and birth order on aggressive behavior on young male children. *Psychological Reports,* 1979, *44,* 1223–1229.

Boss, P.   A clarification of the concept of psychological father presence in families experiencing ambiguity of boundary. *Journal of Marriage and the Family,* February 1977, 141–151.

Boss, P. G.   The relationship of psychological father presence, wife's personal qualities and wife/family dysfunction in families of missing fathers. *Journal of Marriage and the Family,* 1980, *42*(3), 541–549.

Bowlby, J. *Attachment and Loss* (Vol. 1). *Attachment.* New York: Basic Books, 1969.

Bowlby, J. *Maternal care and infant health.* Geneva: World Health Organization, 1951. (Monograph series, No. 2.)

Bowlby, J. The nature of the child's tie to the mother. *International Journal of Psycho-Analysis,* 1958, *39,* 350–373.

Brandis, W., & Henderson, D. *Social class language and communication.* London: Routledge & Kegan Paul, 1971.

Brandwein, R. A., Brown, C. A., & Fox, E. M. Women and children last: The social situation of divorced mothers and their families. *Journal of Marriage and the Family,* August 1974, 498–514.

Bratter, T. E. Treating alienated, unmotivated, drug-abusing adolescents. *American Journal of Psychotherapy,* 1973, *27,* 585–598.

Brenz, M. Fatherless families in the public assistance program. In *The significance of the father.* New York: Family Service Association of America, 1959.

Brim, O. G. Family structure and sex role learning by children: A further analysis of Helen Koch's data. *Sociometry,* 1958, *21,* 1–16.

Briscoe, W., Smith, J. B., Robins, E., Marten, S., & Gaskin, F. Divorce and psychiatric disease. *Archives of General Psychiatry,* July 1973, *29,* 119–125.

Broderick, C. B. Preadolescent sexual behavior. *Medical Aspects of Human Sexuality,* 1968, *2,* 20–29.

Bronfenbrenner, U. The psychological costs of quality and equality in education. *Child Development,* 1967, *38,* 909–925.

Brown, D. G. Sex-role preference in young children. *Psychological Monographs,* 1956, *70*(14, Whole No. 421).

Brown, F. Childhood bereavement and subsequent psychiatric disorder. *British Journal of Psychiatry,* 1966, *112,* 1035–1041.

Brown, F. Depression and childhood bereavement. *British Journal of Psychiatry,* 1961, *107,* 754–777.

Brubacher, J., & Rudy, W. *Higher education in transition: A history of American colleges and universities, 1636–1968.* New York: Harper and Row, 1968.

Bruhn, J. G. Broken homes among attempted suicides and psychiatric outpatients: A comparative study. *Journal of Medical Science,* 1962, *108,* 772–779.

Bumpass, L. L. Marriage and childbearing. In A. E. Fisher (Ed.), *Science Monographs of Women's Worlds* (NIMH supported research on women), 1978, DHEW pub. no. (ADM) 78-660, Rockville, Maryland.

Bunch, J., & Barraclough, B. The influence of parental death anniversaries upon suicide dates. *British Journal of Psychiatry,* 1971, *118,* 621–626.

Burchinal, L. G. Characteristics of adolescents from unbroken, broken, and reconstituted families. *Journal of Marriage and the Family,* February 1964, 44–51.

Burkart, J., & Whatley, A. E. The unwed mother: Implications for family life educators. *Journal of School Health,* September 1973, *43*(7), 451–454.

Burke, P. J. Leadership role differentiation. In C. G. McClintock (Ed.), *Experimental social psychology.* New York: Holt, Rinehart & Winston, 1972.

Burnes, K. Patterns of WISC scores for children of two socioeconomic classes and races. *Child Development,* 1970, *41,* 493–499.

Buros, O. K. (Ed). *The eighth mental measurements yearbook.* Lincoln: University of Nebraska, Buros Institute of Mental Measurements, 1978.

Burton, R. V., & Whiting, J. W. M. The absent father and cross-sex identity. *Merrill-Palmer Quarterly,* 1961, *7*(2), 85–95.

Butts, R. Y., & Sporakowski, M. J. Unwed pregnancy decisions: Some background factors. *Journal of Sex Research,* May 1974, *10*(2), 110–117.

Caplan, M. G., & Douglas, V. I. Incidence of parental loss in children with depressed mood. *Journal of Child Psychology and Psychiatry,* 1969, *10,* 225–232.

Carkhuff, R. R., & Berenson, B. G. The utilization of black functional professionals to reconstitute troubled families. *Journal of Psychology,* 1972, *38,* 92–93.

Carlsmith, L. Effect of early father absence on scholastic aptitude. *Harvard Educational Review,* 1964, *34,* 3–21.

Carlsmith, L. Some personality characteristics of boys separated from their father during World War II. *Ethos,* Winter 1973, *38,* 466–477.

Carpenter, T. S., & Busse, T. V. Development of self concept in Negro and white welfare children. *Child Development,* 1969, *40,* 935–939.

Carroll, M. P. The sex of our gods. *Ethos,* Spring 1979, *7*(1), 37–50.

Carter, H., & Glick, P. C. *Marriage and divorce: A social and economic study.* Cambridge: Harvard University Press, 1970.

Castellano, V., & Dembo, M. H. The relationship of father absence in antisocial behavior to social egocentrism in adolescent Mexican-American females. *Journal of Youth and Adolescence,* 1981, *10*(1), 77–84.

Chapman, M. Father absence, stepfathers, and the cognitive performance of college students. *Child Development,* 1977, *48,* 1155–1158.

Chodoff, P. A critique of Freud's theory of infantile sexuality. *American Journal of Psychiatry,* November 1966, *123*(5), 507–518.

Chodorow, N. *The reproduction of mothering: Psychoanalysis and the sociology of gender.* Berkeley: University of California Press, 1978.

Cobliner, W. G. Social factors in mental disorders: A contribution to the etiology of mental illness. *Genetic Psychology Monographs,* 1963, *67,* 151–215.

Cohen, G. Absentee husbands in spiralist families. *Journal of Marriage and the Family,* August 1977, 595–604.

Cohler, B. J., Grunebaum, H. U., Weiss, J. L., & Moran, D. L. The children attitudes of two generations of mothers. *Merrill-Palmer Quarterly,* 1971, *17,* 3–17.

Colcord, J. C., Lenroot, K. F., Shulman, H. M., & Maller, J. B.   Discussion of "Are broken homes a causative factor in juvenile delinquency?" *Social Forces,* 1932, *10*(4), 525–527.

Cole, J. B.   Culture: Negro, black, and nigger. *The Black Scholar,* June 1970, 40–45.

Coletta, N. D.   The impact of divorce: Father absence or poverty. *Journal of Divorce,* Fall 1979, *3*(1), 27–35.

Colley, T.   The nature and origin of psychological sexual identity. *Psychological Review,* 1959, *66,* 165–177.

Colier, L., Mitchell, L. K., Sandidge, V., & Smith, R.   The effect of the father-absent home on "lower class" black adolescents. *Educational Quest,* 1973, *17*(1), 11–14.

Colletta, N. D.   The impact of divorce: Father absence or poverty? *Journal of Divorce,* 1979, *3*(1), 27–35.

Collins, B. E., & Raven, B. H.   Group structure: Attraction, coalitions, communication, and power. In G. Lindzey and E. Aronson (Eds.), *Handbook of social psychology* (Vol. 4). Reading, Mass.: Addison-Wesley, 1968.

Collins, G.   A new look at life with father. In H. E. Fitzgerald and T. H. Carr (Eds.), *Human development 82/83.* Guilford, Connecticut: the Dushkin Publishing Group, Inc., 1982.

Collins, M. A.   Achievement, intelligence, personality and selected school-related variables in Negro children from intact and broken families attending parochial school in central Harlem (Doctoral dissertation, Fordham University, 1969). *Dissertation Abstracts International,* 1969, *29,* 5280A–5281A.

Condry, J., & Condry, S.   Sex difference: A study of the eye of the beholder. In S. Chess & A. Thomas (Eds.), *Annual progress in child psychiatry and child development.* New York: Brunner/Mazel Pub., 1977.

Condry, J. C., & Simon, M. A.   Characteristics of peer and adult-oriented children. *Journal of Marriage and the Family,* 1974, *36,* 543–554.

Cooper, D.   *The death of the family.* New York: Pantheon Books, 1970.

Coriat, I. H.   Dental anxiety: Fear of going to the dentist. *Psychoanalytic Review,* 1946, *33,* 365–367.

Corrigan, E. M.   The child at home: Child-rearing practices of the unwed mother compared to other mothers. In *Illegitimacy: Changing services for changing times.* New York: National Council on Illegitimacy, 1970.

Covell, K., & Turnbull, K.   The long-term effects of father absence in childhood on male university students' sex-role identity and personal adjustment. *Journal of Genetic Psychology,* 1982, *141,* 271–276.

Crain, A. J., & Stamm, C. S.   Intermittent absence of fathers and children's perceptions of parents. *Journal of Marriage and the Family,* August 1965, 344–347.

Crawford, A. G.   The stability of man's family of origin, its causes, and its effects on his achievement: A test of Moynihan's theory. *Dissertation Abstracts International,* October 1976, *37*(4A), 2442.

Cronenwett, L. R.   Father participation in child care: A critical review. *Research in Nursing and Health,* 1982, *5*, 63–72.

Crumley, F. E., & Blumenthal, R. S.   Children's reaction to temporary loss of the father. *American Journal of Psychiatry,* July 1973, *130*(7), 778–779.

Curtis, F. L. S.   Observations of unwed pregnant adolescents. *American Journal of Nursing,* January 1974, *74*(1), 100–102.

Cutright, P.   Components of change in the number of female heads ages 15–44: United States, 1940–1970. *Journal of Marriage and the Family,* 1974, *34*, 714–721.

Dads.   Louisville *Courier-Journal & Times,* Sunday, June 17, 1979, G-1&2; G-16 &17.

Daly, M.   *Beyond God the father: Toward a philosophy of women's liberation.* Boston: Beacon Press, 1973.

D'Andrade, R. G.   Father absence, identification, and identity. *Ethos,* Winter 1973, *38*, 440–445.

Dasen, P. K. (Ed.).   *Piagetian psychology: Cross-cultural contributions.* New York: Halsted, 1977.

DaSilva, G.   The role of the father with chronic schizophrenic patients: A study in group therapy. *Canadian Psychiatric Journal,* 1963, *8*, 190–203.

Dauber, B., Zalar, M., & Goldstein, P.   Abortion counseling and behavioral change. *Family Planning Perspectives,* 1972, *4*, 23–27.

Deaton, H. S.   An analytic intervention in the life of a girl growing up in a chaotic environment: "Why are my glasses so hot?" *Journal of Child Psychotherapy,* 1979, *5*, 69–87.

Dennehy, C. M.   Childhood bereavement and psychiatric illness. *British Journal of Psychiatry,* 1966, *112*, 1049–1069.

Deutsch, M.   Minority group and class status as related to social and personality factors in scholastic achievement. *The Society for Applied Anthropology,* 1960, *70*(12), 1958–1962.

Dollard, J., & Miller, N.   *Personality and psychotherapy: An analysis in terms of learning, thinking and culture* (1st ed.). New York: McGraw-Hill, 1950.

Donini, G. P.   An evaluation of sex-role identification among father-absent and father-present boys. *Psychology: A Journal of Human Behavior,* 1967, *4*(3), 13–16.

Donne, J., & Blake, W.   [*The complete poetry and selected prose of John Donne and the complete poetry of William Blake.*] (S. Hillyer, Ed.) New York: Modern Public Library, 1941.

Dorpat, T. L., Jackson, J. K., & Ripley, H. S.   Broken homes and attempted and completed suicide. *Archives of General Psychiatry,* February 1965, *12*, 213–216.

Douglas, J. W. Broken families and child behavior. *Journal of the Royal College of Physicians,* April 1970, *4,* 203–210.

Drake, C. T., & McDougall, D. Effects of the absence of a father and other male models on the development of boys' sex roles. *Developmental Psychology,* 1977, *13*(5), 537–538.

Dubois, W. F. B. *The souls of black folk.* Greenwich, Conn.: Fawcett Publications, Inc., 1961.

Duke, M. P., & Lancaster, W. A note on locus of control as a function of father absence. *Journal of Genetic Psychology,* 1976, *129,* 335–336.

Dunn, Lloyd M. Peabody Picture and Vocabulary Test, American Guidance Services, Inc., 1959.

Dunn, L. M., & Markwardt, F. C. *Peabody Individual Achievement Test ages 5–18.* American Guidance Service, 1970.

Earle, A. M., & Earle, B. V. Early maternal deprivation and later psychiatric illness. *American Journal of Orthopsychiatry,* 1961, *31,* 181–185.

Earl, L., & Lohmann, N. Absent fathers and black male children. *Social Work,* September 1978, *23*(5), 413–415.

Earls, F. The fathers (not the mothers): Their importance and influence with infants and young children. *Psychiatry,* August 1976, *39,* 209–226.

Earls, F., Jacobs, G., Goldfein, D., et al. Concurrent validation of a behavior problems scale to use with 3-year-olds. *Journal of the American Academy of Child Psychiatry,* 1982, *21,* 47–57.

Eisenberg, J., Henderson, R., Kuhlmann, W., & Hill, J. P. Six- and ten-year olds' attribution of punitiveness and nurturance to parents and other adults. *Journal of Genetic Psychology,* 1967, *111*(2), 233–240.

Eisenstadt, J. M. Parental loss and genius. *American Psychologist,* 1978, *33*(3), 211–223.

Eisner, V. Effect of parents in the home on juvenile delinquency. *Public Health Reports,* October 1966, *81*(10), 905–910.

Elkin, H. Aggressive and erotic tendencies in army life. *American Journal of Sociology,* 1946, *51,* 408–413.

Elliot, F. R. Occupational commitments and paternal deprivation. *Child: Care, Health and Development,* 1978, *4,* 305–315.

Elliot, M. A., & Merrill, F. E. *Social disorganization* (3rd ed.). New York: Harper & Row, 1950.

Epstein, A. S., & Radin, N. Motivational components related to father behavior and cognitive functioning in preschoolers. *Child Development,* 1975, *46,* 831–839.

Erikson, E. H. *Childhood and society.* New York: Norton, 1963.

ETS, The Basic Skills Assessment Program, 1976.

Evans-Pritchard, E. E. *Kinship and marriage among the Nuer.* Oxford: Oxford University Press, 1951.

Eysenck, H. J. Masculinity–femininity, personality and sexual attitudes. *Journal of Sex Research,* May 1971, 7(2), 83–88.

Fagen, S. A., Janda, E. J., Baker, S. L., Fisher, E. G., & Cove, L. A. *Impact of father absence in military families: II. Factors relating to success of coping with crisis.* Paper presented at the meeting of the American Psychological Association, Washington, D.C., September 1967.

Fagot, B. Sex differences in toddlers' behavior and parental reaction. *Developmental Psychology,* 1974, 10, 554–558.

Fanon, F. *Black skins, white masks.* New York: Grove Press, 1967.

Father's influence on son's masculine role not primary. *Roche report: Frontiers of Psychiatry,* May 1, 1980, 3.

Feiner, J. Family therapy and public practice in mental health. In J. L. Carleton & U. R. Mahlendorf (Eds.), *Dimensions of Social Psychiatry.* Princeton: Science Press, 1979.

Ferenczi, S. [*Thalassa: A theory of genitality*] (H. A. Bunker, trans.). New York: W. W. Norton, 1968. (Originally published, 1923.)

Festinger, T. B. Unwed mothers and their decisions to keep or surrender children. *Child Welfare,* 1971, 50(5), 253–263.

Field, T. Interaction behaviors of primary versus secondary caretaker fathers. *Developmental Psychology,* 1978, 14(2), 183–184.

Fleck, J. R., Fuller, C. C., Malin, S. Z., Miller, D. H., & Acheson, K. R. Father psychological absence and heterosexual behavior, personal adjustment and sex-typing in adolescent girls. *Adolescence,* 1980, 15(60), 847–860.

Fleisher, B. M. The effect of income on delinquency. *American Economic Review,* 1966, 56(1), 118–137.

Floyd, J., & Viney, L. L. Ego identity and ego ideal in the unwed mother. *British Journal of Medical Psychology,* 1974, 47, 273–281.

Forer, L. The rights of children. In F. Rebelsky & L. Dorman (Eds.), *Child development and behavior* (2nd Ed.). New York: Alfred A. Knopf, Inc., 1973.

Fowler, P. C., & Richards, H. C. Father absence, educational preparedness and academic achievement: A test of the confluence model. *Journal of Educational Psychology,* 1978, 70(4), 595–601.

Franck, K., & Rosen, E. A. A projective test of masculinity–femininity. *Journal of Consulting Psychology,* 1949, 13, 247–256.

Franke, L., et al. The children of divorce. *Newsweek,* February 11, 1980.

Freedheim, D. K. An investigation of masculinity and parental role patterns. Unpublished doctoral dissertation, Duke University, 1960.

Freud, A., & Burlingham, D. T. *Infants without families: The case for and against residential nurseries.* New York: Medical War Books, International Universities Press, 1944.

Freud, S. [*Collected papers of Sigmund Freud*] (E. Jones, Ed.). New York: Basic Books, 1950.

Freud, S.   Eine Kindheitserinnerung des Leonardo da Vinci [Leonardo da Vinci and a memory of his childhood]. (Original 1919.) (Trans. by A. and J. Strachey.) London: Hogarth, 1956. *Collected Papers,* Vol. 3.

Freud, S.   [*New introductory lectures on psychoanalysis*] (J. Strachey, Ed. and trans.). New York: Norton, 1965. (Originally published, 1933.)

Freud, S.   [Totem and taboo (Vol. 13).] [*The standard edition of the complete psychological works of Sigmund Freud*] (J. Strachey, Ed. and trans.). New York: Norton, 1976.

Freudenthal, K.   Problems of the one-parent family. *Social Work,* 1959, *4,* 44–48.

Fromm, E.   Individual and social origins of neurosis. *American Sociological Review,* 1944, *9,* 380–384.

Frommer, E. A., & O'Shea, G.   Antenatal identification of women liable to have problems in managing their infants. *British Journal of Psychiatry, 123,* 149–156.

Furman, E.   *A child's parent dies: Studies in childhood bereavement.* New Haven: Yale University Press, 1974.

Gadpaille, W. J.   Brief guide to office counseling: A mother rearing a young son alone. *Medical Aspects of Human Sexuality,* February 1974, 199–200.

Galenson, E., & Roiphe, H.   Some suggested revisions concerning early female development. In M. Kirkpatrick (Ed.), *Women's sexual development.* New York: Plenum Press, 1980.

Gans, H. J.   *The urban villagers: Group and class in the life of Italian-Americans.* New York: Free Press of Glencoe, 1962.

Gans, H. J.   The uses of poverty: The poor pay all. *Social Policy,* July/August, 1971, 20–24.

Gardiner, H. W., & Suttipan, C. S.   Parental tolerance of aggression: Perceptions of preadolescents in Thailand. *Psychologia,* 1977, *20,* 28–32.

Gardner, G. E.   Separation of the parents and the emotional life of the child. *Mental Hygiene,* 1956, *40,* 53–64.

Gardner, R.   *The boys' and girls' book about divorce.* New York: Bantam Books, 1970.

Gauthier, Y.   The mourning reaction of a ten-year-old boy. *Canadian Psychiatric Association Journal,* 1966, *11,* 307–308.

Gay, M. J., & Tonge, W. L.   The late effects of loss of parents in childhood. *British Journal of Psychiatry,* 1967, *113,* 753–759.

Gershansky, I. S., Hainline, L., & Goldstein, H. S.   Effects of onset and type of fathers' absence on children's levels of psychological differentiation. *Perceptual and Motor Skills,* 1980, *51,* 1263–1268.

Gershansky, I. S., Hainline, I., & Goldstein, H. S.   Maternal differentiation, onset and type of father's absence and psychological differentiation in children. *Perceptual and Motor Skills,* 1978, *46,* 1147–1152.

Gesell, A., & Amatruda, C. S. *Developmental diagnosis* (2nd ed.). New York: Hoeber-Harper, 1947.

Giele, J. Z. Changes in the modern family: Their impact on sex roles. *American Journal of Orthopsychiatry,* October 1971, *41*(5), 757–766.

Gittleman, R. The role of psychological tests for differential diagnosis in child psychiatry. *Journal of the American Academy of Child Psychiatry,* 1980, *19,* 413–438.

Glasser, P., & Navarre, E. Structural problems of the one-parent family. *Journal of Social Issues,* 1965, *21,* 98–109.

Glasser, P. H., & Glasser, L. N. (Eds.). *Families in crisis.* New York: Harper & Row, 1970.

Glassman, C. Women and the welfare system. In R. Morgan (Ed.), *Sisterhood is powerful.* New York: Vintage Press, 1970.

Glautz, O. Family structure, fate control, and counter-normative political beliefs among lower-class black students. *College Student Journal,* Summer 1976, *10*(2), 121–126.

Glick, I. Practical considerations. In D. Reiss & H. Hoffman (Eds.), *The American family: Dying or developing?* New York: Plenum Press, 1979.

Glick, P. C. Marriage and marital stability among blacks. *Milbank Memorial Fund Quarterly,* April 1970, *48*(2), 99–126.

Glueck, E. T. A preview of "family environment and delinquency." *International Journal of Orthopsychiatry,* October 1971, *41*(5), 757–766.

Glueck, S., & Glueck, E. *Delinquents and non-delinquents in perspective.* Cambridge, Mass.: Harvard University Press, 1968.

Glueck, S., & Glueck, E. *Physique and delinquency.* New York: Kraus Reprint Co., 1956.

Glueck, S., & Glueck, E. *Unraveling juvenile delinquency.* New York: Commonwealth Fund, 1950.

Godenne, G. Unwed mothers. *International encyclopedia of psychiatry, psychology, psychoanalysis and neurology* (Vol. II). New York: Aesculapius Publishers, 1977.

Goldfarb, W. Psychological privation in infancy and subsequent adjustment. *American Journal of Orthopsychiatry,* 1945, *15,* 247–255.

Goldstein, H. S. Internal controls in aggressive children from father-present and father-absent families. *Journal of Counseling and Clinical Psychology,* 1972, *39*(3), 512.

Goldstein, H. S., & Gershansky, I. Psychological differentiation in clinic children. *Perceptual and Motor Skills,* 1976, *42,* 1159–1162.

Goldstein, H. S., & Peck, R. Maternal differentiation, father absence and cognitive differentiation in children. *Archives of General Psychiatry,* September 1973, *29,* 370–373.

Goldstein, J., Freud, A., & Solnit, A. J. *Beyond the best interests of the child.* New York: The Free Press, 1973.

Goldstein, M. Z. Fathering—A neglected activity. *American Journal of Psychoanalysis,* 1977, *37*, 325–336.

Gooblar, H. M. Double-bind: Aspects of the communicational style of the father-absent family. *Dissertation Abstracts International,* 1979, *39*(8-B), 4030.

Goodenough, F. *Measurement of intelligence by drawings.* New York: Harcourt, Brace & World, 1926.

Goodnow, J. J. The nature of intelligent behavior: Questions raised by cross-cultural studies. In L. B. Resnick (Ed.), *The nature of intelligence.* Hillsdale, N.J.: Erlbaum, 1976, chap. 9.

Gordon, S. What makes a good father. *Harper's Bazaar,* July 1975, 52; 86.

Gorer, G. *The American people: A study of national character.* New York: Norton, 1948.

Gottfried, A. W., & Brody, N. Interrelationships between and correlates of psychometric and Piagetian scales of sensorimotor intelligence. *Developmental Psychology,* 1975, *11*, 379–387.

Graves, P. L. Infant behavior and maternal attitudes: Early sex differences in West Bengal, India. *Journal of Cross-Cultural Psychology,* 1978, *9*(1), 45–60.

Green, R. Case conference, effeminate behavior in young boys. *Medical Aspects of Human Sexuality,* 1978, *13*(2), 119–120.

Greenacre, P. *The quest for the father.* New York: International Universities Press, 1963.

Greenstein, J. M. Father characteristics and sex typing. *Journal of Personality and Social Psychology,* 1966, *3*(3), 271–277.

Gregory, I. Retrospective data concerning childhood loss of a parent. *Archives of General Psychiatry,* October 1966, *15*, 362–367.

Gregory, I. Studies of parental deprivation in psychiatric patients. *American Journal of Psychiatry,* 1958, *114*, 432–442.

Gross, E. Plus ça change? The sexual structure of occupations over time. *Social Problems,* 1968, *16*, 198–208.

Grossberg, S. H., & Crandall, L. Father loss and father absence in preschool children. *Clinical Social Work Journal,* 1978, *6*(2), 123–134.

Grygier, T., Chesley, J., & Tutters, E. W. Parental deprivation: A study of delinquent children. *British Journal of Criminology,* July 1969, *9*(3), 209–253.

Gutman, H. G. *The black family in slavery and freedom: 1750–1925.* New York: Pantheon Books, 1976.

Hacker, A. Divorce a la mode. *New York Review of Books,* May 8, 1979, *26*(7), 23–27.

Hahn, J. *Random reflections on the squire of Derrymore, matrifocal families, and other trivia.* Unpublished paper, University of Florida, 1972.

Hainline, L., & Feig, E.   The correlates of childhood father absence in college age women. *Child Development,* 1978, *49*(1), 37–42.

Hall, J. A., & Halberstadt, A. G.   Masculinity and femininity in children: Development of the Children's Personal Attributes Questionnaire. *Developmental Psychology,* 1980, *16*, 270–280.

Hamilton, M.   *Father's influence on children.* Chicago: Nelson-Hall, 1977.

Harris, D. B.   *Children's drawings as measures of intellectual maturity: A revision and extension of the Goodenough Draw-a-Man Test.* New York: Harcourt Brace Jovanovich, 1963.

Harris, J.   *The working mother: The effect upon home and family.* Paper presented at the meeting of the Occupational Health Session of the Health Congress, Eastbourne, April 1970.

Hartley, Ruth E.   Children's concepts of male and female roles. *Merrill-Palmer Quarterly,* 1960, *6*, 83–91.

Hathaway, S. R., & Monachesi, E. D.   *Adolescent personality and behavior.* Minneapolis: University of Minnesota Press, 1963.

Haworth, M. R.   Parental loss in children as reflected in projective responses. *Journal of Projective Techniques and Personality Assessment,* 1964, *28,* 31–45.

Heacock, D. R., & Seale, C.   *Presence or absence of the father and its significance in adolescent boys admitted to a general psychiatric hospital.* Paper presented at the 45th annual meeting of the American Orthopsychiatric Association, Chicago, March 1968.

Heckel, R. V.   The effects of fatherlessness on the preadolescent female. *Mental Hygiene,* 1963, *47*, 69–73.

Heckscher, B. T.   Household structure and achievement orientation in lower-class Barbadian families. *Journal of Marriage and the Family,* 1967, *29*, 521–526.

Heilbrun, A. B.   An empirical test of the modeling theory of sex-role learning. *Child Development,* 1965, *36*, 789–799.

Heilbrun, A. B.   Perceived maternal child rearing experience and the effects of vicarious and direct reinforcement on males. *Child Development,* 1970, *41*, 253–262.

Heilbrun, A. B., & Norbert, N.   Sensitivity to maternal censure in paranoid and nonparanoid schizophrenics. *Journal of Nervous and Mental Disease,* 1971, *152*(1), 45–49.

Heilbrun, A. R.   Maternal child rearing and creativity in sons. *Journal of Genetic Psychology,* 1971, *119*, 175–179.

Helper, M. H.   Learning theory and sex concept. *Journal of Abnormal Social Psychology,* 1955, *51*, 184–194.

Henderson, E. H., & Long, B. H.   Academic expectancies of black and white teachers for black and white first graders. *Proceedings of the 81st annual con-*

vention of the American Psychological Association, 1973, *8,* 685–686 (Summary).

Henderson, J. On fathering (The nature and functions of the father role). *Canadian Journal of Psychiatry,* 1980, *25,* 403–427.

Hendricks, L. E., Howard, C. S., & Caesar, P. P. Help-seeking behavior among select populations of black unmarried adolescent fathers: Implications for human service agencies. *American Journal of Public Health,* 1981, *71*(7), 733–739.

Herzog, E. Families out of wedlock (Chap. 7). In O. Pollack & A. S. Friedman (Eds.), *Family dynamics and female sexual delinquency.* Palo Alto: Science & Behavior Books, Inc., 1969.

Herzog, E., & Lewis, H. Children in poor families: Myths and realities. *American Journal of Orthopsychiatry,* April 1970, *40*(3), 375–387.

Herzog, E., & Sudia, C. E. Children in fatherless families. In B. M. Caldwell & H. N. Ricciuti (Eds.), *Review of child development research* (Vol. 3). *Child development and social policy.* Chicago: The University of Chicago Press, 1970.

Herzog, E., & Sudia, C. E. Fatherless homes: A review of research. *Children,* September/October 1968, *15*(5), 177–182.

Herzog, J. D. Father-absence and boys' school performance in Barbados. *Human Organization,* Spring 1974, *33*(1), 71–83.

Herzog, J. M. Sleep disturbance and father-hunger in 18- to 28-month-old boys: The Erlkönig syndrome. *Psychoanalytic Study of the Child,* 1980, *35,* 219–233.

Hetherington, E. M. A developmental study of the effects of sex of the dominant parent on sex-role preference, identification, and imitation in children. *Journal of Personality and Social Psychology,* 1965, *2*(2), 188–194.

Hetherington, E. M. Effects of father absence on personality development in adolescent daughters. *Developmental Psychology,* 1972, *7,* 313–326.

Hetherington, E. M. Effects of paternal absence on sex-typed behaviors in Negro and white preadolescent males. *Journal of Personality and Social Psychology,* 1966, *4*(1), 87–91.

Hetherington, E. M. Girls without fathers. *Psychology Today.* February 1973, 47–52.

Hetherington, E. M., Cox, M., & Cox, R. The development of children in mother-headed families. In D. Reiss & H. Hoffman (Eds.), *The American family: Dying or developing?* New York: Plenum Press, 1979.

Hetherington, E. M., Stouwie, R. J., & Ridberg, E. H. Patterns of family interaction and child-rearing attitudes related to three dimensions of juvenile delinquency. *Journal of Abnormal Psychology,* 1971, *78*(2), 160–176.

Hill, O. W., & Price, J. S. Childhood bereavement and adult depression. *British Journal of Psychiatry,* 1967, *113,* 743–751.

Hillenbrand, E. D. Father absence in military families. *Family Coordinator,* October 1976, 451–458.

Hisop, I. G. Childhood deprivation: An antecedent of the irritable bowel syndrome. *Medical Journal of Australia,* 1979, *1,* 372–374.

Hoffman, M. L. Father absence and conscience development. In F. Rebelsky & L. Dorman (Eds.), *Child development and behavior.* New York: Alfred A. Knopf, 1973.

Hogbin, H. I. A New Guinea childhood: From weaning till the eighth year in Wogeo. *Oceania,* June 1946, *16,* 275–296.

Hogkiss, M. The influence of broken homes and working mothers. *Smith College Studies in Social Work, III,* March 1933, 259–274.

Hollingshead, A. B., & Redlich, F. C. Social stratification and schizophrenia. *American Sociological Review,* 1954, *19,* 302–306.

Hollingshead, A. B., & Redlich, F. C. *Social class and mental illness.* New York: John Wiley & Sons, 1958.

Holman, P. Some factors in the etiology of maladjustment in children. *Journal of Mental Science,* 1953, *99,* 654–688.

Hopkinson, G., & Reed, G. F. Bereavement in childhood and depressive psychosis. *British Journal of Psychiatry,* 1966, *112,* 459–469.

Horn, J. L. Human abilities: A review of research and theory in the early 1970s. *Annual Review of Psychology,* 1976, *27,* 437–485.

Horne, A. M. Aggressive behavior in normal and deviant members of intact versus mother-only families. *Journal of Abnormal Child Psychology,* 1981, *9*(2), 283–290.

Houston, S. Father-absence and the development of sex role. *Australian Journal of Social Issues,* 1973, *8*(3), 209–216.

Howells, J. G. Child-parent separation as a therapeutic procedure. *American Journal of Psychiatry,* 1963, *119,* 922–928.

Howells, J. G. Fallacies in child care: 1. That "separation" is synonymous with "deprivation." *Acta Paedopsychiatrica,* 1970, *37.1,* 3–14.

Howells, J. G., & Layng, J. Child-parent separation: Its causes, and care of the child during separation. *Medical Officer,* 1956b, *96,* 269–271.

Howells, J. G., & Layng, J. Separation experiences and mental health: A statistical study. *Lancet,* August 6, 1955, 285–288.

Howells, J. G., & Layng, J. The effect of separation experiences on children given care away from home. *Medical Officer,* 1956a, *95,* 345–352.

Hunt, J. G., & Hunt, L. L. Race, daughters and father loss: Does absence make the girl stronger? *Social Problems,* 1977, *25,* 90–102.

Hunt, J. McV., & Kirk, G. E. Criterion-referenced tests of school readiness: A paradigm with illustrations. *Genetic Psychology Monographs,* 1974, *90,* 143–182.

Hunt, J. McV. The utility of ordinal scales inspired by Piaget's observations. *Merrill-Palmer Quarterly*, 1976, *22*, 31–45.

Hunt, L. L., & Hunt, J. G. Race and the father-son connection: The conditional relevance of father absence for the orientations and identities of adolescent boys. *Social Problems*, October 1975, *23*(1), 35–52.

Huttunen, M. O., & Niskanen, P. Prenatal loss of father and psychiatric disorders. *Archives of General Psychiatry*, April 1978, *35*, 429–431.

Hylton, L. Trends in adoption, 1958–1962. *Child Welfare*, July 1965, 377–386.

Hyman, H. H., & Reed, J. S. "Black matriarchy" reconsidered: Evidence from secondary analysis of sample surveys. *Public Opinion Quarterly*, 1969, *33*(3), 346–354.

Ilgenfritz, M. P. Mothers on their own—widows and divorcees. *Journal of Marriage and the Family*, 1961, *23*(1), 38–41.

Illsley, R., & Thompson, B. Women from broken homes. *Social Review*, 1961, *9*(1), 27–54.

Information Please Almanac, 1983. 37th Edition. New York: A & W Publishers, 1982.

Jackson, D. N., & Paunonen, S. V. Personality structure and assessment. *Annual Review of Psychology*, 1980, *31*, 503–551.

Jackson, R. M., & Meara, N. M. Father identification, achievement and occupational behavior of rural youth: 5-year follow-up. *Journal of Vocational Behavior*, 1977, *10*, 82–91.

Jacobson, E. The return of the lost parent. *Canadian Psychiatric Association Journal*, 1966, *11*, S259–S266.

Jenkins, R. L. The varieties of children's behavior problems and family dynamics. *American Journal of Psychiatry*, April 1968, *124*(10), 1440–1445.

Jenkins, R. L., & Boyer, A. Effects of inadequate mothering and inadequate fathering on children. *International Journal of Social Psychiatry*, Winter 1969, *16*, 72–78.

Jenkins, S. Divorce. *Children Today*, March/April 1978, 17–20; 48.

Jensen, A. R. How much can we boost IQ and scholastic achievement? *Harvard Educational Review*, 1969, *39*, 11–23.

Johnson, B. L. Marital and family characteristics of workers, 1970–78. *Monthly Labor Review*, April 1979, 49.

Johnson, M. M. Sex role learning in the nuclear family. *Child Development*, 1963, *34*, 319–333.

Josselyn, I. M. Cultural forces: Motherliness and fatherliness. *American Journal of Orthopsychiatry*, 1956, *26*, 264–271.

Jung, C. G. *Man and his symbols.* New York: Dell/Laurel, 1968.

Jung, C. G. [*Memories, dreams, reflections*] (A. Jaffee, Ed.). New York: Random House, 1965.

Kagan, J.   The child in the family. *Daedalus,* Spring 1977, *106*(2), 33–56.

Kagel, M. A., White, R. M., & Coyne, J. C.   Father-absent and father-present families of disturbed and nondisturbed adolescents. *American Journal of Orthopsychiatry,* April 1978, *48*(2), 342–352.

Kamerman, S. B., & Kahn, A. J.   *Family policy.* New York: Columbia University Press, 1978.

Kanzer, M.   Writers and the early loss of parents. *Journal of Hillside Hospital,* 1953, *11,* 148–151.

Kaplan, H. B.   Self-derogation and childhood family structure: Family size, birth order, and sex distribution. *Journal of Nervous and Mental Disease,* 1970, *151* (1), 13–23.

Kardiner, A., & Ovesey, L.   *The mark of oppression.* Cleveland: World Publishing Co., 1962.

Katz, M. M., & Konner, M. J.   The role of the father: An anthropological perspective. In Lamb, M. E. (Ed.), *The role of the father in child development,* Second Edition, 155–185. New York: Wiley, 1981.

Kauffman, J. M.   Family relations test responses of disturbed and normal boys: Additional comparative data. *Journal of Personality Assessment,* April 1971, *35,* 128–138.

Kaufman, A. S.   The relationship of WPPSI IQs to SES and other background variables. *Journal of Clinical Psychology,* 1973, *29,* 354–357.

Kearney, H. R.   Feminist challenges to the social structure and sex roles. *Psychology of Women Quarterly,* 1979, *4*(1), 16–31.

Keeler, W. R.   Children's reaction to the death of a parent. In P. H. Hoch & J. Zubin (Eds.), *Depression.* New York: Grune & Stratton, 1954.

Kellam, S. G., Branch, J., Brown, C. H., & Russell, G.   *Why teenagers come for treatment: A ten-year prospective study in Woodlawn.* Paper presented at the meeting of the American Psychiatric Association, Chicago, May 1979.

Kellam, S. G., Ensminger, M. E., & Turner, R. J.   Family structure and the mental health of children. *Archives of General Psychiatry,* September 1977, *34,* 1012–1022.

Keller, P. A., & Murray, E. J.   Imitative aggression with adult male and female models in father present Negro boys. *Journal of Genetic Psychology,* 1973, *122,* 217–221.

Kelly, J. A., & Worell, J.   New formulations of sex roles and androgyny: A critical review. *Journal of Consulting and Clinical Psychology,* 1977, *45,* 1101–1115.

Kelly, J. B., & Wallerstein, J. S.   The effects of parental divorce: Experiences of the child in early latency. *American Journal of Orthopsychiatry,* January 1976, *46*(1), 20–32.

Kemper, T. D., & Reichler, M. L.   Father's work integration and types of frequency of rewards and punishments administered by fathers and mothers in adolescent sons and daughters. *Journal of Genetic Psychology,* 1976, *129,* 207–219.

Kestenbaum, C. J., & Bird, H. R.   A reliability study of the Mental Health Assessment Form for school-age children. *Journal of the American Academy of Child Psychiatry, 17*(2), 1978, 338–355.

Kestenbaum, C. J., & Stone, M. H.   The effects of fatherless homes upon daughters: Clinical impressions regarding paternal deprivation. *Journal of the American Academy of Psychoanalysis,* 1976, *4*(2), 171–190.

Kety, S. S., Rosenthal, D., Wender, P. H., & Schulsinger, F.   Mental illness in the biological and adoptive families of adopted schizophrenics. *American Journal of Psychiatry,* September 1971, *128*(3), 302–306.

King, K.   Adolescent perception of power structure in the Negro family. *Journal of Marriage and the Family,* November 1969, *31*(4), 751–755.

Klein, C.   *The single parent experience.* New York: Avon Books, 1973.

Kluckhohn, C.   *Mirror for man.* New York: McGraw-Hill, 1949.

Koch, H. L.   Attitudes of children toward their peers as related to certain characteristics of their siblings. *Psychological Monographs,* 1956, *70*(19, Whole No. 326).

Koch, H. L.   Sissiness and tomboyishness in relation to sibling characteristics. *Journal of Genetic Psychology,* 1956, *88,* 231–244.

Koch, H. L.   The relation of certain family constellation characteristics and the attitudes of children toward adults. *Child Development,* 1955, *52,* 3–50.

Koch, H. L.   The relation of primary mental abilities in five- and six-year olds to sex of child and characteristics of his siblings. *Child Development,* 1954, *25,* 210–223.

Koch, M. B.   Anxiety in preschool children from broken homes. *Merrill-Palmer Quarterly,* 1961, *7*(4), 225–231.

Kogelschatz, J., Adams, P. L., & Tucker, D. McK.   Family styles of fatherless households. *Journal of the American Academy of Child Psychiatry,* 1972, *11*(2), 365–383.

Kohlberg, L.   The development of moral stages: Uses and abuses. *Proceedings, 1973 Invitational Conference on Testing Problems, Educational Testing Service,* 1974, 1–8.

Kohlberg, L.   A cognitive–developmental analysis of the children's sex-role concept and attitudes. In E. Maccoby (Ed.), *The development of sex differences.* Stanford: Stanford University Press, 1968.

Kohlberg, L., & Zigler, E.   The impact of cognitive maturity on the development of sex-role attitudes in the years 4–8. *Genetic Psychological Monographs,* 1967, *75,* 84–165.

Kohn, M., & Carroll, E. E.   Social class and the allocation of parental responsibilities. *Sociometry,* December 1960, 389.

Koller, K. M.   Parental deprivation, family background and female delinquency. *British Journal of Psychiatry,* 1971, *118,* 319–327.

Koller, K. M., & Castanos, J. N.   Family background in prison groups: A comparative study of parental deprivation. *British Journal of Psychiatry,* 1970, *117,* 371–380.

Koller, K. M., & Williams, W. T.   Early parental deprivation and later behavioural outcomes: Cluster analysis study of normal and abnormal groups. *Australian and New Zealand Journal of Psychiatry,* 1974, *8,* 89–96.

Kolvin, I., Garside, R. F., & Kidd, J. S. H.   IV. Parental personality and attitude and childhood psychoses. *British Journal of Psychiatry,* 1971b, *110,* 402–406.

Kolvin, I., Ounsted, C., Richardson, L. M., & Garside, R. F.   III. The family and social background in childhood psychoses. *British Journal of Psychiatry,* 1971a, *118,* 396–402.

Kopf, D. E.   Family variables and school adjustment of eighth-grade father-absent boys. *Family Coordinator,* 1970, *19*(2), 145–150.

Kraft, I. A.   Group therapy with children and adolescents. In Sholevar, G. P., Benson, R. M., & Blinder, B. J. (Eds.), *Emotional Disorders in Children and Adolescents: Medical and Psychological Approaches to Treatment.* New York: Spectrum, 1980.

Krammer, S., & Prall, R.   The role of the father in the preoedipal years. *American Psychoanalytic Association Journal,* 1978, *26*(1), 143–161.

Kravitz, H., Trossman, B., & Feldman, R. B.   Unwed mothers: Practical and theoretical considerations. *Canadian Psychiatric Association Journal,* December 1966, *11*(6), 456–464.

LaBarre, M., Jessner, L., & Ussery, L.   The significance of grandmothers in the pathology of children. *American Journal of Orthopsychiatry,* 1960, *30,* 175–185.

LaBarre, W.   *The human animal.* Chicago: The University of Chicago Press, 1954.

Lamb, M. E.   Interactions between eight-month-old children and their fathers and mothers. In M. E. Lamb (Ed.), *The role of the father in child development.* New York: John Wiley & Sons, 1976b.

Lamb, M. E.   The role of the father: An overview. In M. E. Lamb (Ed.), *The role of the father in child development.* New York: John Wiley & Sons, 1976a.

Lamb, M. E. (Ed.).   *The role of the father in child development.* New York: John Wiley & Sons, 1976c.

Lancet.   Parental deprivation and mental health. London, August 6, 1966.

Land, H., & Parker, R.   United Kingdom. In S. B. Kamerman & A. J. Kahn (Eds.), *Family Policy.* New York: Columbia University Press, 1978.

Landis, J. T.   A comparison of children from divorced and nondivorced unhappy marriages. *Family Life Coordinator,* 1962, *11*(3), 61–65.

Landis, J. T.   The trauma of children when parents divorce. *Marriage and Family Living,* 1960, *22*(1), 7–13.

Landy, F., Rosenberg, B. G., & Sutton-Smith, B.   The effect of limited father absence on cognitive development. *Child Development,* 1969, *40,* 941–944.

Lang, D. M., Papenfuhs, R., & Walters, J.   Delinquent females' perceptions of their fathers. *Family Coordinator,* October 1976, 475–481.

Langer, T.   Broken homes and mental disorder. *Public Health Reports,* November 1963, *78*(11), 921–926.

Langer, T. S., Gersten, J. D., et al.   A screening inventory for assessing psychiatric impairment in children 6 to 8. *Journal of Consulting and Clinical Psychology,* 1976, *44,* 286–296.

Laosa, L. M., Swartz, J. D., & Diaz-Guerrero, R.   Perceptual-cognitive and personality development of Mexican and Anglo-American children as measured by human figure drawings. *Developmental Psychology,* 1974, *10,* 131–139.

Lasch, C.   *The culture of narcissism: American life in an age of diminishing expectations.* New York: W. W. Norton & Co., 1979.

Layman, E. M.   Discussion. Symposium: Father influence in the family. *Merrill-Palmer Quarterly,* 1961, *7,* 107–111.

Lecorgne, L. L., & Laosa, L. M.   Father absence in low-income Mexican-American families: Children's social adjustment and conceptual differentiation of sex role attributes. *Developmental Psychology,* 1976, *12*(5), 470–471.

Leichty, M. M.   The effect of father-absence during early childhood upon the oedipal situation as reflected in young adults. *Merrill-Palmer Quarterly,* 1960, *6,* 212–217.

Leik, R. K.   Instrumentality and emotionality in family interaction. *Sociometry,* 1963, *26,* 131–145.

Leiter, R. G.   *Leiter International Performance Scale.* Chicago: C. H. Stoelting Co., 1948.

LeMasters, E. E.   The passing of the dominant husband-father. In H. P. Dreitzel (Ed.), *Family, marriage, and the struggle of the sexes.* New York: Macmillan, 1972.

Leonard, S. W.   How first-time fathers feel toward their newborns. *The American Journal of Maternal Child Nursing,* November/December 1976, 361–365.

Lerner, S. H.   Effects of dissertion on family life. *Social Casework,* 1954, *35,* 3–8.

Lessing, E. E., Zagorin, S. W., & Nelson, D.   WISC subtest and IQ score correlates of father absence. *Journal of Genetic Psychology,* December 1970, *117*(2), 181–195.

Levine, C.   When father's a traveling man. *Parents Magazine,* 1977, *42,* 54; 75–76.

Levy, D. M.   *Maternal overprotection: Treatment, prognosis, psychopathology* (Vol. IX). New York: Columbia University Press, 1943.

Levy-Shiff, R.   The effects of father absence on young children in mother-headed families. *Child Development,* 1982, *53,* 1400–1405.

Lewin, P.   *Home and self-concept factors related to differential academic achievement of teenagers in one-parent, father-absent families from two social classes.* Unpublished doctoral dissertation, Cornell University, 1969.

Lidz, T., Cornelison, A. R., Fleck, S., & Terry, D.   The intrafamilial environment of schizophrenic patients: II. Marital schism and marital skew. *American Journal of Psychiatry,* 1954, *114,* 241–248.

Lidz, T., Fleck, S., Cornelison, A., & Terry, D. The intrafamilial environment of the schizophrenic patients: IV. Parental personalities and family interaction. *American Journal of Orthopsychiatry*, 1958, *28*, 764–776.

Lidz, T., Parker, B., & Cornelison, A. The role of the father in the family environment of the schizophrenic patient. *American Journal of Orthopsychiatry*, 1956, *26*, 126–132.

Liebow, E. Attitudes toward marriage and family among black males in Tally's corner. *Milbank Memorial Fund Quarterly*, April 1970, *38*(2), 151–180.

Liebow, E. *Tally's corner: A study of Negro streetcorner men.* Boston: Little Brown and Co., 1967.

Lifshitz, M. Long range effects of father's loss: The cognitive complexity of bereaved children and their school adjustment. *British Journal of Medical Psychology*, 1976, *49*, 189–197.

Liljeström, R. Sweden. In S. B. Kamerman & A. J. Kahn (Eds.), *Family policy*. New York: Columbia University Press, 1978.

Llorens, L. A. Black culture and child development. *American Journal of Occupational Therapy*, 1971, *25*(3), 144–148.

Loeb, J. The personality factor in divorce. *Journal of Consulting Psychology*, 1966, *30*(6), 562.

Longarbaugh, R. Mother behavior as a variable moderating the effects of father absence. *Ethos*, 1975, *40*, 456–465.

Lott, B. Who wants the children? *American Psychologist*, July 1973, 573–582.

Louisville *Courier-Journal & Times.* U.S. agency says 20% of children now live in one-parent households, August 9, 1982.

Lourie, R. S. Personality development and the genesis of neurosis. *Clinical Proceedings of Children's Hospital*, Washington, D.C., June 1967, *23*(6), 167–182.

Lourie, R. S. The first three years of life: An overview of a new frontier of psychiatry. *The American Journal of Psychiatry*, May 1971, *127*(71), 1457–1463.

Lowery, D. W. Classroom dependency and modeling behavior of father-absent and father-present pre-school boys with a male teacher. *Dissertation Abstracts International*, 1978, *39*(2-A), 759.

Luepnitz, D. A. Children of divorce. *Law and Human Behavior*, 1978, 2(2), 167–179.

Lynn, D. B. Fathers and sex-role development. *The Family Coordinator*, October 1976, 403–409.

Lynn, D. B. *The father: His role in child development.* Belmont, CA: Wadsworth Publishing Co., 1974.

Lynn, D. B., & Sawrey, W. L. The effects of father absence on Norwegian boys and girls. *Journal of Abnormal and Social Psychology*, 1964, *69*, 258–262.

Maccoby, E. E., & Jacklin, C. N. *The psychology of sex differences.* Stanford: Stanford University Press, 1974.

Macdonald, M. W.   Criminally aggressive behavior in passive, effeminate boys. *American Journal of Orthopsychiatry,* 1938, *8,* 70–78.

Machover, K.   *Personality projection in the drawing of the human figure: A method of personality investigation.* Springfield, Ill.: Charles C. Thomas, 1949.

Mackie, J. B., Lloyd, D. N., & Rafferty, F.   The father's influence on the intellectual level of black ghetto children. *American Journal of Public Health,* June 1974, *64*(6), 615–616.

Madow, L., & Hardy, S. E.   Incidence and analysis of the broken family in the background of neurosis. *American Journal of Orthopsychiatry,* 1947, *17,* 521–528.

Mahler, M. S., & Goslinger, R. J.   On symbiotic child psychosis: Genetic, dynamic and restitutive aspects. *Psychoanalytic Study of the Child,* 1955, *10,* 195–212.

Mallan, L. B.   Young widows and their children: A comparative report. *Social Security Bulletin.* Washington, D.C.: U.S. Government Printing Office, May 1975.

Malone, C. A.   Some observations on children of disorganized families and problems of acting out. *Journal of the American Academy of Child Psychiatry,* 1963, *2,* 22–39.

Marsella, A. J., Dubanoski, R. A., & Mohs, K.   The effects of father presence and absence upon maternal attitudes. *Journal of Genetic Psychology,* 1974, *125,* 257–263.

Martin, C. D.   Psychological problems of abortion for unwed teenage girls. *Genetic Psychology Monographs,* 1973, *88,* 23–110.

Martindale, C.   Father's absence, psychopathology, and poetic eminence. *Psychological Reports,* 1972, *31,* 843–847.

Masters, W. H., & Johnson, V.   *Homosexuality in perspective.* Boston: Little, Brown & Co., 1979.

Matarazzo, J. D.   *Wechsler's measurement and appraisal of adult intelligence* (5th Ed.). Baltimore: Williams & Wilkins, 1972.

Matarazzo, Joseph D., & Weins, Arthur N.   Black intelligence test of cultural homogeneity & Wechsler Adult Intelligence Scale scores of black and white police applicants. *Journal of Applied Psychology,* 1977, *62*(1), 57–63.

Maxwell, A. E.   Discrepancies between the pattern of abilities for normal and neurotic children. *British Journal of Psychiatry,* 1961, *107,* 300–307.

McClelland, D. C., & Watt, N. F.   Sex-role alienation in schizophrenia. *Journal of Abnormal Psychology,* 1968, *73*(3), 226–239.

McCord, J., McCord, W., & Thurber, E.   Effects of maternal employment on lower-class boys. *Journal of Abnormal and Social Psychology,* 1963, *67*(2), 177–182.

McCorkle, L., Elias, A., & Bixby, F. L.   *The Highfields story: An experimental project for youthful offenders.* New York: Holt, Rinehart & Winston, 1968.

McCubbin, H. I., Dahl, B. B., Lester, G. R., Benson, D., & Robertson, M. L.   Coping repertoires of families adapting to prolonged war-induced separations. *Journal of Marriage and the Family,* August 1976, 461–471.

McDermott, J. F.   Divorce and its psychiatric sequelae in children. *Archives of General Psychiatry,* November 1970, *23,* 421–427.

McDermott, J. F.   Parental divorce in early childhood. *American Journal of Psychiatry,* April 1968, *124*(10), 1424–1432.

McKay, M. J., & Richardson, H.   Personality differences between one-time and recidivist unwed mothers. *Journal of Genetic Psychology,* 1973, *122,* 207–210.

Mead, M.   *Sex and temperament.* New York: William Morrow & Co., 1935.

Mead, S. L., & Rekers, G. A.   Role of the father in normal psychosexual development. *Psychological Reports,* 1979, *45,* 923–931.

Medico-Legal Society. Notes of proceedings of an extra meeting of the society held at the royal society of medicine. *Medico-Legal Journal,* 1969, *37,* 23–37.

Meerloo, J. A. M.   The psychological role of the father: The father cuts the cord. *Child and Family,* Spring 1968, 102–116.

Meiss, M.   The oedipal problem of a fatherless child. *Psychoanalytic Study of the Child,* 1952, *7,* 216–229.

Messer, A. A.   The "Phaedra complex." *Archives of General Psychiatry,* August 1969, *21,* 213–218.

Miller, L. C.   School behavior checklist: An inventory of deviant behavior for elementary school children. *Journal of Consulting and Clinical Psychology,* 1972, *22,* 134–144.

Miller, L.   Louisville behavior checklist for males 6–12 years of age. *Psychological Reports 21,* 1967, 285–296.

Millen, L., & Roll, S.   Relationships between sons' feelings of being understood by their fathers and measures of the sons' psychological functioning. *Journal of Genetic Psychology,* 1977, *130,* 10–25.

Miller, R.   The development of competence and behaviour in infancy. [Doctoral dissertation, University of the Witwatersrand (South Africa), 1977.] *Dissertation Abstracts International,* 1977, *38*(10-B), 5066B.

Miller, S. M.   Guest editorial. *Social Policy,* March/April 1980, 2–3.

Miller, W. B.   Lower class culture as a generating milieu of gang delinquency. *Journal of Social Issues,* 1958, *14*(3), 5–19.

Minuchin, S., Montalvo, B., Guerney, B. G., Rosman, B., & Schumer, F.   *Families of the slums.* New York: Basic Books, 1967.

Mischel, W.   Delay of gratification, need for achievement, and acquiescence in another culture. *Journal of Abnormal and Social Psychology,* 1961, *62*(3), 543–552.

Mischel, W.   Preference for delayed reinforcement: An experimental study of a cultural observation. *Journal of Abnormal and Social Psychology,* 1958, *56,* 57–61.

Mischel, W.   Sex-typing and socialization. In P. Mussen (Ed.), *Manual of child psychology.* New York: John Wiley & Sons, 1970.

Mitchell, D., & Wilson, W.   Relationship of father absence to masculinity and popularity of delinquent boys. *Psychological Reports,* 1967, *20,* 1173–1174.

Moerk, E. L.   Like father like son: Imprisonment of fathers and the psychological adjustment of sons. *Journal of Youth and Adolescence,* 1973, *2*(4), 303–312.

Moffitt, T. E.   Vocabulary and arithmetic performance of father-absent boys. *Child Study Journal,* 1981, *10*(4), 233–241.

Monahan, T. P.   Broken homes by age of delinquent children. *Journal of Social Psychology,* 1960, *51,* 387–397.

Monahan, T. P.   Family status and the delinquent child: A reappraisal and some new findings. *Social Forces,* 1957, *35,* 250–258.

Mondale, W. F.   Introducing a special report: The family in trouble. *Psychology Today,* May 1977, 39.

Money, J., & Erhardt, A. A.   *Man and woman, boy and girl: The differentiation and dimorphis of gender identity from conception to maturity.* Baltimore: Johns Hopkins University Press, 1972.

Montagu, A.   *Natural superiority of women* (rev. ed.). New York: Macmillan, 1968.

Montare, A., & Boone, S. L.   Agression and paternal absence: Racial-ethnic differences among inner-city boys. *Journal of Genetic Psychology,* 1980, *137,* 223–232.

Morris, L.   Estimating the need for family planning services among unwed teenagers. *Family Planning Perspectives,* Spring 1974, *6*(2), 91–97.

Moss, H. A.   Sex, age and state as determinants of mother-infant interaction. *Merrill-Palmer Quarterly,* 1967, *13,* 19–36.

Moss, P., & Pleuris, I.   *Mental distress in mothers of pre-school children in inner London.* Undated paper from the Thomas Coram Research Unit, University of London.

Moulton, R. W., Burnstein, E., Liberty, P. G., & Altucher, N.   Patterning of parental affection and disciplinary dominance as a determinant of guilt and sex typing. *Journal of Personality and Social Psychology,* 1966, *4*(4), 356–363.

Mowrer, O. H.   Identification: A link between learning theory and psychotherapy. In *Learning theory and personality dynamics.* New York: Ronald Press, 1950.

Moynihan, D. P.   *The Negro family: The case for national action* (the Moynihan Report). U.S. Department of Labor, Office of Policy Planning and Research, 1965.

Mumbauer, C. C., & Miller, J. O.   Socio-economic background and cognitive functioning in preschool children. *Child Development,* 1970, *41,* 471–480.

Munro, A.   Childhood parent-loss in a psychiatrically normal population. *British Journal of Preventive Socialized Medicine,* 1965, *19,* 69–79.

Munro, A.   Parental deprivation in depressive patients. *British Journal of Psychiatry*, 1966, *112*, 443–457.

Munro, A., & Griffiths, A. B.   Further data on childhood parent-loss in psychiatric normals. *Acta Psychiatrica Scandinavia*, 1968, *44*(4), 385–400.

Murdock, G. P., & White, D. R.   Standard cross-cultural sample. *Ethnology*, 1969, *8*(4), 329–369.

Murphy, S. A.   *A social worker's view of family policy in the United States.* Unpublished paper, University of Louisville, 1979.

Mussen, P., & Distler, L.   Masculinity, identification and father-son relationships. *Journal of Abnormal Psychology*, November 1960, *59*, 350–356.

Nabokov, V.   *Lolita.* Greenwich, Conn.: C. Fawcett Publications, Inc., 1959.

Naiman, J.   A comparative study of unmarried and married mothers: Preliminary Report. *Canadian Psychiatric Association Journal*, 1966, *11*, 465–469.

Nash, J.   The father in contemporary culture and current psychological literature. *Child Development*, 1965, *36*, 261–297.

National Institute of Mental Health. *Yours, mine, and ours: Tips for stepparents*, DHEW pub. no (ADM) 78-676. Washington, D.C.: U.S. Government Printing Office, 1978.

Nelsen, E. A., & Maccoby, E. E.   The relationship between social development and differential abilities on the scholastic aptitude test. *Merrill-Palmer Quarterly*, 1966, *12*, 269–289.

Nettelbladt, P., Uddenberg, N., & Englesson, I.   Father-child relationship: Background factors in the father. *Acta Psychiatrica Scandinavia*, 1980, *61*, 29–42.

Neubauer, P. B.   The one-parent child and his oedipal development. *Psychoanalytic Study of the Child*, 1960, *15*, 286–309.

Neumann, E.   [On the moon and matriarchal consciousness. In *Dynamic aspects of the psyche*] (H. Nagel, trans.). New York: Analytical Psychology Club, 1956. (Originally published, 1950.)

New study contradicts other research. Louisville *Courier-Journal & Times*. Sunday, June 26, 1983, A-6.

Newman, G., & Denman, S. B.   Felony and paternal deprivation: A sociopsychiatric view. *International Journal of Social Psychiatry*, 1971, *17*(1), 65–71.

Nichol, H.   The death of a parent. *Canadian Psychiatric Association Journal*, 1964, *9*, 263–271.

Nimkoff, M. F., & Middleton, R.   Types of family and types of economy. *American Journal of Sociology*, November 1960, *LXVI*(3), 215–225.

Nye, F. I.   Child adjustment in broken and in unhappy unbroken homes. *Marriage and Family Living*, 1957, *19*(4), 356–361.

Nye, F. I.   *Family relationships and delinquent behavior.* New York: John Wiley & Sons, 1958. (Reprinted 1973 by Greenwood Press, Westport, Connecticut.)

Nye, F. I., Short, J. F., & Olson, V. J.   Part II. Family structure and delinquent behavior. 3. Socio-economic status and delinquent behavior. In F. I. Nye (Ed.),

Family relationships and delinquent behavior. New York: John Wiley & Sons, 1958.

Oates, W. Personal recollection. University of Louisville, 1980.

O'Donoghue, P. D. The role of the father in infant and pre-oedipal development: A review of literature. *Maternal-Child Nursing Journal,* Fall 1978, 7(3), 155–162.

Olds, S. W. When mommy goes to work. In H. E. Fitzgerald & T. H. Carr (Eds.), *Human development 82/83.* Guildford, Connecticut: Dushkin Publishing Group, Inc., 1982.

Oltman, J. E., McGarry, J. J., & Friedman, S. Parental deprivation and the "broken home" in dementia praecox and other mental disorders. *American Journal of Psychiatry,* March 1952, 108(9), 685–694.

Orlofsky, Jacob L. Sex-role orientation. In *Encyclopedia of Clinical Assessment* Vol. 2, Robert Henley Woody (Ed.). San Francisco: Jossey-Bass, 1980, 656–672.

Orshansky, M. The shape of poverty in 1966. *Social Security Bulletin* [Department of Health, Education & Welfare, 31(3)]. Washington, D.C.: U.S. Government Printing Office, March 1968.

Oshman, H. P., & Manosevitz, M. Death fantasies of father-absent and father-present late adolescents. *Journal of Youth and Adolescence,* 1978, 7(1), 41–48.

Oshman, H. P., & Manosevitz, M. Father absence: Effects of stepfathers upon psychosocial development in males. *Developmental Psychology,* 1976, 12(5), 479–480.

Osofsky, H. J., & Osofsky, J. D. Adolescents as mothers: Results of a program for low-income pregnant teenagers with some emphasis upon infants' development. *American Journal of Orthopsychiatry,* October 1970, 40(5), 825–834.

Osofsky, H., Osofsky, J. D., Kendall, N., & Rajan, R. Adolescents as mothers: An interdisciplinary approach to a complex problem. *Journal of Youth and Adolescence,* 1973, 2(3), 223–249.

Ostrovsky, E. S. *Father to the child.* New York: G. P. Putnam, 1959.

Overall, J. K. Associations between marital history and the nature of manifest psychopathology. *Journal of Abnormal Psychology,* 1971, 78(2), 213–221.

Parental deprivation and mental health. *Lancet,* August 6, 1966, 325.

Parish, T. S. The impact of divorce on the family. *Adolescence,* 1981a, 16(63), 577–580.

Parish, T. S. The relationship between years of father absence and locus of control. *Journal of Genetic Psychology,* 1981b, 138, 301–302.

Parish, T. S., & Copeland, T. F. The relationship between self-concepts and evaluations of parents and stepfathers. *Journal of Psychology,* 1979, 101, 135–138.

Parish, T. S. The relationship between factors associated with father loss and delinquency. *Journal of the American Academy of Child Psychiatry,* 1978, 17, 224–238.

Parish, T. S., & Kappes, B. M.   Impact of father loss on the family. *Social Behavior and Personality*, 1980, *8*(1), 107–112.

Parish, T. S., & Nunn, G. D.   Children's self-concepts and evaluations of parents as a function of family structure and process. *Journal of Psychology*, 1981, *107*, 105–108.

Parish, T. S., & Parish, J.   The role of environmental factors in the development of moral judgment. In T. S. Parish (Ed.), *Critical Issues in Human Behavior*, Lexington, Massachusetts: Ginn, 1979.

Parish, T. S., & Taylor, J. C.   The impact of divorce and subsequent father-absence on children's and adolescents' self-concepts. *Journal of Youth and Adolescence*, 1979, *8*(4), 427–432.

Parker, G.   Parental deprivation and depression in a non-clinical group. *Australian and New Zealand Journal of Psychiatry*, 1979, *13*(1), 51–55.

Parker, S., & Kleiner, R. J.   Characteristics of Negro mothers in single-headed households. *Journal of Marriage and the Family*, 1966, *28*, 507–513.

Parker, S., Smith, J., & Ginat, J.   Father absence and cross-sex identity, the puberty rites controversy revisited. *American Ethnologist*, November 1975, *2*(4), 687–706.

Parsons, T., & Bales, R. F.   *Family, socialization, and interaction process*. Glencoe, Ill.: The Free Press, 1955.

Pasamanick, B.   A child is being beaten. *American Journal of Orthopsychiatry*, 1971, *41*(4), 540–556.

Pasamanick, B., & Knobloch, H.   Complications of pregnancy and neuropsychiatric disorder. *Journal of Obstetrics and Gynaecology of the British Empire*, 1959, *66*, 753–755.

Payne, D. E., & Mussen, P. H.   Parent-child relations and father identification among adolescent boys. *Journal of Abnormal and Social Psychology*, 1956, *52*, 358–362.

Pedersen, F. A.   Relationships between father-absence and emotional disturbance in male military dependents. *Merrill-Palmer Quarterly*, 1966, *12*, 321–331.

Pedersen, F., & Robson, K.   Father participation in infancy. *American Journal of Orthopsychiatry*, April 1969, *39*(3), 366–372.

Pedersen, F., Rubenstein, J., & Yarrow, L.   Infant development in father-absent families. *Journal of Genetic Psychology*, 1979, *135*, 51–61.

Person, E., & Ovesey, L.   The transsexual syndrome in males. I. Primary transsexualism. *American Journal of Psychotherapy*, 1974, *28*, 4–20.

Peterson, D. R., Becker, W. C., Hellmer, L. A., Shoemaker, D. J., & Quay, H. C.   Parental attitudes and child adjustment. *Child Development*, 1959. *30*, 119–130.

Peterson, D. R., Quay, H. C., & Cameron, G. C.   Personality and background factors in juvenile delinquency as inferred from questionnaire responses. *Journal of Consulting Psychiatry*, 1959, *23*, 395–399.

Petrullo, L., & Bass, M.　*Leadership and interpersonal behavior.* New York: Holt, Rinehart & Winston, Inc., 1961.

Pettigrew, T. F.　*A profile of the Negro American.* Princeton: D. VanNostrand Company, Inc., 1964.

Petursson, E.　A study of parental deprivation and illness in 291 psychiatric patients. *International Journal of Social Psychiatry,* 1961, *7,* 97–105.

Phelan, H. M.　The incidence and possible significance of the drawing of female figures by sixth-grade boys in response to the Draw-a-Person test. *Psychiatric Quarterly,* 1964, *38,* 488–503.

Phelps, D. W.　Parental attitudes toward family life and child behavior of mothers in two-parent and one-parent families. *Journal of School Health,* 1969, *39,* 413–416.

Philadelphia County Board of Assistance. *A Report on dependent children families: Annual report.* Philadelphia: Author, 1963.

Pienciak, R.　Sexual, racial bias still pervades business, study says. Louisville *Courier-Journal & Times,* Sunday, January 21, 1980, A-16.

Pietropinto, A., & Simenaur, J.　Husbands and wives: A nation-wide survey of marriage (reviewed by Andrew Hacker in Divorce a la mode). *New York Review of Books,* May 3, 1979, *26*(7), 23–27.

Pincus, L., & Dare, C.　*Secrets in the family.* New York: Pantheon Books, 1978.

Pitts, F. N., Meyer, J., Brooks, M., & Winokur, G.　Adult psychiatric illness assessed for childhood parental loss, and psychiatric illness in family members—a study of 748 patients and 250 controls. *American Journal of Psychiatry,* June 1965, *12*(Suppl.), i–x.

Piven, F. F., & Cloward, R. A.　*Regulating the poor: The functions of public welfare.* New York: Pantheon Books, 1971.

Plateris, A.　*Children of divorced couples: United States* (National Center for Health Statistics, Series 21, No. 18). Washington, D.C.: U.S. Government Printing Office, 1970.

Platt, R.　The myth and reality of the "matriarch": A case report in family therapy. *Psychoanalytic Review,* 1970, *57,* 203–223.

Polier, J. W.　External and internal roadblocks to effective child advocacy. *Child Welfare,* 1977, *56,* 497–508.

Pollack, O.　Family structure: Its implications for mental health (Chap. 3). In O. Pollack & A. S. Friedman (Eds.), *Family dynamics and female sexual delinquency.* Palo Alto: Science and Behavior Books, Inc., 1969.

Pollack, O., & Friedman, A. S.　*Family dynamics and female sexual delinquency.* Palo Alto: Science and Behavior Books, Inc., 1969.

Pollack, S.　Child of divorce. *Mademoiselle,* May 1968, *67,* 172; 215–219.

Pope, H.　Negro-white differences in decisions regarding illegitimate children. *Journal of Marriage and the Family,* November 1969, *31*(4), 756–764.

Popplewell, J. W., & Sheikh, A. A.   The role of the father in child development: A review of the literature. *International Journal of Social Psychology*, 1978, *25*, 267–284.

Powdermaker, H.   *Life in Lesu.* New York: W. W. Norton Co., 1933.

Poznanski, E., Maxey, A., & Marsden, G.   Clinical implications of maternal employment: A review of research. *Journal of the American Academy of Child Psychiatry*, October 1970, *9*(4), 741–761.

Profile of broken families. *Statistical bulletin of the metropolitan life insurance company*, December 1970, *51*, 8–9.

Proshansky, H., & Newton, P.   The nature and meaning of Negro self-identity (Chap. 5). In M. Deutsch, I. Katz, & A. R. Jensen (Eds.), *Social class, race, and psychological development.* New York: Holt, Rinehart & Winston, 1968.

Rabban, M.   Sex-role identification in young children in two diverse social groups. *Genetic Psychology Monographs*, 1950, *42*, 81–158.

Rabin, A. I.   Some psychosexual differences between kibbutz and non-kibbutz Israeli boys. *Journal of Projective Techniques*, 1958, *22*, 328–332.

Rachman, A. W.   The role of "fathering" in group psychotherapy with adolescent delinquent males. *Corrective and Social Psychiatry*, 1974, *20*(4), 11–22.

Rank, O.   The trauma of human birth and its importance for psychoanalytic therapy. *Psychoanalytic Review*, July 1924, *11*(3), 241–245.

Raskin, A., Crook, T., & Herman, K.   Psychiatric history and symptom differences in black and white depressed inpatients. *Journal of Counseling and Clinical Psychology*, 1975, *43*(1), 73–80.

Ratcliffe, Kevin J., & Ratcliffe, Melanie W.   The Leiter Scales: A review of validity findings. *American Annals of the Deaf*, 1979, *124*(1), 38–44.

Rebelsky, F.   Infancy in two cultures. *Nederlands Tijaschrift voor de psychologie*, 1967, *22*, 379–385.

Rebelsky, F., & Hanks, C.   Fathers' verbal interaction with infants in the first three months of life. *Child Development*, 1971, *42*, 63–68.

Reiber, V.   Is the nurturing role natural to fathers? *American Journal of Maternal Child Nursing*, December 1976, 366–371.

Reinhold, R.   Marriage-go-round: Study shows dramatic climb in divorces. Louisville *Courier-Journal & Times*, Sunday, July 8, 1979, G-13.

Reis, M., & Gold, D.   Relation of paternal availability to problem solving and sex-role orientation in young boys. *Psychological Reports*, 1977, *40*, 823–829.

Reiss, A. J.   Social correlates of psychological types of delinquency. *American Sociological Review*, 1952, *17*, 710–718.

Report of the Harvard Child Health Project Task Force: Toward a primary medical care system responsive to children's needs. Cambridge, Mass.: Ballinger Publishing Company, 1977.

Report of the national advisory commission on civil disorders. Washington, D.C.: U.S. Government Printing Office, 1967, *129*, 337–338.

Reyes, T. F.   Father absence and the social behavior of pre-school children. *Dissertation Abstracts International,* 1978, *39*(1-A), 185–186.

Reynolds, W.   *The American father: A new approach to understanding himself, his woman, his child.* New York: Paddington Press, 1978.

Richards, H. C., & McCandless, B. R.   Socialization dimensions among five-year-old slum children. *Journal of Educational Psychology,* February 1972, *63,* 44–56.

Richards, M., Dunn, J., & Antonis, B.   Caretaking in the first year of life: The role of fathers' and mothers' social isolation. *Child: Care, Health & Development,* 1977, *3,* 23–36.

Richman, N., & Graham, P.   A behavioral screening questionnaire for use with 3-year-old children, preliminary findings. *Journal of Child Psychology and Psychiatry,* 1971, *12,* 5–33.

Riessman, F.   Low-income culture: The strengths of the poor. *Journal of Marriage and the Family,* 1964, *26*(4), 417–421.

Rimoldi, H. J.   A note on Raven's Progressive Matrices Test. *Educational and Psychological Measurement,* 1948, *8,* 347–352.

Risen, M. L.   Relation of lack of one or both parents to school program. *Elementary School Journal,* 1939, *39,* 528–531.

Roach, D. A.   Some social variables in conceptual style preference. *Perceptual and Motor Skills,* 1980, *50,* 452–454.

Robins, L. N.   *Deviant Children Grown Up: A Sociological and Psychiatric Study of Sociopathic Personality.* Baltimore: Williams & Wilkins, 1966.

Robson, K., & Moss, H.   Patterns and determinants of maternal attachment. *Journal of Pediatrics,* December 1970, *77*(6), 976–985.

Rodman, H., Nichols, F. R., & Voydanoff, P.   Lower-class attitudes toward "deviant" family patterns: A cross-cultural study. *Journal of Marriage and the Family,* May 1969, *31*(2), 315–321.

Rohrer, J. H., & Edmonson, M. S.   *The eighth generation grows up: Cultures and personalities of New Orleans Negroes.* (Co-authors: H. Lief, D. Thompson, & W. Thompson under the editorship of Gardner Murphy). New York: Harper Torch Books, 1964. (Originally published in 1960 under the title *The eighth generation* by Harper & Brothers.)

Rorschach, H.   (Transl. by P. Lemkau & B. Kronenburg.) *Psychodiagnostics: A diagnostic test based on perception.* Berne: Huber, 1942. (1st German ed., 1921; U.S. distributor, Grune & Stratton.)

Rosen, L.   Matriarchy and lower class Negro male delinquency. *Social Problems,* 1969, *17*(2), 175–189.

Rosenberg, B. G., & Sutton-Smith, B.   The measurement of masculinity and femininity in children. *Child Development,* 1959, *30,* 373–380.

Rosenberg, B. G., & Sutton-Smith, B.   Family interaction effects on masculinity–femininity. *Journal of Personality and Social Psychology,* 1968, *8,* 117–120.

Rosenberg, M. *Society and the adolescent self image.* Princeton: Princeton University Press, 1965.

Rosenfeld, J. M., Rosenstein, S., & Raab, M. Sailor families: The nature and effects of one kind of father absence. *Child Welfare,* January 1973, *52*(1), 33–44.

Rosenthal, D., Wender, P. H., Kety, S. S., Weiner, J., & Schulsinger, F. The adopted-away offspring of schizophrenics. *American Journal of Psychiatry,* September 1971, *128*(3), 307–310.

Ross, H., & Sawhill, I. *Time of transition: The growth of families headed by women.* Washington, D.C.: The Urban Institute, 1975.

Ross, J. M. Fathering: A review of some psychoanalytic contributions and paternity. *International Journal of Psycho-Analysis,* 1979, *60,* 317–327.

Rossi, A. S. A biosocial perspective on parenting. *Daedalus,* Spring 1977, *106*(2), 1–31.

Rotter, J. B. Generalized expectancies for internal versus external control of reinforcement. *Psychological Monographs,* 1966, *80* (1, whole no. 609).

Rouman, J. School childrens' problems as related to parental factors. *Journal of Educational Research,* 1956, *50,* 105–112.

Rubenstein, B. O., & Levitt, M. Some observations regarding the role of fathers in child psychotherapy. *Bulletin of the Menninger Clinic,* 1957, *21,* 16–27.

Rubin, L. B. Working-class marriages. In A. E. Fisher (Ed.), *Science Monographs of Women's Worlds* (NIMH supported research on women), 1978, DHEW pub. no. (ADM) 78–660, 51–54, Rockville, Maryland.

Rubin, R. H. Adult male absence and the self-attitudes of black children. *Child Study Journal,* 1974, *4*(1), 33–46.

Russell, I. L. Behavior problems of children from broken homes and intact homes. *Journal of Educational Sociology,* 1957, *31,* 124–129.

Russo, N. F. Overview: Sex roles, fertility and the motherhood mandate. *Psychology of Women Quarterly,* 1979, *4*(1), 7–15.

Rutter, M. Maternal deprivation, 1972–1978: New findings, new concepts, new approaches. *Child Development,* June 1979, *50*(2), 283–305.

Rutter, M. *Maternal deprivation reassessed.* Harmondsworth, England: Penguin, 1972.

Rutter, M. Psycho-social disorders in childhood, and their outcome in adult life. *Journal of the Royal College of Physicians of London,* April 1970, *4*(3), 211–218.

Rutter, M., & Graham, P. J. The reliability and validity of the psychiatric assessment of the child: I. Interview with the child. *British Journal of Psychiatry,* *114,* 563–579.

Sachs, L. J. The maid: Her importance in child development. *Psychoanalytic Quarterly,* 1971, *40,* 469–484.

Salk, L. The critical nature of the post-partum period in the human for the establishment of the mother-infant bond: A controlled study. *Diseases of the Nervous System,* November 1970, *31*:Suppl., 110–116.

Saluter, A. *1977 marital status and living arrangements reports* (Current Population Reports, series P-20, no. 323). Washington, D.C.: U.S. Government Printing Office, April 1978.

Samuda, R. J. *Psychological testing of American minorities: Issues and consequences.* New York: Dodd, Mead, 1975.

Santrock, J. W. Effects of father absence on sex-typed behaviors in male children: Reason for the absence and age of onset of the absence. *Journal of Genetic Psychology,* 1977, *130,* 3–10.

Santrock, J. W. Parental absence, sex typing, and identification. *Developmental Psychology,* 1970, *2*(2), 264–272.

Santrock, J. W. Relation of type and onset of father absence to cognitive development. In F. Rebelsky & L. Dorman (Eds.), *Child development and behavior.* New York: Alfred A. Knopf, 1973.

Santrock, J. W., & Tracy, R. L. Effects of children's family structure status on the development of stereotypes by teachers. *Journal of Educational Psychology,* 1978, *70*(5), 754–757.

Sarrell, P., & Davis, C. The young unwed primapara: A study of 100 cases with 5 year follow-up. *American Journal of Obstetrics and Gynecology,* 1966, *95,* 722.

Sauer, R. J. Absentee father syndrome. *The Family Coordinator,* April 1979, 245–249.

Saving the family. *Newsweek,* May 15, 1978, 63–90.

Sawhill, I. V. Economic perspectives on the family. *Daedalus,* Spring 1977, *106* (2), 115–125.

Schaffer, H. R. *The growth of sociability.* Harmondsworth, England: Penguin Books, 1971.

Schanegold, M. The relationship between father-absence and encopresis. *Child Welfare,* 1977, *56*(6), 385–394.

Schlesinger, B. The one-parent family: An overview. *The Family Life Coordinator,* October 1966, *15,* 133–138.

Schorr, A. L. *Poor kids: A report on children in poverty.* New York: Basic Books, Inc., 1966.

Schorr, A. L., & Moen, P. The single parent and public policy. *Social Policy,* March/April 1979, 15–21.

Schrut, A., & Michels, T. Suicidal divorced and discarded women. *Journal of the American Academy of Psychoanalysis,* 1974, *2*(4), 329–347.

Schvenveldt, J. D., Freyer, M., & Ostler, R. Concepts of "badness" and "goodness" of parents as perceived by nursery school children. *Family Coordinator,* 1970, *19,* 98–103.

Sciara, F. J., & Jantz, R. K.   Father absence and its apparent effect on the reading achievement of black children from low income families. *Journal of Negro Education,* 1974, *43*(2), 221–227.

Scully, D.   Unpublished data for Ph.D. thesis. Department of Sociology, University of Illinois, Chicago Circle Campus, 1975.

Sears, P. S.   Doll play aggression in normal young children: Influence of sex, age, sibling status, father's absence. In H. S. Conrad (Ed.), *Psychological Monographs: General and applied,* 1951, *65*(6, whole no. 323).

Seegmiller, B. R.   Sex-role differentiation in preschoolers: Effects of maternal employment. *Journal of Psychology,* 1980, *104*, 185–189.

Seligman, R., Gleser, G., Rauh, J., & Harris, L.   The effect of earlier parental loss in adolescence. *Archives of General Psychiatry,* October 1974, *31*, 475–479.

Seplin, C. D.   A study of the influence of the fathers' absence for military service (thesis abstract). *Smith College Studies in Social Work,* 1952, *22*, 123–124.

Shaw, C. R., & McKay, J. D.   Are broken homes a causative factor in juvenile delinquency? *Social Forces,* 1932, *10*(4), 514–525.

Shaw, P.   A study of social problems in a group of young women treated with brief psychotherapy. *Journal of Medical Psychology,* 1977, *50*, 155–161.

Shill, M.   TAT measures of gender identity (castration anxiety) in father-absent males. *Journal of Personality Assessment,* 1981, *45*(2), 136–146.

Shinn, M.   Father absence and children's cognitive development. *Psychological Bulletin,* 1978, *85*(2), 295–324.

Shoicket, S. G.   *Affinal relationships of the divorced mother.* New York: Columbia University Press, 1968.

Sholevar, P. (Ed.).   *Treatment of emotional disorders in children and adolescents* (Vol. 1). New York: Basic Books, Inc., 1980.

Siegman, A. W.   Father-absence during childhood and antisocial behavior. *Journal of Abnormal Psychology,* 1966, *71*, 71–74.

Sigusch, V., & Schmidt, G.   Lower-class sexuality: Some emotional and social aspects in West German males and females. *Archives of Sexual Behavior,* 1971, *1*(1), 29–44.

Silverman, P., & Englander, S.   The widow's view of her dependent children. *Omega,* 1975, *6*(1), 3–20.

Skarsten, S.   Family desertion in Canada. *Family Coordinator,* January 1974, *23*, 19–25.

Slawson, D.   Personal communication, March 23, 1979.

Slawson, J.   *The delinquent boy.* Boston: Richard G. Badger, 1926.

Slosson, R. L.   *Slosson Intelligence Test.* Aurora, New York: Slosson Educational Publications, Inc. (1st Ed. 1961, 2nd Ed., 1981).

Slosson, R. L.   Reply [to Swanson, M. S., & Jacobson, A.: Evaluation of the S.I.T. for Screening Children with Learning Disabilities. *Journal of Learning Disabilities, 3*(6), 318–320, 1970]. *Journal of Learning Disabilities, 3*(9), 466, 1970.

Smith, C., & Lloyd, B.   Maternal behavior and perceived sex of infant: Revisited. *Child Development*, 1978, *49*, 1263–1265.

Smith, T. E.   Social class and attitudes towards fathers. *Sociology and Social Research*, 1969, *53*, 217–226.

Soloman, D., Hirsch, J. G., Scheinfeld, D. R., & Jackson, J.   Family characteristics and elementary school achievement in an urban ghetto. *Journal of Counseling and Clinical Psychology*, 1972, *39*(3), 462–466.

Solow, R. A., & Adams, P. L.   Custody by agreement: Child psychiatrist as child advocate. *Journal of Psychiatry and Law*, Spring 1977, 77–100.

Song, R. H.   Self-concept variables of delinquent boys from intact homes and broken homes. *Psychologia*, 1969, *12*, 150–152.

Spence, J. T., & Helmreich, R. L.   *Masculinity and femininity: Their psychological dimensions, correlates, and antecedents.* Austin: University of Texas Press, 1978.

Spitz, R. A.   Anaclitic depression: An inquiry into the genesis of psychiatric conditions in early childhood. II. *Psychoanalytic Study of the Child*, 1946, *2*, 313–352.

Spitz, R. A.   Fundamental education. In M. M. Piers (Eds.), *Play and development.* New York: Norton, 1972.

Spitz, R. A.   Hospitalism: An inquiry into the genesis of psychiatric conditions in early childhood. *Psychoanalytic Study of the Child*, 1945, *1*, 53–74.

Stein, Z., & Susser, M.   Widowhood and mental illness. *British Journal of Preventive Socialized Medicine*, 1969, *23*, 106–110.

Stenger, R. L.   The Supreme Court and illegitimacy: 1968–1977. *Family Law Quarterly*, Winter 1978, *XI*(4), 365–405.

Stephens, N., & Day, H. D.   Sex-role identity, parental identification, and self-concept of adolescent daughters from mother-absent, father-absent, and intact families, *Journal of Psychology*, 1979, *103*, 193–202.

Stephens, W.   Judgments by social workers on boys and mothers in fatherless families. *Journal of Genetic Psychology*, 1961, *99*, 59–64.

Stern, E. E.   Single mothers' perceptions of the father role and of the effects of father absence on boys. *Journal of Divorce*, 1980 *4*(2), 77–84.

Sterne, R. S.   *Delinquent conduct and broken homes: A study of 1,050 boys.* New Haven, Conn.: College & University Press, 1964.

Stewart, M. S.   *A chance for every child* (Public Affairs Pamphlet No. 333). The Public Affairs Committee, February 1970.

Stillman, A.   Leadership: P.W.P.'s permanent crisis. *The Journal,* February/March 1965, *7*(2), 4–8.

Sticht, T. G. (Ed.).   *Reading for working: A functional literacy anthology.* Alexandria, Va.: Human Resources Research Organization, 1975.

Stodolsky, S. S., & Lesser, G.   Learning patterns in the disadvantaged. *Harvard Educational Review*, 1967, *37*, 546–593.

Stoller, R. J. Boyhood gender aberrations: Treatment issues. *Journal of the American Psychoanalytic Association,* 1978, *26*(3), 541–558.

Stolorow, R. D., & Lachmann, F. M. Early object loss and denial: Developmental considerations. *Psychoanalytic Quarterly,* 1975, *44,* 596–611.

Stone, M. *When God was a woman.* New York: Dial Press, 1976.

Sugar, M. Group therapy for pubescent boys with absent fathers. *Journal of the American Academy of Child Psychiatry,* July 1967, *6*(3), 49–67.

Sugar, M. (Ed.). *The Adolescent in Group and Family Therapy.* New York: Brunner/Mazel, 1975.

Sullivan, H. S. *Personal psychopathology: Early formulations.* New York: W. W. Norton & Company, 1972.

Sunday daddy. *Look Magazine,* 1967, *31,* 23–29.

Sussman, M. B. The family today. *Children Today,* March/April 1978, 7(2), 32–37.

Susz, E., & Marberg, H. M. Autistic withdrawal of a small child under stress. *Acta Paedopsychiatrica,* 1978, *43,* 149–158.

Sutherland, H. E. G. The relationship between I. Q. and size of family in the case of fatherless children. *Journal of Genetic Psychology,* 1930, *38,* 161–170.

Sutton-Smith, B. The interaction of father absence and siblings presence on cognitive abilities. *Child Development,* 1969, *40,* 941–944.

Sutton-Smith, B., Rosenberg, B. G., & Landy, F. Father-absence effects in families of different sibling compositions. *Child Development,* 1968, *39,* 1213–1221.

Szasz, T. *The myth of mental illness: Foundations of a theory of personal conduct* (rev. ed.). New York: Harper and Row, 1974.

Taft, J. *Otto Rank: A biographical study based on notebooks, letters, collected writings, therapeutic achievements and personal associations.* New York: Julian Press, 1958.

Taylor, P. *A woman of means* (1st ed.). New York: Harcourt, Brace, 1950.

Tcheng-Laroche, F., & Prince, R. H. Middle income, divorced female heads of families: Their lifestyles, health and stress levels. *Canadian Journal of Psychiatry,* 1979, *23,* 35–42.

Teele, J. E., & Schmidt, W. M. Illegitimacy and race: National and local trends. *Milbank Memorial Fund Quarterly,* April 1970, *48*(2), 127–150.

TenHouten, W. D. The black family: Myth and reality. *Psychiatry,* 1971, *34* (224), 145–173.

Terman, L. M. *The measurement of intelligence.* Boston: Houghton Mifflin, 1916.

Terman, L. M., & Merrill, M. A. *Measuring intelligence.* Boston: Houghton Mifflin, 1937.

Terman, L. M., & Merrill, M. A. *Stanford-Binet Intelligence Scale: Manual for the third revision, Form L-M.* Boston: Houghton Mifflin, 1960.

Terman, L. M., & Miles, C. C. *Sex and personality: Studies in masculinity and femininity.* New York: McGraw-Hill, 1936.

Their hearts belong to daddy. *Time,* July 6, 1970, 41.

The social and economic status of the black population in the United States: An historical view, 1790–1978 (CPR Series P-23, No. 80). Washington, D.C.: U.S. Government Printing Office, 1979.

Thomes, M. M. Children with absent fathers. *Journal of Marriage and the Family,* 1968, *30,* 89–96.

Thurstone, L. L. Creative talent. *Proceedings of the 1950 Invitational Conference on Testing Problems, Educational Testing Service,* 1951, 55–69. (Reprinted in A. Anastasi [Ed.], *Testing problems in perspective.* Washington, D.C.: American Council on Education, 1966, 414–428.)

Tobias, C. The home visit in child psychiatry. *Child Psychiatry and Human Development,* 1979, *10*(2), 77–84.

Torrance, E. P. *Rewarding creative behavior.* Englewood Cliffs, N.J.: Prentice-Hall, 1965.

Trachtman, R. S. Father absence during the oedipal phase of development. A study of post oedipal development and adaption in father absent and father present boys. *Dissertation Abstracts International,* 1978, *39A,* 3846.

Trunnell, T. L. The absent father's children's emotional disturbances. *Archives of General Psychiatry,* August 1968, *19,* 180–188.

Tuck, S. Working with black fathers. *American Journal of Orthopsychiatry,* April 1971, *41*(3), 465–472.

Tuckman, J., & Regan, R. A. Intactness of the home and behavioral problems in children. *Journal of Child Psychology and Psychiatry,* 1966, *7,* 225–233.

Ucko, L. E., & Moore, T. Parental roles as seen by young children in doll play. *Vita Humana,* 1963, *6,* 213–242.

U.S. Bureau of the Census. Marital status and living arrangements: March 1977. *Current population reports* (Series P-20, No. 323). Washington, D.C.: U.S. Government Printing Office, 1978.

U.S. Bureau of the Census. Unpublished data from current population survey, March 1980.

U.S. Department of Health and Human Services. Supplemental instructions for preparing application for training grant continuation support (Form PHS 2498-2), 1979.

U.S. Department of Health, Education & Welfare. Divorce and divorce rates: United States. [DHEW Publication No. (PHS) 78-1907]. *Vital and health statistics* (Series 21, No. 29). Washington, D.C.: U.S. Government Printing Office, 1978.

U.S. Department of Labor. *Bureau of labor statistics news.* Washington, D.C.: U.S. Government Printing Office, 1978.

U.S. Department of Labor. *Employment in perspective: Working women, Report 587.* Washington, D.C.: U.S. Government Printing Office, February 1980.

Usdin, G. (Ed.). *Schizophrenia: Biological and psychological perspectives.* Larchmont, N.Y.: Brunner/Mazel Publishers, 1975.

Valentine, C. A. *Culture and poverty: Critique and counter-proposals.* Chicago: University of Chicago Press, 1968.

Visher, E. B., & Visher, J. S. *Stepfamilies: A guide to working with stepparents and stepchildren.* New York: Brunner/Mazel, 1979.

Voth, M. M. *The castrated family.* Kansas City: Sheed Andrews & McMell, Inc., 1977.

Vroegh, K., Jenkin, N., Black, M., & Hendrick, M. Discriminant analysis of preschool masculinity and femininity. *Multivariate Behavioral Research,* 1967, *2,* 299–313.

Vroegh, K. S. The relationship of sex of teacher and father presence-absence to academic achievement. *Dissertation Abstracts International,* 1972, *33*(10-A), 5669.

Wakefield, W. M. Awareness, affection, and perceived similarity in the parent–child relationship. *The Journal of Genetic Psychology,* 1970, *117,* 91–97.

Waldman, E., Grossman, A. S., Hayghe, H., & Johnson, B. L. Working in the 1970's: A look at the statistics. In *Young workers and families: A special section* (Special Labor Force Report 233, U.S. Department of Labor). Washington, D.C.: U.S. Department Printing Office, 1979.

Waldron, J. A., & Whittington, R. The stepparent/stepfamily. *Journal of Operational Psychiatry,* 1979, *10*(1), 47–50.

Wallace, E. R. Freud and Leonardo. *Psychiatric Forum,* 1979, *8*(1), 1–10.

Wallerstein, J. S., & Kelly, J. B. Effects of divorce on the visiting father–child relationship. *American Journal of Psychiatry,* December 1980, *137*(12), 1534–1539.

Ward, J. Dads: Stepfather knows it's not easy to live as a stepchild. Louisville *Courier-Journal & Times,* Sunday, June 15, 1980, G-6.

Watt, N. F., & Nicholi, A. Early death of a parent as an etiological factor in schizophrenia. *American Journal of Orthopsychiatry,* July 1979, *49*(3), 465–473.

Weber, M. [*From Max Weber: Essays in Sociology*] (H. Gerth & C. W. Mills, Eds. and trans.). New York: Oxford University Press, 1946.

Wechsler, D. *The measurement of adult intelligence.* Baltimore: Williams & Wilkins, 1939.

Wechsler, D. *The measurement and appraisal of adult intelligence* (4th ed.). Baltimore: Williams & Wilkins, 1958.

Weeks, A., & Smith, M. G. Juvenile delinquency and broken homes in Spokane, Washington. *Social Forces,* October 1939, *18,* 48–55.

Weinraub, M., & Frankel, J. Sex differences in parent-infant interaction during free play, departure, and separation. *Child Development,* 1977, *48,* 1240–1249.

Weiss, R. S. *Going it alone.* New York: Basic Books, Inc., 1979.

Weissman, Myrna, Orvaschel, Helen, & Sholonskas, Diane. Assessment of psychopathology and behavioral problems in childhood—A review of scales suitable for epidemiological and clinical research, 1967–79. NIMH publication (ADN)80-1037, 1980.

Weitzman, L., & Dixon, R.   Alimony as an instrument of justice. In A. E. Fisher (Ed.), *Science Monographs of Women's Worlds* (NIMH supported research on women), 1978, DHEW pub. no (ADM) 78-660, Rockville, Maryland.

Wertham, F.   *A sign for Cain: An exploration of human violence.* New York: Warner Paperback Library, 1966.

West, M. M., & Konner, M. J.   The role of the father: An anthropological perspective (Chapter 5). In M. E. Lamb (Ed.), *The role of the father in child development.* New York: John Wiley & Sons, 1976.

Westley, W. A., & Epstein, N. B.   *The silent majority.* San Francisco: Jossey-Bass, 1969.

Westman, J.   Role of child psychiatry in divorce. *Archives of General Psychiatry,* November 1970, *23,* 416–420.

White-Coleman, G.   *Trends analysis and dynamisms of completed suicides and dynamisms of attempted suicides in Jefferson County, Kentucky.* Unpublished doctoral dissertation, 1979.

Whiting, B. B., & Whiting, J. W. M.   *Children of six cultures: A psycho-cultural analysis.* Cambridge, Mass.: Harvard University Press, 1975.

Whiting, J. W. M., Kluckhohn, R., & Anthony, A.   The function of male initiation ceremonies at puberty. In E. E. Maccoby, T. M. Newcomb, & E. L. Hartley (Eds.), *Readings in Social Psychiatry.* New York: Holt, Rinehart & Winston, 1958.

Wilkinson, C. B., & O'Connor, W. A.   Growing up male in a black single-parent family. *Psychiatric Annals,* July 1977, 7(7), 50–51; 55–59.

Willard, L. S.   A comparison of Culture Fair Test scores with group and individual intelligence test scores of disadvantaged Negro children. *Journal of Learning Disabilities,* 1968, *1,* 584–589.

Willie, C. V.   The relative contribution of family status and economic status to juvenile delinquency. *Social Problems,* 1967, *101*(14), 326–335.

Wilson, I. C., Alltop, L. B., & Buffaloe, W. J.   Parental bereavement in childhood: MMPI profiles in a depressed population. *British Journal of Psychiatry,* 1967, *113,* 761–764.

Wimperis, V.   *The unmarried mother and her child.* London: George Allen and Union Ltd., 1960.

Winn, D., & Halla, R.   Observations of children who threaten to kill themselves. *Canadian Psychiatric Association Journal,* 1966, *11,* 5283–5294.

Wisdom, J. O.   The role of the father in the mind of parents, in psychoanalytic theory and in the life of the infant. *International Review of Psycho-Analysis,* 1976, *3,* 231–239.

Wohlford, P., Santrock, J. W., Berger, S. E., & Liberman, D. Older brothers' influence on sex-typed, aggressive, and dependent behavior in father-absent children. *Developmental Psychology, 1971, 4,* 124–134.

Wolfenstein, M. How is mourning possible? *The Psychoanalytic Study of the Child,* 1966, *21,* 93–123.

Woodward, W. R. Scientific genius and loss of a parent. *Science Studies,* 1974, *4,* 265.

Worell, J. Sex roles and psychological well-being: Perspectives on methodology. *Journal of Consulting and Clinical Psychology,* 1978, *46,* 777–791.

Wylie, H. L., & Delgado, R. A. A pattern of mother–son relationship involving the absence of the father. *American Journal of Orthopsychiatry,* 1959, *29,* 644–649.

Wylie, P. *Generation of vipers.* New York: Farrar & Rinehart, Inc., 1942.

Wylie, R. C. Children's estimates of their school work ability as a function of sex, race, and socioeconomic level. *Journal of Personality,* 1963, *31,* 203–224.

Young, F. W. The function of male initiation ceremonies: A cross-cultural test of an alternative hypothesis. *American Journal of Sociology,* 1962, 379–396.

Young, L. *Out of wedlock: A study of the problems of the unmarried mother and her child.* New York: McGraw-Hill, 1954.

Zelditch, M. Role differentiation in the nuclear family: A comparative study. In T. Parsons & R. F. Bales (Eds.), *Family, socialization, and interaction process.* Glencoe, Ill.: The Free Press, 1955.

Zunich, M. Lower-class mothers' behavior and attitudes toward child rearing. *Psychological Reports,* 1971, *29,* 1051–1058.

Index

Upward-bound, lifestyle of black family, 47

Urban, life styles of black family, 45–48

Variables, needing control, 129, 131–132, 153, 163, 170

Venus figures, and female deities, 22

Victim, blaming, 338

Vietnam War, 119, 343

Violence, 342
  culture of, 47–48

Visit, to noncustodial parent by child, 342

Visitation practices, 27

WAIS, 280

Wechsler Intelligence Scale for Children (WISC), 133

Wechsler Preschool and Primary Scale of Intelligence (WPPSI), 276, 280

Wechsler scales, 280, 281

Welfare Department, 345, 350

Welfare system, 70–75

Welfare worker, 332

Whites:
  delinquency among, 195
  illegitimacy among, 107–108
  male domination among, 39

Wide Range Achievement Test (WRAT), 279

Widowhood, *see* Death of father

Widow-to-Widow program, 99

Wife beating, and narcissism in family life, 59

WISC, 280

WISC-R, 280

Women:
  alternative lifestyles of, 60
  denigration of, 23
  fear of, 24
  oppression of, 57
  vengeance for oppression, 53

Work, temporary absence due to, 117–119

Working class:
  family structure of, 32–37
  parental role division in, 54
  role of father, 54

Working with poor black fathers, 51

Working mothers, 75–79, 165–166, 313, 316

Work patterns:
  and race, 38–39
  and social class, 32–35

Work relationships, in lower class, 36

Youth Movement, and role of father, 55

Zero Population Growth, 316